Endodontic Radiology, Second Edition

Endodontic Radiology, Second Edition

Edited by

Bettina Basrani, DDS, PhD

Specialist in Endodontics
Associate Professor (Tenured)
Co-Director, MSc Program in Endodontics
Discipline of Endodontics
Faculty of Dentistry
University of Toronto
Toronto, Ontario, Canada

WILEY-BLACKWELL

A John Wiley & Sons, Inc., Publication

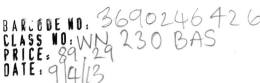
This edition first published 2012 © 2012 by John Wiley & Sons, Inc.

First Edition, Radiología en Endodoncia by Enrique Basrani © 2002 AMOLCA

Wiley-Blackwell is an imprint of John Wiley & Sons, formed by the merger of Wiley's global Scientific, Technical and Medical business with Blackwell Publishing.

Editorial offices: 2121 State Avenue, Ames, Iowa 50014-8300, USA
                The Atrium, Southern Gate, Chichester, West Sussex, PO19 8SQ, UK
                9600 Garsington Road, Oxford, OX4 2DQ, UK

For details of our global editorial offices, for customer services and for information about how to apply for permission to reuse the copyright material in this book please see our website at www.wiley.com/wiley-blackwell.

Library of Congress Cataloging-in-Publication Data
Endodontic radiology / edited by Bettina Basrani. – 2nd ed.
        p. ; cm.
    Rev. ed. of: Radiologia en endodoncia / [ed. por] Enrique Basrani. c2003.
    Includes bibliographical references and index.
    ISBN 978-0-470-95849-0 (hardcover : alk. paper)
    I. Basrani, Bettina.   II. Radiología en endodoncia.
    [DNLM: 1. Dental Pulp Cavity–radiography.   2. Root Canal Therapy–methods.   3. Periapical Diseases–radiography. WN 230]
    617.6342059–dc23

                                        2012005062

A catalogue record for this book is available from the British Library.

Wiley also publishes its books in a variety of electronic formats. Some content that appears in print may not be available in electronic books.

Set in 9.5/11.5 pt Palatino by Toppan Best-set Premedia Limited
Printed and bound in Singapore by Markono Print Media Pte Ltd

1   2012

"Every great dream begins with a dreamer. Always remember, you have within you the strength, the patience, and the passion to reach for the stars to change the world."
Harriet Tubman

This book is dedicated to my children, Jonathan and Daniel, to encourage them to follow their dreams with conviction and hard work, and especially with love.

Contents

About the Editor   ix
Contributors   x
Foreword   xiv
Preface   xvi
Acknowledgments   xvii

Part 1: General Principles and Techniques   3

1   General Principles of Radiology
    in Endodontics   5
    Anda Kfir and Bettina Basrani

2   Intraoral Radiographic Principles
    and Techniques   18
    Mindy Cash and Bettina Basrani

3   Special Situations   39
    Bettina Basrani

4   Intraoral Digital Imaging   43
    Ernest W. N. Lam

5   Radiographic Considerations Before the
    Endodontic Treatment Is Initiated   49
    Calvin D. Torneck

6   Radiographic Analysis of Anomalous
    Tooth Forms and Morphological
    Variations Related to Endodontics   54
    Jeffrey M. Coil

Part 2: Endodontic Disease   79

7   Radiographic Expression of
    Endodontic Disease   81
    Calvin D. Torneck

8   Image Interpretation of Periapical
    Abnormalities   101
    Ernest W. N. Lam

9   Radiographic Interpretation
    of Traumatic Injuries   129
    Nestor Cohenca

10 Radiographic Analysis of Acquired
    Pathological Dental Conditions   153
    Amir Azarpazhooh

11 Radiographic Analysis of Periodontal
    and Endodontic Lesions   166
    Jim Yuan Lai and Bettina Basrani

12 Radiographic Imaging in Implant
    Dentistry   177
    Amir Azarpazhooh and Jim Yuan Lai

**Part 3: Sequence of
Endodontic Treatment**   **191**

13 Radiographic Considerations during
    the Endodontic Treatment   193
    Bettina Basrani

14 Electronic Apex Locators and
    Conventional Radiograph in
    Working Length Measurement   218
    *Gevik Malkhassian, Andres Plazas,
    and Yosef Nahmias*

15 Vertical Root Fractures: Radiological
    Diagnosis   235
    Anil Kishen and Harold H. Messer

16 Healing of Chronic Apical
    Periodontitis   251
    Dag Ørstavik

Part 4: Teaching and Research   **267**

17 Radiographic Consideration for
    Endodontic Teaching   269
    Bettina Basrani

18 Micro-Computed Tomography
    in Endodontic Research   278
    Mana Mirfendereski and Ove Peters

Part 5: Advanced Techniques   **285**

19 Alternative Imaging Systems in
    Endodontics   287
    Elisabetta Cotti and Girolamo Campisi

20 Introduction to Cone Beam
    Computed Tomography   304
    Ernest W. N. Lam

21 Interpretation of Periapical Lesions
    Using Cone Beam Computed
    Tomography   307
    *Carlos Estrela, Mike Reis Bueno,
    and Ana Helena Gonçalves Alencar*

Part 6: Clinical Cases   **329**

22 Clinical Cases   331
    Le O'Leary

23 Clinical Impact of Cone Beam
    Computed Tomography in Root
    Canal Treatment   367
    Carlos Bóveda Z.

Index   416

To download figures and tables from this book, please visit www.wiley.com/go/basrani.

About the Editor

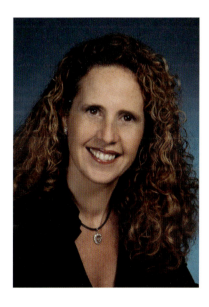

Dr. Bettina Basrani is Tenured Associate Professor and Co-Director, MSc Program in Endodontics on the Faculty of Dentistry, University of Toronto, in Ontario, Canada. Dr. Basrani received her D.D.S. degree from the University of Buenos Aires and a Specialty Diploma in Endodontics and Ph.D. from Maimonides University in Buenos Aires, Argentina. A long-time educator and researcher, she began her teaching career at the University of Buenos Aires. In 2000, she moved to Canada to serve as Head of the Endodontic Program at Dalhousie University, Halifax, Nova Scotia. In 2004, she moved to Toronto, where she has continued her academic and clinical work, nurturing two careers in parallel—those of educator/researcher and practicing clinician. Internationally recognized as a leading authority in endodontics and as an excellent lecturer, effectively combining clinical and scientific information, Dr. Basrani has received many teacher awards throughout her career and has international courses and lectures, over 30 peer-reviewed scientific publications, textbook chapters, and abstracts to her credit. She serves as an Editorial Board Member for the *Journal of Endodontics* and *International Endodontic Journal*. Dr. Basrani is a member of many endodontics societies around the world, and also serves on the special committee to develop researchers of the American Association of Endodontics. She makes her home in Toronto, where she is married to Canadian psychiatrist Dr. Howard Alter and spends her leisure time taking their sons, Jonathan and Daniel, to soccer practices, chess tournaments, skating lessons, and piano recitals.

Contributors

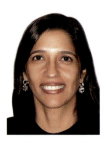

Ana Helena Gonçalves Alencar, DDS, MSc, PhD
Professor of Endodontics
Department of Oral Science
Federal University of Goiás
Goiânia, GO, Brazil

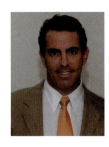

Carlos Bóveda Z.
DDS, Specialist in
    Endodontics
Private Practice
Limited to Endodontics
Centro de Especialidades
    Odontológicas
Caracas, Venezuela

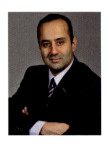

Amir Azarpazhooh, DDS, MSc, PhD, FRCD(C)
Assistant Professor
Discipline of Dental Public
    Health and Discipline of
    Endodontics
Faculty of Dentistry
University of Toronto
Toronto, Ontario, Canada

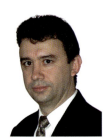

Mike Reis Bueno, DDS, MSc, PhD
Professor of Semiology and
    Stomatology
University of Cuiabá
Cuiabá, MT, Brazil

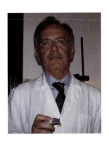

Girolamo Campisi, MD
Specialist in Radiology
University of Cagliari
Italy

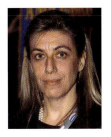

Elisabetta Cotti, DDS, MS
Professor and Chairman
Department of Conservative
    Dentistry and Endodontics
University of Cagliari
Italy

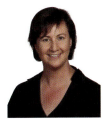

Mindy Cash, BSc, DDS
Lecturer
Oral and Maxillofacial
    Radiology
Faculty of Dentistry
University of Toronto
Toronto, Ontario, Canada

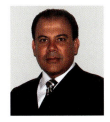

**Carlos Estrela, DDS, MSc,
PhD**
Chairman and Professor of
    Endodontics
Department of Oral Science
Federal University of Goiás
Goiânia, GO, Brazil

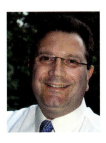

Nestor Cohenca, DDS
Diplomate, American Board
    of Endodontics
Associate Professor,
    Department of Endodontics
Adjunct Associate Professor,
    Department of Pediatric
    Dentistry
School of Dentistry
University of Washington
Seattle, WA, USA

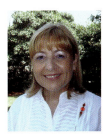

Anda Kfir, DMD
Lecturer
Specialist in Endodontics
Coordinator, Department of
    Endodontology
School of Dental Medicine
Tel-Aviv University
Tel-Aviv, Israel

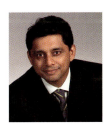

**Anil Kishen, BDS, MDS,
PhD**
Associate Professor
Discipline of Endodontics
Faculty of Dentistry
University of Toronto
Toronto, Ontario, Canada

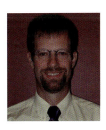

**Jeffrey M. Coil, DMD, MSD,
PhD, FRCD(C), FADI, FACD**
Diplomate, American Board
    of Endodontics
Director of Graduate
    Endodontics
Department of Oral Biological
    & Medical Sciences
Faculty of Dentistry
University of British
    Columbia
Vancouver, British Columbia,
    Canada

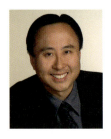

Jim Yuan Lai, DMD, MSc(Perio), MEd, FRCD(C)
Assistant Professor and
   Discipline Head
Periodontology
Faculty of Dentistry
University of Toronto
Toronto, Ontario, Canada

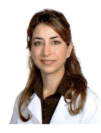

Mana Mirfendereski, BSc, DMD, MSc, FRCD(C)
Discipline of Endodontics
University of Toronto
Toronto, Ontario, Canada

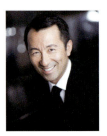

Ernest W. N. Lam, DMD, MSc, PhD, FRCD(C)
Diplomate, American Board
   of Oral and Maxillofacial
   Radiology
Associate Professor and Head
Discipline of Oral and
   Maxillofacial Radiology
Faculty of Dentistry
University of Toronto
Toronto, Canada

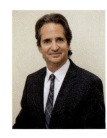

Yosef Nahmias, DDS, MSc
Private Practice
Oakville, Ontario, Canada

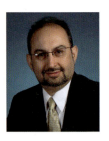

Gevik Malkhassian DDS, MSc, FRCD(C)
Assistant Professor
Discipline of Endodontics
Faculty of Dentistry
University of Toronto
Toronto, Ontario, Canada

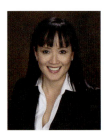

Le O'Leary, DDS
Private Practice
Plano, TX, USA

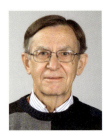

Harold H. Messer, MDSc, PhD
Emeritus Professor
Melbourne Dental School
University of Melbourne
Melbourne, Australia

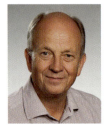

Dag Ørstavik, dr. odont.
Professor and Chairman
Department of Endodontics
Institute of Clinical Dentistry
Faculty of Dentistry
University of Oslo
Oslo, Norway

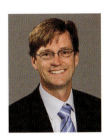

Ove Peters, DMD MS PhD
Diplomate, American Board
   of Endodontics
Professor and Co-Chair
Department of Endodontics
University of the Pacific,
   Arthur A. Dugoni School of
   Dentistry
San Francisco, CA, USA

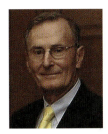

**Calvin D. Torneck DDS, MS,
FRCD**
Diplomate, American Board
   of Endodontics
Professor Emeritus
Discipline of Endodontics
Faculty of Dentistry
University of Toronto
Toronto, Ontario, Canada

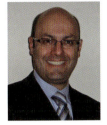

**Andres Plazas DDS,
Endodontist**
Assistant Professor
Discipline of Endodontics
Faculty of Dentistry
University of Toronto

Foreword

The new edition of *Endodontic Radiology* represents a change of generations and the evolutionary process this change encompasses.

The first edition of *Radiologia en Endodoncia* was a unique textbook published in Spanish in 2003. It was edited by Prof. Enrique E. Basrani, Dr. Ana Julia Blank, and Dr. Maria Teresa Cañete, all from the Maimonides University in Buenos Aires, Argentina, and included contributions from 21 prominent educators and clinicians from Latin America and beyond. It was the first textbook to provide readers with a comprehensive digest of all aspects of radiology related to endodontic therapy. It explained radiology from the endodontic perspective, and it explained many aspects of endodontics through the radiology perspective. It captured the state-of-the-art radiographic technologies available to clinicians at the beginning of the 21st century. In addition to a comprehensive, detailed description of the basic "bread-and-butter" applications of radiology in endodontics, the first edition included at its end several brief chapters featuring the "cutting edge" technologies of that period, including digital radiography, electronic image processing, and digital subtraction. Little could be known at that time that within one decade, what was cutting edge would become the bread and butter, and that newer technologies would emerge that would revolutionize the applications of radiology in endodontics.

The second edition of *Endodontic Radiology* in front of you has been authored by Dr. Bettina

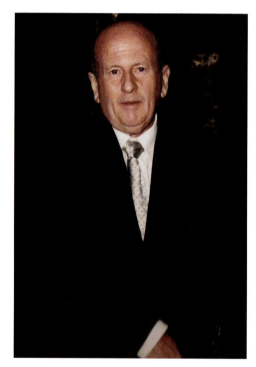

Professor Emeritus Enrique E. Basrani

Basrani, the late Prof. Basrani's daughter. She is the representative of the younger generation, but she remains her father's daughter. An experienced endodontist, she is as dedicated to endodontics and to education as her father was throughout his illustrious career. While in the first edition she coauthored a short chapter with colleagues, she has since taken it upon herself to update her late father's labor of love and to make it current for the contemporary clinician. True to her generation, she has been able to expand international and interdisciplinary collaborations, allowing the reader to benefit from contributions by 19 foremost educators, researchers, and clinicians from Australia, Brazil, Canada, Israel, Italy, Norway, the United States and Venezuela, spanning across four different disciplines of dentistry. With access to this collective international expertise, the reader gains an in-depth and wide-ranging insight into the current state of radiology applications in endodontics.

With the change of generations in authorship, the second edition's content also has evolved greatly from the original published in less than one decade ago. In this respect it provides the clinician an updated, current, and thorough reference to the critical role of radiology in all steps of endodontic therapy. Accurate diagnosis of endodontic diseases and sequellae after traumatic injury to teeth, appreciation of the sites and extent of associated bone loss, insight into the anatomy of teeth, morphology of the endodontic system and resorptive defects, precise execution of endodontic treatment procedures, assessment of treatment outcome, documentation and effective communication of treated cases among dental professionals, all require sophisticated use of radiology at each step. The second edition of *Endodontic Radiology* will guide the clinician toward achieving the required sophistication in applying the most current radiological tools to benefit their patients.

Another aspect of the generation change and evolution is extension of the availability of the information to a much wider readership. Whereas the first edition could only benefit readers versed in Spanish, the second edition of *Endodontic Radiology* published in English will benefit numerous clinicians all over the world.

All clinicians, both general dentists and specialists in different disciplines of dentistry including endodontists, will acquire critical knowledge by reading this current textbook. The acquired knowledge, in turn, will provide the clinicians with the basis for sophisticated use of radiological tools when providing endodontic care to their patients, resulting in upgraded quality of treatment.

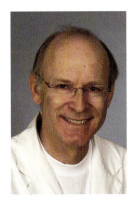

Prof. Shimon Friedman
Head, Discipline of Endodontics
Director, MSc Program in Endodontics
Faculty of Dentistry
University of Toronto
Toronto, Ontario, Canada

Preface

Radiology is an indispensable tool in endodontic practice and provides the clinician with information that is not otherwise accessible. It is also an ever-expanding field driven exponentially by constant changes in technology. It is for these reasons that this textbook, devoted to achieving a mastery of radiographic techniques and understanding in radiographic interpretation as applied to endodontic, is of particular importance to those who teach, study, and practice in this field.

There has been only one textbook dedicated entirely to endodontic radiology that has been published up to now, *Radiologia en Endodoncia*, by my father, Professor Emeritus Dr. Enrique Basrani (1928–2001) in collaboration with his colleagues, Dr. Teresa Cañete and Dr. Ana Blank. Published in Spanish in 2001, it gained wide academic acceptance in many Spanish-speaking countries. This English revised version on the same topic both fills an academic void for those who practice endodontics in non-Spanish-speaking countries and satisfies my personal wish to continue the work originally undertaken by my father. *Radiologia en Endodoncia* was his sixth and last book. He was

a pioneer of our specialty, internationally recognized for his ability to inspire and motivate others to love what he loved: The art of endodontics. Now, eleven years after his untimely death, he is still remembered by his colleagues, peers, and students for his unique vision and passion for knowledge.

The field of endodontic imaging is changing and expanding rapidly, and it is for this reason that several chapters incorporating the application of the newer technologies and the information gained through them have been included in this edition.

This book is not intended to cover in detail every aspect of dental radiology; its purpose is directed toward improving endodontic treatment outcomes by identifying and expanding the link between endodontic practice and radiographic imaging.

Clarity in endodontics is comprehended through the shadows. As Leonard Cohen put it: "That's how the light gets in." Enjoy the book, and I welcome your feedback at any time.

Bettina Basrani

Acknowledgments

I would like to thank the Dean of the University of Toronto, Faculty of Dentistry, Dr. David Mock, for granting me a sabbatical from my position at the Department of Endodontics to pursue writing this book. This decision was enthusiastically supported by the Head of the Endodontic Department, Dr. Shimon Friedman, who has always been ahead of his time and who constantly inspires all of us who work around him with his knowledge and wisdom.

Special recognitions to my collaborators on this project, all keen, clever, and dedicated specialists who contributed the highest quality of knowledge. Some of the collaborators have a lifetime of experience and others are recent graduates; some are pure academicians while others are pure clinicians. I thank them all for the enthusiasm they brought to the project.

I want to acknowledge Dr. Lyon Schwartzben for his invaluable help in editing the early manuscript.

Special thanks to Andrea Cormier and James Fiege from the Media Services Department at the Faculty of Dentistry for their beautiful photographs and diagrams.

My gratitude to Rick Blanchette, Melissa Wahl, and all the team from Wiley-Blackwell, who trusted and honored me with this project and helped me throughout the process.

My final thanks are to my family, starting with my parents Clarita and Enrique Basrani for providing me with the opportunity to be where I am today. They have always been my biggest fans and gave me motivation and inspiration to follow my academic career without limits and with unconditional love. My brother, Dr. Damian Basrani, for his care and support throughout my entire personal life and professional career. To my dear and extraordinary husband, Dr. Howard Alter, for keeping me grounded, and because his encouragement, input, and constructive criticism have been priceless.

Finally, I'd like to conclude by thanking you, the reader of *Endodontic Radiology, Second Edition,* for reading this book, and hope that it has served its purpose of enhancing your clinical practice. Enjoy!

Endodontic Radiology, Second Edition

Part 1

General Principles and Techniques

Chapter 1 General Principles of Radiology in Endodontics

Chapter 2 Intraoral Radiographic Principles and Techniques

Chapter 3 Special Situations

Chapter 4 Intraoral Digital Imaging

Chapter 5 Radiographic Considerations before the Endodontic Treatment Is Initiated

Chapter 6 Radiographic Analysis of Anomalous Tooth Forms and Morphological Variations Related to Endodontics

1 General Principles of Radiology in Endodontics

Anda Kfir and Bettina Basrani

". . . And God said: Let there be light. And there was light. And God saw the light, which it was good; and God divided the light from the darkness . . ." (Genesis 1:3–4, The Bible, King James version)

Endodontics is the branch of dentistry in which radiology plays a critical indispensable role. Radiology illuminates what otherwise would be dark and hidden zones and allows the dentists to visualize areas not accessible by other diagnostic means. It is the use of oral radiographs which enables visualization of the bone around the apices of the teeth, as well as the results of the root canal treatments, and as such it has allowed turning endodontics into a scientific professional entity (Grossman, 1982).

History of dental radiology

The many developments over the years in the field of dental radiology cannot be adequately appreciated without looking back to the discovery of X-radiation.

The cathode tube

The first step occurred in 1870. Wilhelm Hittorf found that a partially evacuated discharged tube could emit rays able to produce heat and cause a greenish-yellow glow when they strike glass. By placing a magnet within easy reach and changing the path of the rays Varley determined that these rays were negatively charged particles and they were later called electrons. It was Goldstein from Germany who called the streams of charged particles "cathode rays." He was followed by William Crooks, an English chemist, who redesigned the vacuum tube which subsequently was known as Hittorf–Crookes tube. In 1894, Philip Lenard studied the cathode rays' behavior with the aid of a tube with an aluminum window. He placed screens with fluorescent salts outside the aluminum window and found that most of the rays could penetrate the window and make the fluorescent screen glow. He noticed that when the tube and screens were separated, the light emitted decreased. When they were separated by 8 cm, the screens would not fluoresce.

Radiographs

Dr. Wilhelm Conrad Roentgen from Würzberg, Germany, studied rays emitted from a tube in a darkened room; he noticed that some crystals of barium platinocyanide from a table nearby became fluorescent The observation was made on the evening of Friday, November 8, 1895. Roentgen understood that the tube was emitting some hitherto unknown kind of ray which produced the fluorescence and called this rays "X-rays" because the nature of the rays was unknown and uncertain. He also noticed that if a metallic object was placed between the tube and screen, it cast a shadow, and he reported a number of "shadow-pictures" he had photographed. One was the shadow of a set of weights in a closed box; another was a piece of metal whose homogeneity was revealed by the X-rays. But the most interesting picture was of the bones of his wife's hand which was exposed to the rays for 15 minutes. This was the first radiograph taken of the human body and represented the beginning of practicing radiology in medicine and dentistry.

Roentgen continued to study the X-rays and found that the beam could be diminished in relation to what was placed in its path. The only material that completely absorbed the beam was lead. He went on with his experiments and finally defined the following features of X-rays: (1) they are able to distinguish between various thicknesses of materials; (2) they cause certain elements to fluoresce; (3) they are made of pure energy with no mass; (4) they go in straight lines; and (5) they are not detectable by human senses. Roentgen's great work revolutionized the diagnostic capabilities of the medical and dental professions, and he was awarded with the first Nobel Prize in Physics in 1901. In modern terms, X-ray radiation is a form of electromagnetic radiation with a wavelength from 0.01 to 10 nm. It is emitted from a metal anode (usually tungsten, molybdenum, or copper) when subjected to a stream of accelerated electrons coming from the cathode.

Dental radiographs

It was Otto Walkhoff, a German dentist, who made the first dental radiograph 14 days after Roentgen's discovery.

He placed a glass photographic plate wrapped in black paper and rubber in his mouth and submitted himself to 25 minutes of X-ray exposure. In that same year, W.J. Morton, a New York physician, made the first dental radiograph in the United States using a skull and also took the first whole body radiograph. A dentist from New Orleans, Dr. C. Edmund Kells, made the first intraoral radiograph on a patient in 1896. Kells exposed his hands to X-rays every day for years by holding the plates and trying to adjust the quality of the beam in order to achieve clear images. Unfortunately, this exposure led to the development of cancer in his hand which resulted in the amputation of his arm, demonstrating the potential risk and harmful effects of X-rays. Three years later (1899), Kells used the X-ray to determine tooth length during root canal therapy.

Radiograph machines

William H. Rollins, a Boston dentist, developed the first dental X-ray unit in 1896, as well as intraoral film holders. He was the first one to publish a paper on the potential dangers of X-rays. Rollins proposed the use of filters to suspend the dangerous parts of the X-ray beam, the use of collimation, and the practice of covering the patient with lead to prevent X-ray penetration. Rollins also pointed out the importance of setting safe and harmful dose limits. In 1913, William D. Coolidge, an electrical engineer, developed a high vacuum tube that contained a tungsten filament, which became the first modern X-ray tube. Further in 1923, Coolidge and the General Electric Corporation immersed an X-ray tube, in oil, inside the head of an X-ray machine. This eliminated the accidental exposure to high voltage shock, cooled the tube, and served as a model for all modern dental X-ray machines. From that time on, the dental X-ray machine did not change much until 1957 when a variable kilovoltage dental X-ray machine was introduced, followed by the long-cone head in 1966.

Dental X-ray film

Dental X-ray films also changed through the years; from the original glass photographic plates,

Table 1.1   Milestones in the history of dental radiography.

1895	Discovery of X-rays	W.C. Roentgen
1896	First dental radiograph	O. Walkhoff
1901	First paper on risks of X-radiation	W.H. Rollins
1913	First prewrapped dental films	Eastman Kodak Company
1913	First X-ray tube	W.D. Coolidge
1923	First dental X-ray machine	Victor X-ray Corporation
1947	Introduction of long-cone Paralleling technique	F.G. Fitzgerald
1957	First variable kilovoltage dental X-ray machine	General Electric

hand-wrapped dental X-ray packets in 1896, to the prewrapped intraoral films manufactured by the Eastman Kodak company which were first introduced in 1913. The current high-speed, double-emulsion films require a very short exposure time and were designed to further reduce X-ray exposure.

The bisecting oral radiographic technique was first introduced in 1904 by Weston Price, and the bite-wing technique was introduced by H. Raper in 1925. The paralleling technique was originally introduced in 1896 by C.E. Kells and reformed in 1947 by F.G. Fitzgerald with the introduction of the long-cone (see Table 1.1) (Cieszynski, 1925).

Hazards of X-ray radiation

Ionizing radiation can have harmful effects. The largest man-made source of exposure of radiation to humans is from medical and dental radiographic examinations. Yet one should keep in mind that we are also exposed to other sources and types of radiation. These include radiation from building materials and luminous goods (i.e., television, computer), as well as natural sources (i.e., cosmic rays, soil).

The risk effects depend on the dose received, the frequency of exposure, and the type of tissue irradiated. In general, tissues whose cells divide frequently are more sensitive to the effects of radiation

than those that are less active. Susceptible cells include hematopoietic cells, immature reproductive cells, young bone cells, and epithelial cells. The more radiation-resistant cells include the cells of bones, muscles, and nerves. Ionizing radiation has the effect of increasing the incidence and severity of DNA defects during mitotic division of cells and also interferes with the normal process of repair of these defects. As a consequence, the behavior of the cells may be altered and predispose them to malignant changes. To protect radiation exposure for patients and operators, the use of radiation is governed by state, national, and international agencies. Based on recommendations of the International Commission for Radiation Protection (ICRP), many countries have introduced the following regulation form on radiation protection: (1) doses should be kept as low as reasonably achievable (ALARA); (2) there should be a net benefit for the patient from the use of radiation; (3) radiation doses should not exceed limits laid down by the ICPR; (4) a shield or lead apron should always be used to protect the thyroid and the pelvis; (5) only dental X-ray equipment that is properly collimated, adequate filtrated, and well calibrated should be used; and (6) the X-ray operator shall stand outside the path of the useful X-ray beam or behind a suitable barrier, and should not hold the film in place for the patient during exposure (NCRP Report, 1970, 1989, 1990, 1988; Richard and Colquit, 1981).

Objectives of dental radiography

Dental radiographs are an essential part of the dental diagnostic process, as they enable the practitioner to see many conditions that are not apparent clinically and which could otherwise go undetected. An oral examination without dental radiographs limits the practitioner to what is seen clinically—the surfaces of teeth and soft tissues. Numerous conditions of the teeth and jaws can only be detected on dental radiographs. Missing teeth, extra teeth, and impacted ones, dental caries, periodontal disease as well as root canal fillings, periapical lesions, cysts, and tumors are among the most common conditions that cannot otherwise be diagnosed or properly detected. Suspected pathological conditions can often be confirmed only on

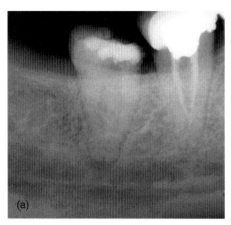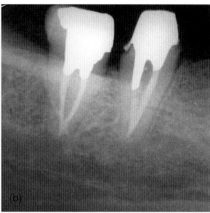

Figure 1.1   (a) Tooth #48 presenting apical lesion. (b) Tooth #48 after root canal treatment presenting healed periapex.

using radiographs. Radiographs often contain a huge amount of information, far more than a written record will usually include. Therefore, initial radiographic examination may provide valuable baseline information about the patient. Follow-up radiographs can then be used to detect and evaluate subsequent changes resulting from treatment, trauma, or disease (Figure 1.1a,b). Patient communication may also greatly benefit from the use of dental radiographs (DeLyre and Johnson, 1995; Haring and Lind, 1996).

X-rays and endodontics

Endodontics is the branch of dentistry that has benefited the most from the introduction of X-rays into everyday dental practice. X-rays allow dentists to visualize areas not accessible by any other diagnostic means such as changes that occur in the bone surrounding the apices of nonvital teeth, intricate root canal anatomy, as well as the ability to follow up the results of endodontic treatment (Gröndahl and Huumonen, 2004). Due to introduction of X-rays, endodontics could turn from an empirical pursuit to a soundly based scientific discipline. Intraoral periapical, occlusal, and panoramic radiographs form the backbone of the endodontic diagnostic process, treatment procedures, and follow-up routine in most of endodontic cases.

Most osteolytic lesions in the jaws result from the pathological changes occurring in the perira-

dicular tissue as a consequence of pulpal infection and necrosis.

The irritants exiting the infected root canal to the periradicular tissues activate both nonspecific inflammatory reactions and specific immune reactions. These not only prevent the spread of infection to the surrounding bone and to remote sites but also result in local bone resorption that can be visualized by radiographic techniques (Stashenko et al., 1998).

The use of radiographs in endodontics is intensive and not limited to the above. They are used to define anatomical features of the roots, such as numbers of roots, their locations, their shape and size, as well as the presence of root canal space. Technical aspects of root canal treatment are greatly assisted by radiographs. These include confirming the length of root canals before instrumentation, determining position of instruments during the procedure and of master cones at the obturation stage. Evaluation of the quality of the root canal filling is based mainly on its radiographic appearance and so is the evaluation of the result of treatment during the follow-up that takes place later. Traumatic injuries to the dentition also make use of radiography for the diagnosis of fractures in the roots and/or the alveolus or for examining the soft tissues for teeth fragment that may have been embedded in them during the traumatic incident. One can hardly imagine endodontic treatment without the assistance of radiography (Cotti and Campisi, 2004; Nair, 1998a; Torabinejad et al., 1985).

Limitations of X-rays in endodontics

With all its benefits, one has to keep in mind that conventional dental radiograph represents merely a two-dimensional (2D) shadow of a three-dimensional (3D) structure (Bender and Seltzer, 1961). As such, it has substantial limitations that should be recognized and taken into consideration when interpreting such records. The buccolingual dimension is not represented in conventional radiographs, thus limiting their interpretation as to the actual 3D size of the radiolucent lesions and their spatial relationship with anatomic landmarks (Cotti and Campisi, 2004; Gröndahl and Huumonen, 2004; Huumonen and Orstavik, 2002). It should also be kept in mind that radiographs do not provide information as to the true nature of the tissue that replaced the bone. Chronic inflammatory lesions cannot reliably be differentiated from cysts or from scar tissue that also mimic osteolytic lesions (Nair, 1998b; Simon, 1980).

For a radiolucent lesion to appear in the radiograph, a substantial amount of bone must have been resorbed; thus, the lack of radiolucency should not be interpreted as absence of bone resorbing process. Furthermore, bone resorption of the cancelous bone surrounding the apex may not be recognized in a periapical radiograph as long as a substantial part of the covering cortical bone has not been resorbed as well (Gröndahl and Huumonen, 2004; Marmary et al., 1999).

Observer bias

Radiographic interpretation is prone to observer bias. Goldman has found that when recall radiographs of endodontic treatment were assessed for success and failure by different radiologists and endodontists, there was more disagreement than agreement between the examiners (Goldman et al., 1972).

Since radiographs are an essential tool in the diagnostic process, they should be carefully analyzed and interpreted with caution.

Digital radiography systems (DRS)

Oral radiographic sensors capable of providing instant images were introduced in 1984 by Dr. Francis Mouyen from Toulouse, France, and formed the basis for the DRS (Mouyen, 1991).

Various digital imaging modalities are available today based on sensors using solid-state technology, such as charge-coupled device (CCD), complementary metal oxide semiconductor (CMOS), or photostimulable phosphor (PSP) technology (Nair and Nair, 2007; Naoum et al., 2003; Wenzel and Gröndahl, 1995). Digital radiography has become an indispensable diagnostic tool in daily dental practice. Requiring a lower radiation dose and providing instantaneous high-resolution digital images make digital radiography especially useful when providing endodontic treatment. Manipulation or processing of the captured image to enhance diagnostic performance makes digital radiography even more versatile in this particular use as it greatly reduces the need to re-expose patients for retakes. In an era of digital archiving, transmission, and long-distance consultation, digital radiography becomes more and more popular. Nevertheless, one should keep in mind that the image is generated using a software program, and as such, it may be subjected to adding or deleting relevant information. The widespread use of these systems, each using their own software, made it important that one software package will be able to adequately handle images produced using another package. The Digital Imaging and Communications in Medicine (DICOM) Standard has therefore been introduced and accepted as the universal standard for digital image transmission and archiving (Calberson et al., 2005; Farman and Farman, 2005). This standard ensures that all images are readable with any viewing software without loss of fidelity or diagnostic information.

Digital images have been shown to perform comparably with conventional intraoral film for a variety of diagnostic tasks (Farman and Farman, 2005; Wenzel and Gröndahl, 1995). However, with continuous upgrading of both software and hardware, and especially with the great advances being made in sensor technology, one may expect great improvement in image quality in the near future.

Characteristics of the radiograph

Radiographic examination is carried out to provide maximum differentiation of tissue structures. A high-quality radiograph is characterized by details which are defined as delineation of the minute structural elements and borders of the objects in the image, by its *density* or the degree of "blackness" on a radiographic film that depends on the amount of radiation reaching a particular area on the film, and by its *contrast* or the ratio between black and white and the different shades of gray on proximate areas of the film. *Distortion* or an unequal magnification of the object causing changes in its size and shape may be another factor affecting the quality of a given radiograph (Anderson, 1974).

Characteristics of a correct radiograph

The requirements for achieving a correct radiograph are as follows:

1. It should record the complete area of interest. The full length of the root and at least 2 mm of periapical bone must be visible.
2. If pathology is evident; the complete rarefaction plus normal bone should be present in the film. In some cases of large areas, an occlusal radiograph or a panoramic radiograph (PAN) maybe needed.
3. Films should have the minimal amount of distortion.
4. Films should have optimal density and contrast.

Defective radiographs

Errors in improperly exposing or processing dental films can produce dental radiographs of nondiagnostic quality. These are known as defective radiographs (Free-Ed.Net, 2006). The dental X-ray specialist should be familiar with the common causes of faulty radiographs and how to prevent them.

1. Underexposed image (Figure 1.2): An image that is too light which may be caused by not enough exposure or not enough development time.
2. Overexposed image (Figure 1.3): An overexposed image, an image that is too dark, may

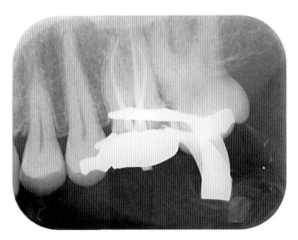

Figure 1.2   Underexposed radiograph.

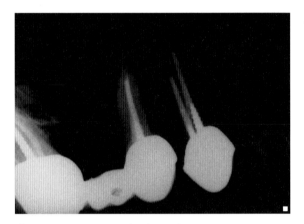

Figure 1.3   Overexposed radiograph.

be caused by very long exposure, or long development time.
3. Blurred image (Figure 1.4): A blurred image is easily recognized by the appearance of more than one image of the object, or objects, on the film. It may be caused by movement of the patient, film, or tube during exposure.
4. Partial image (Figure 1.5): Also known as collimation. A partial image may be caused by failure to immerse the film completely in the developing solution, contact of the film with another film during developing, or improper alignment of the central ray.

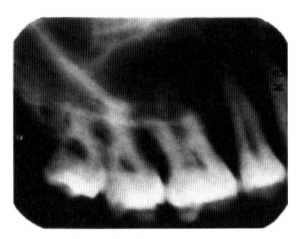

Figure 1.4   Blurry radiograph.

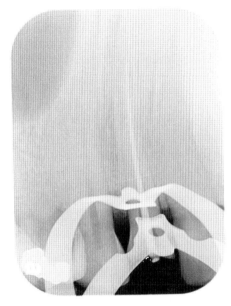

Figure 1.6   Elongated radiograph.

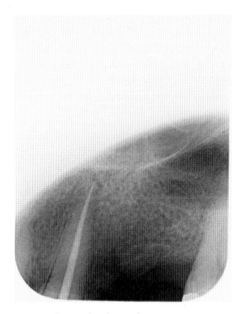

Figure 1.5   Collimated radiograph.

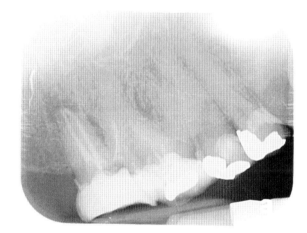

Figure 1.7   Fogged radiograph.

5. Distorted image (Figure 1.6): A distorted image may be caused by improper angulation of the central ray due to bending of the film or sensor.

6. Fogged image (Figure 1.7): A fogged film can be caused by exposure of film to light during storage, or leaving film unprotected (i.e., outside the lead-lined box or in the X-ray room during operation of the X-ray machine) or use of film that has been exposed to heat or chemical fumes, use of improperly mixed or contaminated developer, or defective safelight.

7. Stained or streaked film: Stained or streaked film may be caused by dirty solutions, dirty film holders or hangers, incomplete washing, or solutions left on the workbench.

8. Scratched film: When a film is scratched by film holders or hangers during the development process or when the digital PSP sensor needs to be replaced (Figure 1.8).
9. Lead-foil image (Figure 1.9): A lead-foil image occurs when the embossing pattern from the lead-foil backing appears on the radiograph. The embossing pattern consists of raised diamonds across both ends of the film. This happens when the film is placed in backwards.
10. No image: No image may result if no current was passing through the tube at the time of exposure or if the film was placed in the fixing solution before it was placed in the developing solution.

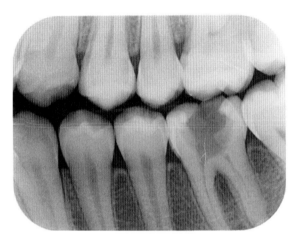

Figure 1.8   Scratched image.

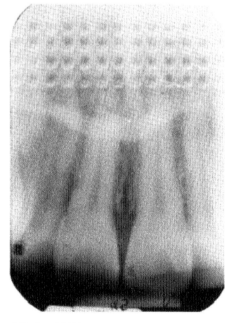

Figure 1.9   Lead foil image.

Control and characteristics of the X-ray machine

The X-ray beam emitted by the generating tube can be controlled and modified by the operator. The milliamperage or the amount of electric charge flowing past a circuit point at a specific time may affect the time required to generate a radiograph. High milliamperage is preferable in order to reduce the exposure time and limit radiation exposure; kilovoltage or the electrical potential difference between the anode and cathode of an X-ray tube is set for dental radiographs in the range between 65 and 90 kVp. Radiographs generated with high kilovoltage will show increased density and reveal more details and information. Exposure time is the parameter most frequently controlled by the operator. It is equivalent to the amount of light allowed to fall on the photographic film or sensor during the process of taking a photograph. Longer exposure time provides denser and darker radiographs. The spread of the X-ray beam is controlled by the collimator which consists of a barrier containing an aperture in the middle. It narrows the X-ray beam and minimizes the formation of secondary diffuse radiation. The collimator thus reduces exposure to excessive ionizing radiation and improves film quality. A filter made as an aluminum barrier is interposed in the path of the beam to eliminate X-rays with low penetrating power and low diagnostic benefit. The distance between target and object is yet another parameter that controls the intensity of the X-ray beam (Anderson, 1974).

Radiographic processing

One of the processing methods in dental radiography is the automatic processor. Most dental facilities use this processing method. With automatic processors, exposed films are immediately loaded to the processors by unwrapping films in the dark room. These processors are equipped with rollers and compartments filled with chemical solutions through which the film advances. At the end of the processing cycle, the film releases.

Another processing method in dental radiography is the manual process. This is done by using the standard time temperature method and a small container consisting of various solutions. The film has to pass through different solutions including developing, rising, fixing, washing, and drying in a temperature-controlled environment. These steps will give better dental radiographic image.

Viewing conditions for radiographs

Accurate diagnosis from radiographs depends upon optimal viewing conditions.

A magnifier-viewer and adequate light are of the utmost importance (Brynolf, 1971). Sensitivity and specificity has been shown to be reduced with inappropriate illumination (Patel et al., 2000). To maximize visual acuity, it is important that the retinal cones of the human eye receive an incident luminance of 100 candela per meter (cdmJ) (CEC, 1990). In diagnostic radiology, viewing boxes with low brightness will reduce the light reaching the eye, limiting visual acuity, and thus reducing the ability to carry out adequate assessment of radiographs. A good viewing box should also demonstrate consistent spatial illumination; otherwise, areas of the image will transmit less light than adjacent areas even when optical densities in the two areas are the same. Also, ambient lighting should be minimized (see Table 1.2) (Abildgaard and Notthellen, 1992).

Radiographic interpretation

Finally, the clinical information that can be derived from a radiograph depends on interpreting what is seen on the film. Such interpretation should be performed systematically. An organized method for evaluation and interpretation of all types of radiographs should be applied on a series Wuehrmann (1970). One structure should be reviewed at a time. For example, the lamina dura is followed around

Table 1.2   Published guidelines on radiological image viewing conditions.

Source of guidelines	Brightness of viewing box (cd m^{-2})	Uniformity of viewing box (%)	Ambient lighting (lux)
WHO (WHO, 1982)	1500–3000	≤15	≤100
CEC (CEC, 1997)	≥1700	≤30	≤5

WHO, World Health Organization; CEC, Commission of European Communities.

the first tooth on the left and then around the next tooth and the next, until the full mouth is scanned. Attention is then turned to the next structure, root form, tooth crowns, and so on. Much of radiographic interpretation is based on differentiation of normal versus abnormal conditions. Radiographical interpretation requires a comprehensive knowledge and familiarity of normal radiographic anatomy and of the oral cavity. Accurate interpretation requires the integration of clinical data, and information provided by the patient with the radiographic data is mandatory.

New horizons in endodontic imaging

Alternative imaging techniques have been introduced over the years to overcome the existing limitations of intraoral radiographs (Abrahams, 2001; Cohenca et al., 2007; Nair and Nair, 2007; Patel et al., 2007, 2009).

Computed tomography (CT)

Computerized axial tomography was first introduced by Hannsfield during the 1970s. CT is an X-ray imaging technique that produces 3D images of an object by using a series of 2D sets of image data and mathematically reconstructing the part under observation in a series of cross sections or planes: axial, coronal, and sagittal (Hannsfield,

1973). CT is exceptional in that it provides imaging of a combination of soft tissues, bone, and blood vessels, and the technique became widely used for the diagnosis of pathologic conditions in maxillary and mandibular bones (Cotti and Campisi, 2004). CT provides valuable information regarding anatomy of the roots and their relation to adjacent anatomical structures such as the maxillary sinus or the inferior alveolar nerve. Information about the thickness of the cortical plates in a given area and their relation to the root apices is of particular interest when endodontic surgery is concerned (Nair and Nair, 2007).

CT also has several drawbacks. On the one hand, it requires high radiation doses and on the other hand, it has a limited low resolution as far as endodontic diagnostic needs are concerned. Scatter from metallic objects presents yet another technological drawback. The high cost of the CT machines which is reflected in the cost of the scans and their limited availability are factors that limit the use of CT in endodontics (Patel, 2009; Patel et al., 2007).

Cone beam computed tomography (CBCT)

The CT is being greatly replaced in endodontics by CBCT (Figure 1.10) (Hashimoto et al., 2003, 2006, 2007). This technology was developed during the 1990s to produce 3D scans of the maxillofacial frame at a considerably lower radiation dose than the CT (Arai et al., 1999; Mozzo et al., 1999). The reduced radiation dose is a result of the rapid scan time, pulsed X-ray beam, and special image receptor sensors. CBCT differs from CT imaging in that the whole volume data are acquired by a single round of the scanner, rotating around the patient's head 180–360 degrees, depending on the CBCT properties. One rotation results in up to 570 projections or exposures. The X-ray beam is cone-shaped (hence the name of the technology) and captures a cylindrical or spherical volume of data called field of view (Patel, 2009; Patel et al., 2007). Voxel size used in CBCT ranges between 0.08 and $0.4\,mm^3$. The radiation dose may be further reduced by decreasing the size of the field of view, increasing the voxel size, and/or reducing the number of projection images during the rotation of the X-ray beam around the patient.

CBCT is usually served by unique software in which the images are displayed simultaneously in the three planes: axial, saggital, and coronal. Moving the cursor on one image simultaneously enables reconstruction in all three planes, allowing for dynamic evaluation of the area involved

CBCT is increasingly used in endodontics, allowing for the earlier detection of periapical disease as compared to conventional radiographs and in assessing the true size, extent, nature, and position of periapical and other resorptive lesions. Diagnosing root fractures and evaluation of root canal anatomy are also greatly enhanced by CBCT (Bartling et al., 2007; Estrela et al., 2008; Huumonen et al., 2006; Mora et al., 2007; Patel and Dawood, 2007; Rigolone et al., 2003; Velvart et al., 2001). It is extremely useful when planning apical microsurgery.

This new technology is still far from being perfect. At present, the spatial resolution of CBCT images is at the range of 2 line-pairs per millimeter, compared to that of conventional radiography which is in order of 15–20 line-pairs per millimeter (Patel, 2009).

Scattering caused by high-density neighboring structures such as enamel, gutta-percha, metal posts, and restorations is another unsolved problem with CBCT images, together with the need to perfectly stabilize the patient for as long as 15–20 seconds (Estrela et al., 2008; Minami et al., 1996).

Magnetic resonance imaging (MRI)

MRI combines the use of a magnetic field and radio waves. During an MRI exam, a magnetic field is created. Different atoms in the body absorb radio waves at different frequencies under the influence of the magnetic field. The absorption is measured and reconstructed by the software into images of the area examined (Haring and Lind, 1996). MRI is a completely noninvasive technique, since it uses radio waves and is not affected by metallic restorations (Abildgaard and Notthellen, 1992; Hashimoto et al., 2003). MRI was used in dentistry to investigate the tissues of the temporomandibular joint and salivary glands (Goto et al., 2007). It may also help to determine the nature of the tissue in periapical lesions when planning surgical inter-

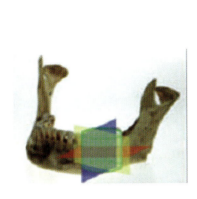
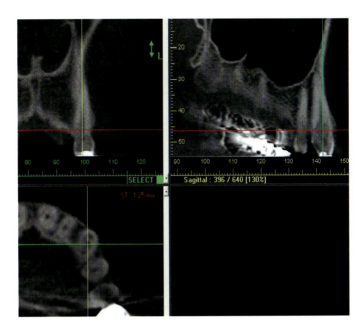

Figure 1.10   3D+cross sections of CBCT.

vention (Cotti and Campisi, 2004; Goto et al., 2007; Minami et al., 1996). The high cost of the unit scans, the limited availability, and the poor resolution of the scans limit the use of this technology in endodontics.

Ultrasound

Ultrasound is an imaging technology based on the reflection of ultrasound waves called "echos," generated by a synthetic crystal. When the ultrasound beam comes across the interface between tissues possessing different acoustic properties, the echo is reflected back to the crystal. The echoes are then transformed into light signals and then into moving images on a monitor. Ultrasound imaging is considered to be a safe technique and is easy to perform. Its use in endodontics may allow detection of periapical lesions and in determining whether vacuolization exists within the lesion, thus possibly allowing for differentiation between cysts and granulomas. Interpretation of the results of this diagnostic technology requires extensive experience.

References

The Bible. King James version. Genesis. Chapter 1:3–4.

CEC. (1990) Quality criteria for diagnostic radiographic images. Working document (2nd ed.), XII/173/90: CEC, Brussels, Belgium.

Abildgaard, A. and Notthellen, J.A. (1992) Increased contrast when viewing radiographic images. *Radiology*, 185, 475–478.

Abrahams, J.J. (2001) Dental CT imaging: a look at the jaw. *Radiology*, 219, 334–345.

Anderson, P.C. (1974) *Dental Radiology*. Delmar Publishers, Albany, NY.

Arai, Y., Tammisalo, E., Iwai, K., Hashimoto, K., and Shinoda, K. (1999) Development of a compact computed tomographic apparatus for dental use. *Dentomaxillofac Radiol*, 28, 245–248.

Bartling, S.H., Majdani, O., Gupta, R. et al. (2007) Large scan field, high spatial resolution flat-panel detector based volumetric CT of the whole human skull base and for maxillofacial imaging. *Dentomaxillofac Radiol*, 36, 317–327.

Bender, I.B. and Seltzer, S. (1961) Roentgenographic and direct observation of experimental lesions in bone. *J Am Dent Assoc*, 87, 708–716.

Brynolf, I. (1971) Improved viewing facilities for better roentgenodiagnosis. *Oral Surg Oral Med Oral Pathol*, 32, 808–811.

Calberson, F., Hommez, G., and De Moor, R. (2005) Fraudulent use of digital radiographs: secret reality or fiction? *Rev Belge Med Dent*, 60, 58–67.

CEC. Criteria for acceptability of radiological (including radiotherapy) and nuclear installations. Radiation Protection No. 91. Luxembourg, 1997. Commission of the European Communities.

Cieszynski A. (1925) The position of the dental axis in the jaws and the exact adjustment of the chief ray in the intraoral method with regard to maxillary irregularities: Table of angle dimensions for the chief ray. *Int J Orthod*, 11, 742.

Cohenca, N., Simon, J.H., Roges, R., Morag, Y., and Malfaz, J.M. (2007) Clinical indications for digital imaging in dento-alveolar trauma: Part 1. Traumatic injuries. *Dent Traumatol*, 23, 95–104.

Cotti, E. and Campisi, G. (2004) Advanced radiographic techniques for the detection of lesions in bone. *Endod Top*, 7, 52–72.

DeLyre, W.R. and Johnson, O.N. (1995) Patient education. In: M. Cohen, ed., *Essentials of Dental Radiography for Dental Assistance and Hygienists*, 5th ed., pp. 365–371. Julie Levin Alexander, Norwalk, CT.

Estrela, C., Bueno, M.R., Leles, C.R., Azevedo, B., and Azevedo, J.R. (2008) Accuracy of cone beam computed tomography and panoramic radiography for the detection of apical periodontitis. *J Endod*, 34, 273–279.

Farman, A.G. and Farman, T.T. (2005) A comparison of 18 different x-ray detectors currently used in dentistry. *Oral Surg Oral Med Oral Pathol Oral Radiol Endod*, 99, 485–489.

Free-Ed.Net. (2006) Fundamentals of dental radiography. Accessed October 26, 2011. www.free-ed.net/free-ed/MedArts/DentalRad01.asp

Goldman, M., Pearson, A.H., and Darzenta, N. (1972) Endodontic success—who's reading the radiograph? *Oral Surg Oral Med Oral Pathol*, 33, 432–437.

Goto, T.K., Nishida, S., Nakamura, Y. et al. (2007) The accuracy of three-dimensional magnetic resonance 3D vibe images of the mandible: an in vitro comparison of magnetic resonance imaging and computed tomography. *Oral Surg Oral Med Oral Pathol Oral Radiol Endod*, 103, 550–559.

Gröndahl, H.-G. and Huumonen, S. (2004) Radiographic manifestations of periapical inflammatory lesions. *Endod Top*, 8, 55–67.

Grossman, L.I. (1982) A brief history of endodontics. *J Endod*, 8, Special Issue, 36.

Hannsfield, G.N. (1973) Computerized transverse axial scanning (tomography) 1. Description of system. *Br J Radiol*, 46, 1016–1022.

Haring, J.I. and Lind, L.J. (1996) *Dental radiography: Principles and Techniques*. W.B. Saunders Company, St. Louis, MO.

Hashimoto, K., Yoshinori, Y., Iwai, K. et al. (2003) A comparison of a new limited cone beam computed tomography machine for dental use with a multidetector row helical CT machine. *Oral Surg Oral Med Oral Pathol Oral Radiol Endod*, 95, 371–377.

Hashimoto, K., Kawashima, S., Araki, M., Sawada, K., and Akiyama, Y. (2006) Comparison of image performance between cone-beam computed tomography for dental use and four-row multidetector helical CT. *J Oral Sci*, 48, 27–34.

Hashimoto, K., Kawashima, S., Kameoka, S. et al. (2007) Comparison of image validity between cone beam computed tomography for dental use and multidetector row helical computed tomography. *Dentomaxillofac Radiol*, 36, 465–471.

Huumonen, S., Kvist, T., Grondahl, K., and Molander, A. (2006) Diagnostic value of computed tomography in re-treatment of root fillings in maxillary teeth. *Int Endod J*, 39, 827–833.

Huumonen, S. and Orstavik, D. (2002) Radiological aspects of apical periodontitis. *Endod Top*, 1, 3.

Marmary, Y., Kotler, T., and Heling, I. (1999) The effect of periapical rarefying osteitis on cortical and cancellous bone. A study comparing conventional radiographs with computed tomography. *Dentomaxillofac Radiol*, 28, 267–271.

Minami, M., Kaneda, T., Ozawa, K., Yamamoto, H., Itai, Y., Ozawa, M., Yoshikwa, K., and Sasaki, Y. (1996) Cystic lesions of the maxillomandibular region: MR imaging distinction of odontogenic keratocysts and ameloblastomas from other cysts. *Am J Roentgenol*, 166, 943–949.

Mora, M.A., Mol, A., Tyndall, D.A., and Rivera, E. (2007) In vitro assessment if local tomography for the detection of longitudinal tooth fractures. *Oral Surg Oral Med Oral Pathol Oral Radiol Endod*, 103, 825–829.

Mouyen, F. (1991) Evaluation of the new radiovisiography system image quality. *Oral Surg Oral Med Oral Pathol*, 72, 627–631.

Mozzo, P., Procacci, C., Tacconi, A., Martini, P.T., and Andreis, I.A. (1999) A new volumetric CT machine for dental imaging based on the cone-beam technique: preliminary results. *Eur Radiol*, 8, 1558–1564.

Nair, M.K. and Nair, U.P. (2007) Digital and advanced imaging in endodontics: a review. *J Endod*, 33, 1–6.

Nair, P.N.R. (1998a) Pathology of apical periodontitis. In: D. Orstavik and T.R. Pitt Ford, eds., *Essential Endodontology: Prevention and Treatment of Apical Periodontitis*. Blackwell Science Ltd, Oxford.

Nair, P.N. (1998b) New perspectives on radicular cysts: do they heal? *Int Endod J*, 31, 155–160.

Naoum, H.J., Chandler, N.P., and Love, R.M. (2003) Conventional versus storage phosphor-plate digital images to visualize the root canal system contrasted with a radiopaque medium. *J Endod*, 29, 349–352.

NCRP Report. National Council on Radiation Protection and Measurements, Bethesda, MD Dental X-Ray Protection, No. 35, 1970.

NCRP Report. Quality Assurance for Diagnostic Imaging Equipment, No. 99, 1988.

NCRP Report. Radiation Protection for Medical and Allied Health Personnel, No. 105, 1989.

NCRP Report. Implementation of the Principle of as Low as Reasonably Achievable (ALARA) for Medical and Dental Personnel, No. 107, 1990.

Patel, N., Rushton, V.E., Macfarlane, T.V., and Horner, K. (2000) The influence of viewing conditions on radiological diagnosis of periapical inflammation. *Br Dent J*, 189, 40–42.

Patel, S. (2009) New dimensions in endodontic imaging: part 2. Cone beam computed tomography. *Int Endod J*, 42, 463–475.

Patel, S. and Dawood, A. (2007) The use of cone beam computed tomography in the management of external cervical resorption lesions. *Int Endod J*, 40, 730–737.

Patel, S., Dawood, A., Whaites, E., and Pitt Ford, T. (2007) The potential applications of cone beam computed tomography in the management of endodontic problems. *Int Endod J*, 40, 818–830.

Patel, S., Mannocci, F., Wilson, R., Dawood, A., and Pitt Ford, T. (2009) Detection of periapical bone defects in human jaws using cone beam computed tomography and intraoral radiography. *Int Endod J*, 42, 507–515.

Richard, A.C. and Colquit, T.W.N. (1981) Reduction in dental x-ray exposures during the past 60 years. *J Am Dent Assoc*, 103, 713.

Rigolone, M., Pasqualini, D., Bianchi, L., Berutti, E., and Bianchi, S.D. (2003) Vestibular surgical access to the palatine root of the superior first molar:"low-dose cone-beam" CT analysis of the pathway and its anatomic variations. *J Endod*, 29, 773–775.

Simon, J.H. (1980) Incidence of periapical cysts in relation to the root canal. *J Endod*, 6, 845–848.

Stashenko, P., Teles, R., and D'Souza, R. (1998) Periradicular inflammatory responses and their modulation. *Crit Rev Oral Bio Med*, 9, 498–521.

Torabinejad, M., Eby, W.C., and Naidorf, I.J. (1985) Inflammatory and immunological aspects of the pathogenesis of human periapical lesions. *J Endod*, 11, 479–488.

Velvart, P., Hecker, H., and Tillinger, G. (2001) Detection of the apical lesion and the mandibular canal in conventional radiography and computed tomography. *Oral Surg Oral Med Oral Pathol Oral Radiol Endod*, 92, 682–688.

Wenzel, A. and Grondahl, H.G. (1995) Direct digital radiography in the dental office. *Int Dent J*, 45, 27–34.

WHO (1982) *Quality Assurance in Diagnostic Radiology*. World Health Organisation, Geneva, Switzerland.

Wuehrmann, A.H. (1970) Radiation hygiene and its practice in dentistry as related to film viewing procedures and radiographic interpretation. Council on Dental Materials and Devices. *JADA*, 80, 346–356.

2 Intraoral Radiographic Principles and Techniques

Mindy Cash and Bettina Basrani

In the practice of endodontics, radiographs are diagnostic tests that provide the clinician with important information during all phases of endodontic treatment: from the initial diagnostic assessment, through the treatment phase, and finally during posttreatment monitoring. Radiographic interpretation of intraoral images is limited by the fact that radiographs provide a two-dimensional representation of three-dimensional structures. Misinterpretations may occur due to image distortions and can be minimized by employing standardized techniques, including specific film placement, beam angulation, and image processing to produce images that are good representations of the structures of interest. Radiographic assessment may employ either film or digital receptors. Both intra- and extraoral radiographs are viable prescription options that may be considered alone or in combination. Intraoral imaging techniques provide superior image resolution, allowing the detection of earlier and less apparent changes. While extraoral techniques produce images with a greater field of view, they produce an image with decreased resolution, a result of multiple superimpositions.

In the everyday practice of endodontics, intraoral radiography utilizing a combination of different techniques and views generally provides the practitioner with sufficient information that can be used as an adjunct to their other diagnostic investigations, to provide a specific diagnosis, and to help provide guidance throughout the procedure. Several different intraoral views are available for use.

These include the periapical, bitewing, and occlusal views.

Intraoral radiography

1. The periapical radiograph
   Techniques:
   - The bisecting angle technique
   - The long cone paralleling technique
2. The bite-wing radiograph
3. The occlusal radiograph
   Types:
   - Periapical type occlusal radiographs
     - Maxillary anterior occlusal
     - Maxillary lateral occlusal
     - Mandibular anterior occlusal

Endodontic Radiology, Second Edition. Edited by Bettina Basrani.
© 2012 John Wiley & Sons, Inc. Published 2012 by John Wiley & Sons, Inc.

- Cross-sectional type occlusal radiographs
  - ➢ Maxillary cross-sectional (vertex) occlusal
  - ➢ Mandibular cross-sectional (standard) occlusal
    - ▪ Anterior
    - ▪ Posterior (lateral)

Intraoral radiography employs common steps in the production of a quality image.

These include patient preparation, infection control protocol, and radiation hygiene along with preparation, stabilization, positioning, exposure, and processing of the receptor, and finally, image evaluation and radiographic interpretation. Differences between the techniques are based on the principles dictating the receptor positioning and the type of stabilizing equipment used for positioning the receptor and aligning the PID (position-indicating device also known as the "cone"). Several different types of intraoral radiographs provide the practitioner with multiple viewing options that can be used alone or in combination, to help to overcome the challenge of interpreting three-dimensional structures, using two-dimensional imaging modalities.

Factors common to all intraoral techniques:

Patient preparation

The patient is seated in an upright position in the dental chair. The patient is instructed to remove eyeglasses, all removable dental appliances, and any metallic piercings or jewelry that may be in the path of the X-ray beam. Metallic objects that have been left in place will attenuate the X-ray beam to produce radiopaque shadows (superimpositions) on the image, which may obscure important structures. The patient is covered with a lead apron and thyroid collar.

Infection control protocol

During the production of radiographs, the operator should wear gloves and adhere to all standard infection control procedures.

Radiation hygiene

Radiographic prescription should be based on the standardized guidelines (The selection of patients for dental radiographic examinations, American Dental Association, 2011) in accordance with the ALARA (as low as reasonably achievable) principle of radiation hygiene.

Receptor preparation

Either digital or film type receptors can be used to capture the image when exposing an intraoral radiograph. Different types of digital receptors include solid state charge-coupled device (CCD), complementary metal oxide semiconductor (CMOS), and photostimulatable phosphor (PSP). It is important to note that for infection control purposes, digital receptors must be wrapped in single-use plastic sleeves prior to intraoral placement, while film type receptors come from the manufacturer as a prepackaged sterile unit (Figure 2.1).

For intraoral radiographs, both digital and film type receptors are available in ANSI sizes 0, 1, 2, and 4 (ranging in size from smallest to largest). The receptor size is selected considering the specific area of interest. In general, the size 1 receptor is chosen for evaluation of the anterior teeth, while the size 2 receptor is used in the posterior regions, specifically from the distal of the canine posteriorly. The size 4 receptor is used exclusively for the occlusal type radiograph and is employed in relationship to the teeth that is unique. The size 0 receptor is reserved for use in pediatric patients or in situations where anatomic considerations limit the ability of adequate placement of a larger receptor (Figure 2.2).

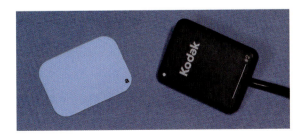

Figure 2.1   From left, PSP and CCD type receptors.

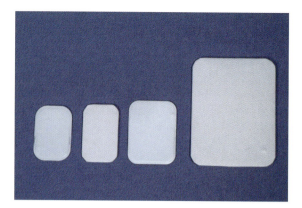

Figure 2.2 From left, ANSI sizes 0, 1, 2, and 4 receptors. (Image courtesy of B. Rakiewicz, BAA, RBP, DPES, Faculty of Dentistry, University of Toronto, 2011.)

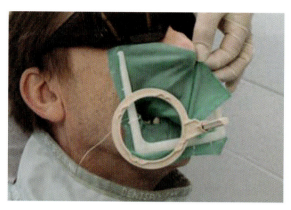

Figure 2.3 Receptor holders specifically designed for endodontics allow imaging during treatment. (Image courtesy of Dr. B.Basrani, Toronto, Canada.)

In addition to the variety of sizes, film type receptors are available in single or double film packets. When the double film packet is used, a duplicate copy of the image is produced, which serves beneficial when a second radiograph is required for consultation with a colleague or in correspondence with an insurance company. Film type receptors are manufactured with different film speeds, which determines the amount of radiation exposure required to produce a radiograph of standard density. To produce an image of comparable density, faster film speeds require lower exposure times when compared to slower film speeds.

It is important that the receptor is always positioned with its active side facing the source of radiation:

- *Films* that are positioned backwards produce an image that is reversed, lighter (less dense) and have a geometric pattern superimposed on one side.
- *PSP* receptors positioned backwards produce no image.
- *CMOS* and *CCD type receptors* have a wire that is attached to their back surface leading directly to a computer monitor, preventing their backward positioning.

Receptor holders

A receptor holder is a device that is placed into the mouth to support the film or sensor, while maintaining the desired position. In endodontics, radiographs that are taken during the treatment phase present a greater stabilizing challenge due to the presence of the rubber dam and clamp. Different holder designs are currently available to help circumvent this problem, and allow proper positioning of the receptor (Figure 2.3). When required, cotton rolls may be used to help to support the holder in position.

If a cotton roll is attached to the surface of the film so that it lies against the lingual surfaces of the teeth, the desired parallelism between film and teeth is achieved, allowing the vertical angulation to be reduced, thus giving rise to improved visualization of the roots and surrounding bone. This method is based on a modification of the bisecting angle technique and results in more parallelism between the teeth and film, thus allowing a reduction in vertical angulation which decreases the incidence of superimposition of the zygomatic process. Clearly, an alternative would be to use a film holder and beam-aiming device.

It is important to emphasize that a holder should be used to support all types of receptors. The practice of engaging the patient in the stabilization process by positioning their thumb or fingers directly in the path of the X-ray beam results in unnecessary patient exposure which, according to the ALARA principle, cannot be justified.

Receptor holders during endodontic procedures

While radiographs are a necessary adjunct in endodontic practice, problems are often encountered. These tend to be related to film placement and stabilization when endodontic instruments, rubber dam, and rubber dam clamps are in position. These problems are encountered most commonly among maxillary teeth and are considered the result of a rigid palate and its accompanying sloping concavity especially in the molar region (Lim and Teo, 1986).

From the earliest days of dental radiography, dentists attempted to standardize radiographic images and techniques. The focus of researchers in the 1950s to the 1970s was to develop a film holder that would hold the film and allow easy and predictable alignment of the X-ray tube. As research projects became more dependent on dental radiographic measurements, the focus shifted to producing reproducible radiographic images, from which highly repeatable measurements could be made. Existing devices have strengths and weaknesses. Readily available devices are adequate for routine clinical use; however, user-friendly and patient-friendly film-holding devices that result in highly reliable and accurate measurements have yet to be introduced (Kazzi et al., 2007).

The routine use of film holders in endodontics ranges from 21.6% (Saunders et al., 1999) to 26% (Chandler and Koshy, 2002). The increasing use of film holders has been shown to have a relationship to those clinicians who routinely use rubber dam (Chandler and Koshy, 2002), those practitioners who are specialists in endodontics (Chandler and Koshy, 2002) and also have a significant relationship to younger practitioners (Saunders et al., 1999).

The EndoRay II (Rinn Dentsply, Weybridge, UK) employing the paralleling technique fits over end-odontic files, rubber dams, and clamps, and is securely held by the patient's bite.

To assemble and use, follow these instructions:

With film centered in the basket, place the assembly over the tooth (with files and clamp) and rest it on adjacent teeth. Release the top or bottom half from the frame of the rubber dam. There is no need to completely remove the rubber dam and frame. The film should be adjacent to the subject tooth and behind the rubber dam. The patient should then bite lightly until the EndoRay II is secure. The EndoRay II is manufactured from a porous plastic material and has a limited life. It must be replaced periodically. For a longer-lasting instrument, always disassemble the three pieces before sterilizing. The EndoRay II should be sterilized in a steam autoclave or chemiclave. Other methods of sterilization are not recommended.

Receptor exposure

Once the receptor is in place and stable, the patient is instructed to maintain position and avoid any movement. The operator leaves the room and stands behind a safe barrier to activate the X-ray unit and expose the receptor. X-ray machine settings are preset prior to receptor positioning and are determined by receptor type, patient size, and X-ray machine.

Receptor processing

The type of receptor used determines the processing method. Film receptors require chemical processing using manual or automatic machines. The resulting image is produced on a coated polyester base that requires a lighted viewing box for evaluation. Digital receptors produce an image that is viewed on a computer monitor. CCD and CMOS receptors are directly linked to a computer monitor where the image can almost instantly be evaluated (within a few seconds) (Versteeg et al., 1997). PSP receptors require a separate scanner that "reads" the receptor and is connected to a computer monitor to produce an image resulting in longer but still rapid processing times (approximately 30 seconds) (Versteeg et al., 1997).

Image evaluation and radiographic interpretation

Both film and digital receptors are initially evaluated for image adequacy. They should provide clear unobstructed images of the teeth and surrounding structures of interest. When using digital receptors image manipulation can be accomplished directly on the computer monitor using the computer's software. Film receptors must be arranged in their correct orientation on a view box. Image evaluation is best done in a darkened room. A radiographic interpretation must be completed for all radiographic images obtained.

Seven basic steps summarize the method used to produce all types of intraoral radiographs. Specific details pertaining to each step and individual variations unique to each specific type of radiograph are discussed under their individual headings.

Intraoral image production
1. Set the exposure time on the X-ray unit
2. Position the patient
3. Prepare and position the receptor
4. Align the PID
5. Expose the receptor
6. Process the receptor
7. Review the image

The periapical radiograph

The periapical radiograph is the most commonly employed radiograph used in the practice of endodontics. When examining a specific tooth, the periapical radiograph should provide an image of the entire tooth from the crown to the apex, including some or all of adjacent teeth, the surrounding bone, and anatomical structures in the vicinity.

Periapical radiographs can help to provide important diagnostic information allowing the detection of new or recurrent caries, the presence of calculus, the status of restorations, the presence and degree of periodontal bone loss, as well as a providing a clear view of the periapical structures (Figure 2.4).

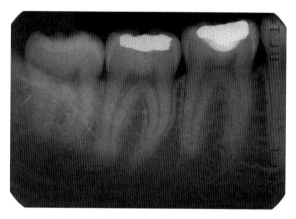

Figure 2.4   A periapical radiograph depicting the mandibular right posterior region.

Two different techniques are available for the production of periapical radiographs; *the bisecting angle technique,* and the more commonly employed *long cone paralleling technique.* Each technique utilizes different methods and equipment, is based on their own specific principles, and result in different limitations in the production of an optimal periapical radiograph.

Concepts unique to each technique

The concepts that are unique to each specific technique are discussed under the individual technique headings. These include a discussion of the technique principles, the types and methods for using the stabilizing the receptor, and the guidelines for aiming the PID.

The bisecting angle technique

Principles

The bisecting angle technique outlines a method to produce an image of an object, minimizing its magnification and distortion, while optimizing its image clarity.

The principles of the technique are based on simple geometry. The rule of isometry states that two triangles are equal if they have two equal angles and share a common side (Figure 2.5).

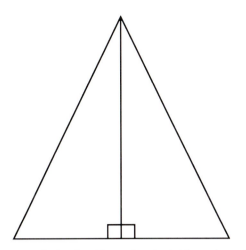

Figure 2.5   A triangle with equal angles is bisected equally, producing two equal triangles that share a common side. (Image courtesy of A. Cormier, BSc, MScBMC, DPES, Faculty of Dentistry, University of Toronto, 2011.)

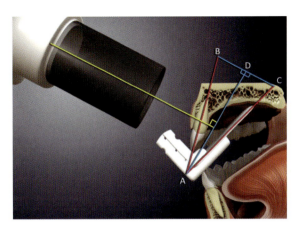

Figure 2.6   The central ray (yellow) is aimed perpendicular to a line that bisects the triangle (blue) formed by the long axis of the tooth and the long axis of the receptor (red lines). (Image courtesy of A. Cormier, BSc, MScBMC, DPES, Faculty of Dentistry, University of Toronto, 2011.)

To apply this principle to intraoral imaging, the receptor (film or sensor) is positioned on the lingual or palatal surface of the mouth, resting against the tooth. The long axis of the receptor meets the long axis of the tooth at point A (tip of the triangle). An imaginary line bisects or divides the triangle into two equal parts (the bisector). The central ray of the X-ray tube must be aligned so that it will strike the bisector at 90 degrees (a right angle). As a result, the rule of isometry can be applied; the two newly produced triangles share a common side and have equal angles, so that the hypotenuse (the side of a right-angled triangle opposite the right angle) AC is equal in length to the hypotenuse of the other triangle AB producing an image of the object that is accurate in length (Haring and Jansen, 2000, pp. 255, 256) (Figure 2.6).

Receptor holders used for the bisecting angle technique and their positioning

- *Styrofoam and rigid plastic stabilizers* (Figure 2.7) are composed of different materials, with a similar design. The occlusal or incisal portion of the receptor rests in a groove located in the horizontal base of the stabilizer. The groove provides alignment and retains the receptor in

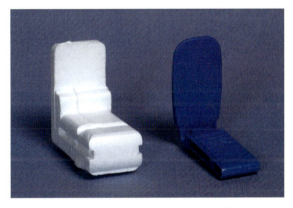

Figure 2.7   Styrofoam and plastic receptor stabilizers. (Images courtesy of B. Rakiewicz, BAA, RBP, DPES, Faculty of Dentistry, University of Toronto, 2011.)

position. The vertical component of the stabilizer supports the vertical component of the receptor, preventing any bending (more commonly a problem when using film type receptors). When positioned lingual or palatal in the mouth, the horizontal base of the stabilizer projects between the occlusal surfaces of the teeth where the patient bites firmly onto it as they close their teeth together, providing stabilization.
- *Hemostat and the Snap-A-Ray® holders* (formerly known as the Eezee-Grip® film holder)

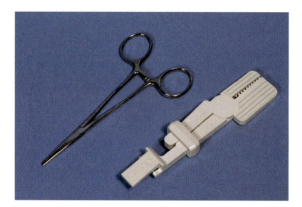

Figure 2.8   Hemostat and Snap-A-Ray® receptor holders. (Images courtesy of B. Rakiewicz, BAA, RBP, DPES, Faculty of Dentistry, University of Toronto, 2011.)

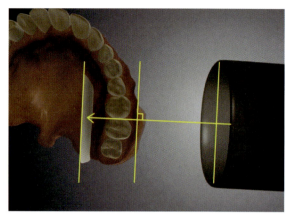

Figure 2.9   When the receptor is correctly positioned (parallel to the buccal surfaces of the teeth), the central ray is aligned perpendicular to it, producing an image that clearly reveals ("opens up") the interproximal contact areas. (Images courtesy of A. Cormier, BSc, MScBMC, DPES, Faculty of Dentistry, University of Toronto, 2011.)

(Figure 2.8) are used in a similar fashion. The open end of each instrument grasps the occlusal portion of the receptor in a horizontal orientation (parallel to the edge), so that when the receptor is positioned palatal or lingual to the teeth, the handle of the devise protrudes out of the mouth. The Snap-A-Ray® has the unique feature of extending a horizontal plate over the occlusal surfaces of the teeth, allowing further stabilization as the patient is instructed to close their teeth together.

Regardless of the type utilized, when in position, the holder aligns the receptor in an upright orientation, as close to the teeth as possible. The shape of the palatal vault or the lingual alveolar bone prevents the receptor/holder combination from aligning parallel to the long axis of the teeth. Instead, an angle is formed at the point where the two long axes intersect.

Aiming the PID

Once the receptor is stabilized intraorally in the desired location, the PID of the dental X-ray unit is aimed. To achieve optimal positioning, three factors must be considered: the horizontal angulations, the vertical angulations, and the aim of the central ray (the centermost ray of the X-ray beam).

- *Horizontal Angulation*
  The horizontal plane of the buccal or labial surfaces of the teeth determines the horizontal angulation. The outer edge of the PID forms a circle. This circle should be aligned parallel to the horizontal plane of the buccal or labial surfaces of the teeth. When correctly positioned, the X-ray beam will strike the horizontal plane of the buccal or labial surfaces of the teeth at a 90-degree or right angle (Figure 2.9).

  When the Snap-A-Ray® or hemostat holder is utilized, the portion that extends out of the patient's mouth is simply an extension of the horizontal plane, and can be used as a guideline to aid in determining the horizontal angulation of the PID.

- *Vertical Angulation*
  The vertical angulation of the PID (see Table 2.1) is determined using the principles of the bisecting angle technique, described earlier. The central ray of the PID is positioned at a 90-degree angle to an imaginary line that bisects the angle formed by the long axis of the tooth and the long axis of the receptor.

  Vertical angulations are divided into "+" and "−" angles depending on the X-ray beam direction, in reference to the horizontal plane. A + angle indicates the downward direction of the

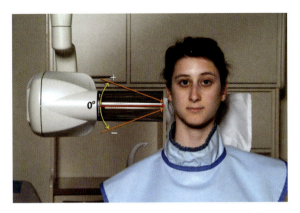

Figure 2.10 When a *positive* angulation is required, the position-indicating device (cone) is rotated about an arc above the horizontal, such that the tube head directs the X-ray beam in a downward direction. Conversely, a *negative* angulation results from the rotation of the position-indicating device below the horizontal directing the X-ray beam in an upward direction. (Image courtesy of B. Rakiewicz, BAA, RBP, DPES, Faculty of Dentistry, University of Toronto, 2011; A. Cormier, BSc, MScBMC, DPES, Faculty of Dentistry, University of Toronto, 2011.)

Table 2.1 Average vertical angles* for the bisecting angle technique using a long PID.

View	Maxilla	Mandible
Molar	+25°	0°
Premolar	+35°	−5°
Canine	+45°	−10°
Incisor	+45°	−15°
Bitewing	+6–8°	

* Note that these angles are based on the patient seated in the dental chair in an upright position, with their head resting against the headrest for support, and their occlusal plane aligned parallel to the floor, when in occlusion.
Source: Langland et al. (2002, p. 123).

X-ray beam, while a − angle refers to an upward beam direction (Figure 2.10).

Guidelines for average vertical angles

- *The Central Ray*
  Finally, the central ray is aimed toward the center of the receptor. As the X-ray beam exits the PID, it begins to diverge. This divergence

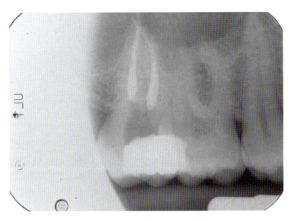

Figure 2.11 A *cone-cut* periapical radiograph occurs when the central ray is not aimed toward the center of the receptor. (Image courtesy of Dr. I. Golosky, Toronto, Canada).

produces a beam with a greater circumference. This larger area beam strikes the active surface of the smaller receptor (sizes 0, 1, and 2), ensuring maximal exposure. Regions of the receptor that are not in the path of the X-ray beam are not exposed to radiation, and therefore, no image is apparent after processing. When the central ray is not centered on the receptor, portions of the receptor are left unexposed and exhibit no image. This positioning error is termed "a cone-cut" and results in an unexposed area on the receptor that outlines the shape of the PID (Figure 2.11).

The long cone paralleling technique

Principles

The long cone paralleling technique is the more commonly used technique to produce an intraoral image. The theory is based on geometric principles of parallelism. Ideally, the concept places the receptor as close to the teeth as possible and parallel to the long axis of the teeth. When the X-ray beam passes through the teeth striking the receptor at a 90-degree angle, it produces an image that is equivalent to the teeth in all dimensions (Figure 2.12).

This ideal theory cannot be applied directly to intraoral radiography, due to several inherent

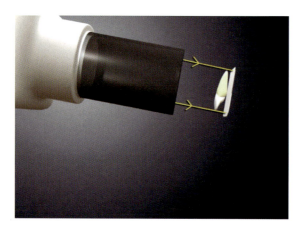

Figure 2.12   With the receptor positioned directly against the tooth, the parallel rays of the X-ray beam produce an accurate representation of the tooth onto the receptor. (Image courtesy of A. Cormier, BSc, MScBMC, DPES, Faculty of Dentistry, University of Toronto, 2011).

factors. The characteristics of the X-ray beam must first be considered. The electron beam produced at the cathode strikes the focal spot on the tungsten target of the anode producing the X-ray beam. The focal spot is not just a spot, but is actually an area. Since X-rays are produced from all areas on the focal spot, the X-rays that strike the object do so at different points, resulting to blurring (decreased sharpness) at the edge of the image. A larger focal spot will produce an image with greater blurring, while a decrease in focal spot size will result in improved sharpness, but greater heat production, causing potential machine overheating concerns (Figure 2.13).

Manufacturers are able to overcome this concern by designing the dental X-ray unit such that the angle between the electron beam and the target is altered, producing a smaller effective focal spot, and thereby improving image sharpness while minimizing the production of heat.

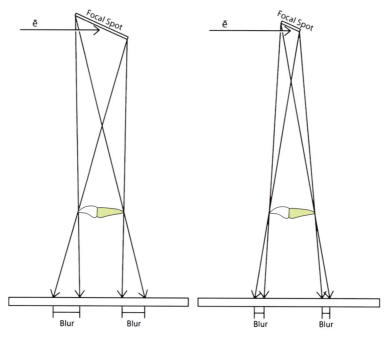

Figure 2.13   The drawings show a comparison of the image blur resulting from two different focal spots sizes. The large focal spot on the left produces an image with a greater area of blur around the edges compared to the smaller focal spot on the right. (Adapted from White and Pharoah, *Oral Radiology Principles and Interpretation*, 2009, p. 87) (Image courtesy of A. Cormier, BSc, MScBMC, DPES, Faculty of Dentistry, University of Toronto, 2011.)

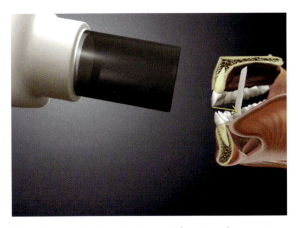

Figure 2.14   Due to anatomic considerations, the receptor must be positioned further into the mouth achieving parallelism between the tooth and the receptor. (Image courtesy of A. Cormier, BSc, MScBMC, DPES, Faculty of Dentistry, University of Toronto, 2011.)

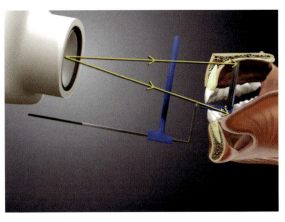

Figure 2.15   The increased distance between the receptor and the tooth results in a magnified image on the receptor, since the X-ray beam diverges as it exits the tube head. (Image courtesy of A. Cormier, BSc, MScBMC, DPES, Faculty of Dentistry, University of Toronto, 2011.)

Furthermore, as the beam exits the X-ray tube, the rays begin to diverge. To achieve parallelism between the receptor and the long axis of the teeth, the receptor must be stabilized in a position at a distance away from the teeth, closer to the center of the mouth (Figure 2.14).

With the receptor positioned at a distance from the teeth (increased focal spot to receptor distance), the X-ray beam penetrates the teeth to expose the receptor, causing the more divergent rays to produce an enlarged or magnified image of the teeth (Figure 2.15).

To compensate for this beam divergence issue, there seem to be two different options. It would seem obvious that if the distance between the receptor and the teeth (receptor to object distance) is decreased, then it would be possible to greatly reduce the negative effects of the diverging beam. This concept is valid and applied wherever possible, but proves difficult to achieve, especially in the maxilla where the curvature of the palate prevents the receptor from resting directly against the teeth in a parallel orientation. Instead, a relatively long PID is attached to the X-ray unit. The longer PID (lead lined) restricts the more divergent rays of the beam, while directing the most central and parallel portion of the X-ray beam at the teeth, thereby reducing magnification while increasing image sharpness (Figure 2.16).

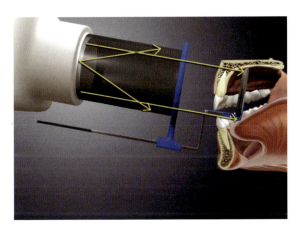

Figure 2.16   The use of a long PID (cone) restricts the more divergent X-rays exiting the tube head, allowing only the most parallel X-rays to interact with the receptor. (Image courtesy of A. Cormier, BSc, MScBMC, DPES, Faculty of Dentistry, University of Toronto, 2011.)

The receptor holder used for the long cone paralleling technique

For the long cone paralleling technique, the Rinn® instrument is used to maintain the receptor in position and aid in directing the X-ray beam. It has three component parts.

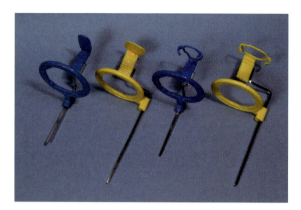

Figure 2.17 Shown from left to right; anterior and posterior Rinn® XCP instruments for film and anterior and posterior Rinn® XCP-DS instruments for digital sensors. (Images courtesy of B. Rakiewicz, BAA, RBP, DPES, Faculty of Dentistry, University of Toronto, 2011.)

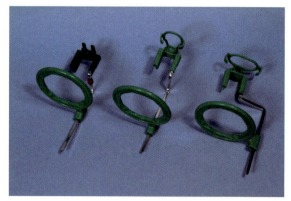

Figure 2.18 Specialized endodontic Rinn XCP (EndoRay) instruments are available for both film and digital receptors. Shown from left to right, universal film (anterior or posterior) Rinn XCP EndoRay instrument; reorientation of the component parts allows universal use, followed by digital anterior and posterior Rinn® XCP EndoRay instruments. (Images courtesy of B. Rakiewicz, BAA, RBP, DPES, Faculty of Dentistry, University of Toronto, 2011.)

- The *stabilizer* component is similar to the holder used with the bisecting angle technique. It has a groove in its horizontal base where the occlusal or incisal portion (dimple on film) of the receptor is inserted. The vertical portion of the stabilizer supports the vertical component of the receptor, preventing bending. The stabilizer base has a horizontal projection that is placed between the occlusal surfaces of the teeth to aid in positioning and stabilization upon closing.
- The *rod* connects the three components and helps to provide a visual guide for the PID. It engages the stabilizer component intraorally, protruding out of the mouth, where it engages the ring component to the unit.
- The *ring* slides along the rod and is positioned close to the cheek to help guide the PID and thereby direct the X-ray beam.

The Rinn instruments are available for both anterior and posterior receptors, permitting the use of the long cone paralleling technique in all regions of the mouth (Figure 2.17). In addition, different models are designed to support both digital and film type receptors (Figure 2.18).

Preparing and positioning the receptor/holder assembly

The appropriate Rinn instrument is selected, considering the receptor type and teeth to be imaged.

In the anterior maxilla and mandible, imaging the anterior teeth from cuspid to cuspid, the size 1 receptor is positioned vertically, and used with the corresponding anterior Rinn instrument. In the posterior regions of the maxilla and mandible, from the distal of the cuspids toward the back of the arch, the size 2 receptor is positioned horizontally and is used with its corresponding posterior Rinn instrument.

Using the correct size receptor in the proper orientation allows production of an image of the entire tooth or teeth along with their supporting structures.

The receptor is inserted into the stabilizing portion of the Rinn instrument in a vertical orientation, with the active side of the receptor directed outward. Positioning the dimple of the film type receptor into the base of the stabilizer ensures that the convex circular area will be projected occlusal to the teeth, usually in the airspace, resulting in an image with an unimpeded view of the desired structures. If the film is not positioned in this manner, an image may be produced where portions of the periapical region are obscured, making thorough examination of the region less than ideal. In addition, it is imperative that the active side of the receptor is directed outward, so that when the instrument is correctly positioned in the patient's mouth, the X-ray beam will strike the active side of the receptor, producing a correctly oriented image with good image characteristics.

Once assembled, the Rinn instrument supporting the receptor is ready to be positioned into the patient's mouth. Considering the area of interest and the local anatomical structures, the assembly is gently rotated into position, so that the occlusal or incisal edges of the teeth are firmly seated onto the horizontal portion of the stabilizer, once the patient has closed their teeth together. It is important for the patient to fully occlude onto the horizontal portion of the stabilizer to ensure maintenance of the assembly position and prevent any movement during exposure. Failure to fully close and maintain position on the assembly may cause movement of the unit, which can result in incomplete receptor coverage in the apical areas as well as an incorrect final position, where the receptor is not aligned parallel with the long axis of the tooth, resulting in image distortions. In the mandible, the height of floor of the mouth may make direct insertion of the assembly uncomfortable for the patient. While the patient's mouth is open, initial insertion of the assembly in a slightly horizontal direction, while gently guiding the device into its final vertical location, may help alleviate any potential discomfort. This method relies on the muscles of the floor of the mouth lowering during the action of closing. Patients with large tongues may make optimal positioning difficult. Gently moving the tongue away from the assembly toward the opposite side of the mouth allows proper seating of the assembly. Sensitive areas of the mouth and some patients may have a gag reflex during the radiologic acquisition process. Definitive receptor placement with minimal adjustments may help to prevent this uncomfortable response.

While positioning the assembly, it is important to ensure that the cheek is released and positioned comfortably over the rod. This prevents the cheek from pushing against the rod and redirecting it, so that the receptor becomes positioned at an angle (not parallel) to the long axis of the teeth. When imaging the posterior regions of the arch, it may prove difficult to accurately position the assembly in a distal enough location to provide image coverage of the entire crown and root area of the most posterior molar. In these unique situations, slightly sliding the receptor distally will ensure adequate imaging of this area. When this alteration is made,

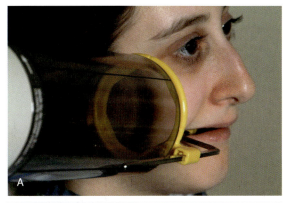

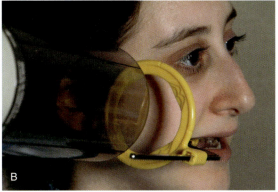

Figure 2.19 (A) The top photograph depicts the ideal PID position in relation to the ring component of the Rinn XCP instrument. (B) In the bottom photograph, the operator slides the receptor posteriorly to capture the posterior region of the maxillary arch. The position of the PID is moved posteriorly in order to direct the central ray toward the center of the receptor, thereby avoiding a "cone-cut." (Images courtesy of B. Rakiewicz, BAA, RBP, DPES, Faculty of Dentistry, University of Toronto, 2011.)

it is important to remember that positioning the PID using the ring as a guide will not deliver radiation to the entire surface of the receptor. To compensate for this alteration, the operator must position the PID at a distance equivalent to the amount of distal movement, thereby ensuring the entire receptor is exposed to the X-ray beam and preventing a "cone-cut" in the distal-most regions (Figure 2.19).

Adjustments to the receptor position, if needed, can be achieved at this point by asking the patient to slightly separate their occluded teeth, just enough to allow the operator to make any small modifications. Once the operator is confident that the assembly is accurately positioned, and fully stabilized by the teeth, the ring is slid along the rod toward, but not touching the patient's cheek. The assembly no longer requires the operator to hold it for support.

Aiming the PID

When positioned correctly, the Rinn assembly accurately positions the horizontal and vertical angulations and the direction of the central ray. The PID is maneuvered into position, using the ring as a guide. The circular open end of the PID is aligned parallel and equal distance from the ring in all areas. Next, the guiding lines on the side of the PID are checked to confirm that they are parallel to the rod of the Rinn assembly. This provides a further check to confirm the vertical angulation of the PID is correct.

Special techniques used during endodontic procedures

The buccal object rule

The rule is also termed as SLOB rule (same lingual opposite buccal). Stated more simply, Ingle's rule is MBD: always shot from Mesial and the Buccal root will move to Distal. As the X-ray tube head is moved from posterior to anterior, objects imaged on the film which are on the lingual aspects (palatal roots or mesial lingual roots or distal lingual roots) will be positioned mesially in the radiograph (the same position as the head tube). Objects located in the buccal aspect will be shifted distally. The palatal root will always shift on the same direction as the tube head. Therefore, the clinician can always determine the direction that the radiograph was taken by looking at the palatal roots of molars.

Roots that are superimposed on a standard radiograph can be visualized when a mesial or distal view is taken. In general, the degree of horizontal angulation necessary to achieve a clear image will depend on the separation of the roots; the more parallel the roots (closer), the greater the alteration should be, while roots with a considerable divergence will require only a modest degree of horizontal angulation. When the horizontal angulation is varied by 20 degrees to mesial, the zygomatic process is "moved" to distal of the first molar, and the distobuccal root is cleared of the palatal root. If we need to isolate the MB root, the head of the radiographic machine will need to be moved to the opposite side (Fava and Dummer, 1997).

The triangular scanning technique

This technique can be used to detect the exact position of root curvatures as well as iatrogenic errors such as ledges, creation of false canals during post space preparation and lateral perforations. The technique involves the exposure of three films, one using the standard angulation and the others using mesial and distal angulations.

To interpret the data available from the three films correctly, it is necessary for each view to draw a diagram with two concentric circles where the outer circle represents the root contour and the inner circle represents the outline of the canal. Each cross-sectional representation of the root is then divided into quadrants by two lines, one vertical dividing the root into mesial and distal halves, the other horizontal dividing the root into buccal and lingual halves. A mesial angulation will superimpose the mesiobuccal (MB) and distolingual (DL) quadrants, while a distal angulation will superimpose the distobuccal (DB) and mesiolingual (ML) quadrants. Data obtained from the three radiographs are transferred to the diagrams to produce a simple representation of the complex three-dimensional architecture of the tooth (Fava and Dummer, 1997).

The bite-wing radiograph

In endodontics, the bite-wing radiograph is often selected as a supplemental radiographic view during the diagnostic phase. The bite-wing radiograph provides a single image depicting the maxillary and mandibular crowns, the interproximal contacts, and the height and relationship of the alveolar crests. It reveals important diagnostic information regarding the status of restorations, the presence of pulp calcifications or resorptions, and the depth of caries, all helping to determine the potential restorability of the tooth, as well as aiding in the planning of a strategy for the root canal procedure.

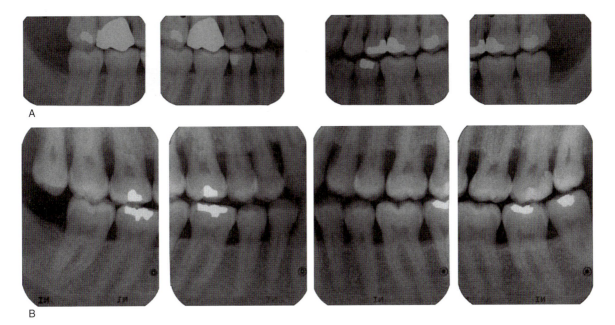

A

B

Figure 2.20   (A) Horizontal bitewings. (B) Vertical bitewings.

Bite-wing radiographs are typically produced with the size 2 receptor in a horizontal orientation, but in situations where the alveolar crests have receded, *horizontal bite-wings* may fail to reveal the alveolar crests. Reorienting the receptor into a vertical position (*vertical bitewing*) will capture the apically positioned alveolar crests on the image (Figure 2.20A,B).

Method

The seven basic steps used to produce intraoral images, as outlined earlier, are applied to produce the bite-wing radiographs.

Receptor holders

To produce a bite-wing radiograph, the receptor must be held in position. Several types of receptor holders are available for use with film type or digital receptors.

- Cardboard bitetabs loops
- Stick on bitetabs
- Rinn XCP and XCP-DS bite-wing instrument (Figure 2.21).

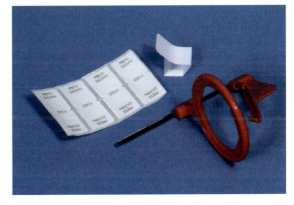

Figure 2.21   Clockwise from left, stick on bite tabs, cardboard bite tab loops and RINN XCP-DS (digital) bitewing instrument. (Images courtesy of B. Rakiewicz, BAA, RBP, DPES, Faculty of Dentistry, University of Toronto, 2011.)

The type of holder is selected and attached appropriately to the receptor.

- When using the *bitetab loop*, the receptor is horizontally inserted into the loop so that the loop wraps around it and the horizontal tab is centered, extending outward from the active side of the receptor.

- *Stick on bitetabs* are attached and centered on the plastic sleeve or outer plastic covering of the active side of the receptor.
- *Rinn XCP and XCP-DS bite-wing instruments* support the correctly inserted receptor to provide rigid stabilization and an aiming ring for the PID.

It is important to correctly attach the bite-wing holder to the receptor. If the horizontal extension is not centered, the resulting image will exhibit a disproportionate amount of each arch and may therefore limit the usefulness of the radiograph.

Attaching the holder so that the horizontal extension is on the incorrect (nonactive) side places the receptor backward in the mouth, producing an image that is reversed, resulting in mounting errors, which can lead to confusion and potential errors in treatment. Film type receptors placed backward will produce a lighter (less dense) image with a geometric superimposition of the embossed lead foil along one side.

Receptor positioning

There are four standard locations for positioning bite-wing radiographs; two on either side of the dental arch. These include the anterior (premolar) bite-wing radiograph and the posterior (molar) bite-wing radiograph (Figure 2.20A,B).

- The *anterior bitewing* is positioned so that the distal aspect of the canine is captured in the image.
- The *posterior bitewing* is positioned more distally in the arch ensuring that the distal aspect of the last erupted molar is evident in the view.

When all four radiographs are prescribed, the maxillary and mandibular crowns of all of the posterior teeth are imaged simultaneously.

To insert the receptor with its holder into position, the patient is instructed to open their mouth while the operator slides the base of the receptor into the lingual aspect of the mandibular arch. The receptor should be aligned parallel and rest against the mandibular teeth. All bite-wing holders have a horizontal portion that extends buccally between

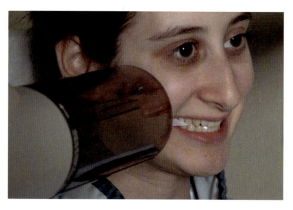

Figure 2.22   Acquiring a bitewing radiograph. (Image courtesy of B. Rakiewicz, BAA, RBP, DPES, Faculty of Dentistry, University of Toronto, 2011.)

the occlusal surfaces of the teeth. The patient is instructed to close their teeth together into their natural biting position. The operator holds the horizontal component during closing so that the receptor position is maintained.

Aiming the PID

- *Vertical angulation*
  With the patient's head stable against the headrest and oriented so that the occlusal plane is parallel to the floor when in occlusion, the vertical plane of the maxillary and mandibular posterior teeth are aligned at a small angle.

  In order for the X-ray beam to strike the receptor at a 90-degree angle (perpendicular), the PID must be rotated to approximately +10 degrees (Figure 2.10). This allows accurate representation of the teeth on the image, with maximal overlapping of the buccal and lingual cusps and surfaces of the alveolar crest.
- *Horizontal angulation*
  The X-ray beam is directed through the interproximal contacts of the adjacent teeth in the view. In this way the beam will strike the receptor at a 90-degree angle (perpendicular), providing a clear view of the interproximal regions free of any superimpositions. If the horizontal angulation of the beam directed incorrectly, the resulting image will display superimpositions

(overlap) of the adjacent proximal surfaces of the teeth, and therefore make evaluation of these areas more problematic.

In general, when exposing the *anterior or premolar bitewing*, the horizontal angulation of the PID should position the central ray at approximately 30-degrees from the mid-sagittal plane or aimed toward the inner canthus of the eye.

For the *posterior or molar bitewing*, the horizontal angulation of the PID should position the central ray at approximately 60 degrees from the mid-sagittal plane or aimed toward the outer canthus of the eye.

- *The central ray* is directed toward the center of the receptor. Imagining the central ray projecting through the bite tab of the holder (when correctly positioned) ensures centering from the top to bottom of the receptor. Instructing the patient to "keep their teeth together and grin" allows the operator to visualize the mesial edge of the receptor and direct the central ray to the midpoint of the receptor in the mesial distal plane (Figure 2.22).

The occlusal radiograph

Occlusal radiographs use size 4 receptors that are larger in size than standard periapical receptors to create two distinct occlusal categories.

These include the following:

- *Periapical type occlusal radiographs*, which are larger versions of standard periapical views, providing visualization of a greater area. PID angulations are based on the principles of the bisecting angle technique.
- *Cross-sectional type occlusal radiographs* provide an image of a region in a different imaging plane (at right angle) to that of the periapical radiograph, thereby allowing visualization of objects and structures in the axial plane. PID angulation is directed parallel to the long axis of the teeth, perpendicular to the active surface of the receptor.

Each category can be further subdivided by the location of the receptor, imaging specifically the anterior or lateral regions of the maxillary or mandibular arches.

Standard occlusal radiographs position the receptor *within the plane of occlusion* (between the occlusal surfaces of the maxillary and mandibular teeth), as opposed to the lingual or palatal positioning of the periapical radiograph. Occlusal radiographs may be used alone or as an adjunct to other imaging modalities to provide the practitioner with valuable diagnostic information.

Types of Occlusal Radiographs
- Periapical type occlusal radiographs (Figure 2.23)
  - ➢ Maxillary anterior occlusal
  - ➢ Maxillary lateral occlusal
  - ➢ Mandibular anterior occlusal
- Cross-sectional type occlusal radiographs (Figure 2.24)
  - ➢ Maxillary cross-sectional (vertex) occlusal
  - ➢ Mandibular cross-sectional (standard) occlusal
    - ◾ Anterior
    - ◾ Posterior (lateral)

Uses for Periapical Type Occlusal Radiographs
- Larger imaging field, allowing more complete visualization of a structure or lesion
- As an alternative to intraoral periapical radiographs in patients with limited opening or severe gag reflexes
- To examine the alveolar processes for the location and extent of fractures
- To produce large periapical type images of the anterior teeth in pediatric patients, using a size 2 receptor

Uses for cross-sectional type occlusal radiographs
- To locate supernumerary, impacted, or unerupted teeth
- To locate foreign bodies
- To provide information about the relationship of structures in the axial plane
- To examine the buccal and lingual cortices for expansion, destruction, or the presence of a periosteal reaction
- To locate and provide information extent of fractures

The seven basic steps used to produce intraoral images, as outlined earlier, are applied to produce

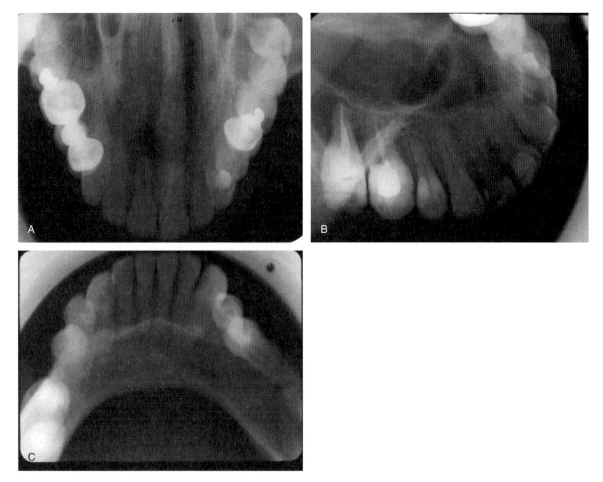

Figure 2.23   (A, B, and C) Periapical type occlusal radiographs (from top left): (A and B) Maxillary anterior and lateral occlusal radiographs; (C) Mandibular anterior occlusal radiograph (bottom).

all of the different types of occlusal radiographs. The major differences when comparing occlusal to other types of intraoral radiography are found in the size of the receptor, its positioning, and the aim of the PID.

All of the different occlusal views provide important and valuable information that is useful for specific diagnostic challenges. In endodontics, occlusal radiographs are an infrequently prescribed category of radiograph. They require the purchasing and maintenance of the size 4 receptors (film or digital sensors) along with their single use plastic sleeves (used for digital systems), as required for infection control. In addition, it is important to understand and apply the principles

of occlusal radiography, the considerations for their prescription, and the techniques involved in creating these views. With proper consideration, occlusal radiographs are a viable prescription option (Tables 2.2 and 2.3).

Extraoral uses for occlusal radiographs

The occlusal radiograph can be used in an extraoral orientation in certain situations. This variation of occlusal radiography positions the receptor in different extraoral locations, determined by the required imaging plane and region of interest.

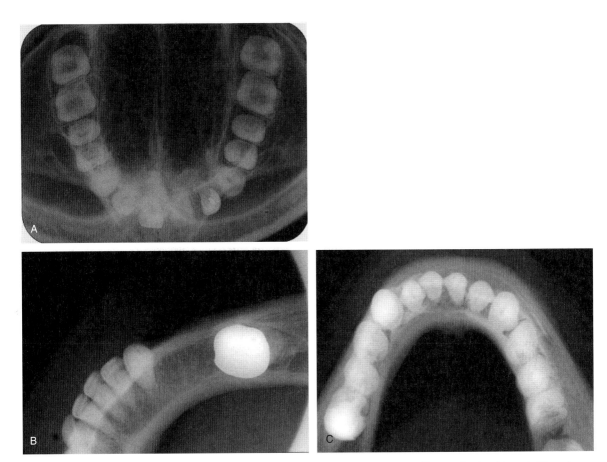

Figure 2.24 (A, B, and C) Cross-sectional type occlusal radiographs (top row): (A) Maxillary occlusal radiograph (Vertex); (from bottom left): (B and C) Mandibular posterior and anterior occlusal radiographs.

Table 2.2 Periapical-type occlusal radiograph.

Maxillary			Mandibular
Active side directed toward	Maxilla		Mandible
	Anterior	Lateral	
Receptor position	Long side centered on midline, parallel to labial surfaces of incisors	Long side parallel to buccal surfaces of posterior teeth	Long side centered on midline, parallel to labial surfaces of incisors
Vertical angulation	+55–65°	+55–65°	−55° from plane of receptor
Horizontal angulation	Long axis of PID perpendicular to front edge of receptor	Long axis of PID perpendicular to front edge of receptor	Long axis of PID perpendicular to front edge of receptor
Central ray			
Guide	Through mid-sagittal plane	Through contacts in premolar region	Through mid-sagittal plane
Anatomical guide	Through middle of nose	Through inner canthus of eye	Through chin

Adapted from Cash and Perschbacher (2010b). DPES Professional-Occlusal Radiographs.

Table 2.3   Cross-sectional type occlusal radiograph.

Maxillary		Mandibular	
Active side directed toward	Maxilla	Mandible	
Receptor position	Long side centered on midline, parallel to labial surfaces of incisors	Anterior	Posterior
Vertical angulation	+110° (Through long axis of max incisors)	−100° from the plane of receptor	Perpendicular to receptor
Horizontal angulation	Open end of PID parallel to receptor	Open end of PID parallel to receptor	Open end of PID parallel to receptor
Central ray			
Guide	Through mid-sagittal plane	Through mid-sagittal plane	Lateral and parallel to mid-sagittal plane
Anatomical guide	Through top of head in anterior region	Under chin	Through inferior border of mandible

- The Profile Occlusal
  The receptor is positioned on the side, and at the level of interest, resting against the cheek, and parallel to the sagittal plane. The receptor can be stabilized in position using a wooden tongue depressor taped to a bite block. The tongue depressor is positioned laterally, within the occlusal plane (patient bites on it). The bite block supports the receptor, maintaining its position. The PID is positioned toward the opposite cheek, with the central ray directed perpendicular and toward the center of the receptor. For the horizontal angulation, the open end of the circular PID is aligned parallel to the receptor. This produces a lateral view (similar to a lateral cephalometric radiograph), allowing visualization of relationship details in the anterior-posterior plane (Figure 2.25).

Extraoral radiography

Extraoral radiographs position the receptor outside of the oral cavity to produce images with a greater field of view. They provide important information about the relationship of structures, while utilizing a less invasive and potentially more comfortable technique. In some ways, the receptor–structure relationship limits these views. The X-ray beam attenuates a multitude of various anatomical structures prior to exposure of the receptor, resulting in poor image resolution due to numerous superimpositions. Various types of extraoral imaging techniques are available to provide many different imaging views. In the practice of endodontics, extraoral imaging is mostly reserved to the panaoramic radiograph. These radiographs are taken regularly to evaluate the relationship of the mandibular canal to the apical region and for presurgical assessment to allow visualization of the sinus floor where evaluation of trabecular height and integrity is required for preimplant consideration.

The panoramic radiograph

The panoramic radiograph presents an image of the maxilla, mandible, and their surrounding structures on a single large radiograph (Figure 2.26). It is a very technique-sensitive radiograph that requires optimal conditions to produce a high-quality radiograph. The patient is prepared by removing all metallic objects that may attenuate the X-ray beam. They are covered with a lead apron and directed to stand in position. They are instructed to bite onto a bite stick attached to the machine, which positions their jaw within an imaginary focal trough. When objects are positioned within the focal trough, and a panoramic image is exposed, the image produced is a good representation of the object, with minimal distortions or magnifications. Both film type and digital sensors are used in panoramic radiography. Film and storage phosphor receptors are encased within a specialized cassette containing intensify-

ing screens that increase receptor sensitivity. CCD receptors are a permanent component within the panoramic machine and therefore do not require the use of a cassette or erasure preparation prior to use. In contrast, storage phosphor sensors must be prepared for exposure by ensuring that any prior image(s) are erased. This can be achieved using the computer software associated with the panoramic unit.

The patient should stand tall, extending their neck, providing maximal extension of the cervical spine. Optimal positioning places the midline of the anterior teeth centered and biting into the groove of the bite block. Horizontal and vertical light lines are used as guides to ensure that the axial and sagittal planes are correctly positioned (Figure 2.27). The ala-tragus line should parallel the horizontal light line, while the canine light line should be aligned vertically through the maxillary canine. Incorrectly positioning the patient outside of the focal trough will produce a distorted image. Supports are adjusted snuggly against the temples to reinforce stability. The patient is instructed to maintain position without any movement, press their tongue against their hard palate, and close their lips.

The operator exits the room and activates and holds the preset exposure button. The receptor and X-ray source rotate around the patient. When complete, the operator re-enters the operatory releasing the patient from position within the panoramic unit and removes the cassette (when used) to process the receptor.

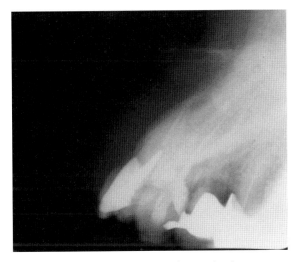

Figure 2.25   Extraoral positioning of an occlusal receptor provides a lateral view of the maxilla in this profile view.

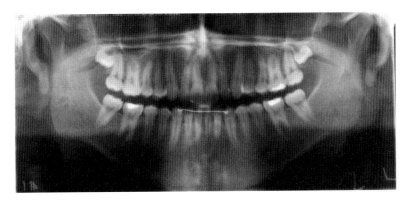

Figure 2.26   A panoramic radiograph.

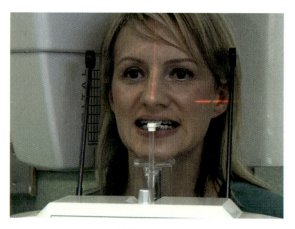

Figure 2.27   The use of light lines as guides when positioning a patient for a panoramic radiograph. (Image courtesy of A. Cormier, BSc, MScBMC, DPES, Faculty of Dentistry, University of Toronto, 2011.)

References

American Dental Association. (2011) The selection of patients for dental radiographic examinations. U.S. Food and Drug Administration Home Page. N.p., n.d. Web. June 21.
www.fda.gov/Radiation-EmittingProducts/
RadiationEmittingProductsandProcedures/
MedicalImaging/MedicalX-Rays/ucm116504.htm

Chandler, N.P., Koshy, S. (2002) Radiographic practices of dentists undertaking endodontics in New Zealand. *Dentomaxillofac Radiol*, 31, 317–321.

Fava, L.R. and Dummer, P.M. (1997) Periapical radiographic techniques during endodontic diagnosis and treatment. *Int Endod J*, 30(4), 250–261.

Haring, J.I. and Jansen, L. (2000) *Dental Radiography Principles and Techniques*, 2nd ed. Saunders, Philadelphia.

Kazzi, D., Horner, K., Qualtrough, A.C., Martinez-Beneyto, Y., and Rushton, V.E. (2007) A comparative study of three periapical radiographic techniques for endodontic working length estimation. *Int Endod J*, 40(7), 526–531. Epub April 24, 2007.

Langland, O., Langlais, R., and Preece, J. (2002) *Principles of dental imaging*, 2nd ed. Williams and Wilkins, Baltimore: Lippincott.

Lim, K.C. and Teo, C.S. (1986) Some problems encountered in endodontic radiography. *Ann Acad Med Singapore*, 15(3), 320–325.

Saunders, W.P., Chestnutt, I.G., Saunders, E.M. (1999) Factors influencing the diagnosis and management of teeth with pulpal and periradicular disease by general dental practitioners. Part 2. *Br Dent J*, 187, 548–554.

Versteeg, C., Sanderink, G., and der Stelt, P.V. (1997) Efficacy of digital intra-oral radiography in clinical dentistry. *J Dent*, 25(3–4), 215–224.

White, S.C. and Pharoah, M.J. (2009) *Oral Radiology Principles and Interpretation*, 6th ed. Mosby, St. Louis.

Further reading

Cash, M. and Perschbacher, S. (2008) DPES professional-periapical radiographic technique-long cone paralleling [homepage on the Internet]. [cited May 31, 2011]. Available from: University of Toronto, Faculty of Dentistry, Department of Oral Radiology Web site: sp.dentistry.utoronto.ca/dpes/pro/procs/Periapical%20Radiographic%20Technique%20-%20Long%20Cone%20Paralleling.aspx

Cash, M. and Perschbacher, S. (2010a) DPES professional-bitewing radiographic technique [homepage on the Internet]. [cited May 31, 2011]. Available from: University of Toronto, Faculty of Dentistry Web site: sp. dentistry.utoronto.ca/dpes/pro/procs/Bitewing%20Radiographic%20Technique.asp

Cash, M. and Perschbacher, S. (2010b) DPES professional-occlusal radiographs [homepage on the Internet]. [cited June 17, 2011]. Available from: University of Toronto, Faculty of Dentistry Web site: sp.dentistry.utoronto.ca/dpes/pro/procs/Occlusal%20Radiographs.aspx

Perschbacher, S. and Cash, M. (2009) DPES professional-panoramic radiographic technique [homepage on the Internet]. [cited June 20, 2011]. Available from: University of Toronto, Faculty of Dentistry Web site: sp.dentistry.utoronto.ca/dpes/pro/procs/Panoramic%20Radiographic%20Technique.aspx

3 Special Situations

Bettina Basrani

Pregnancy

Oral radiography is safe for pregnant patients provided that protective measures such as high speed film and lead apron and a thyroid collar are used. No increase in congenital anomalies or intrauterine growth retardation has been reported for X-ray radiation exposure during pregnancy totaling less than 5–10 cGy, and a full-mouth series of dental radiographs results in only 8×10–4 cGy (National Council on Radiation Protection and Measurements, 2003). A bitewing and panoramic radiographic study generates about one-third the radiation exposure associated with a full-mouth series with E-speed film and a rectangular collimated beam (Freeman and Brand, 1994). Patients who are concerned about radiography during pregnancy should be reassured that in all cases requiring such imaging, the dental staff will practice the ALARA (As Low as Reasonably Achievable) principle and that only radiographs necessary for diagnosis will be obtained (Carlton et al., 2000).

The estimated fetal dose in a single dental exposure is 0.01 mrad. It is known that doses less than 5 rad are not associated with increased congenital malformations; therefore, dental X-ray scans should not be cause for concern. A UK epidemiologic study of a cohort of 7375 mothers did not find a significant association between use of dental X-ray scans and low birth weight or preterm delivery. In addition, a case-control study found no overall increased risk of childhood brain tumors after exposure to prenatal abdominal X-ray scan, which produces many times higher radiation exposure than dental X-ray scans. (Michalowicz et al., 2008)

Radiation therapy

Patients with a malignancy in the oral cavity or perioral region often receive radiation therapy for the treatment of their disease. Although such patients are often apprehensive about receiving additional exposure, dental exposure is insignificant when compared with what they have already received.

In addition to the clinical examination, a thorough radiographic examination is crucial to determine the presence of inflammatory periapical abnormalities, periodontal status, other dental disease, and tumor invasion of mandibular or

Endodontic Radiology, Second Edition. Edited by Bettina Basrani.
© 2012 John Wiley & Sons, Inc. Published 2012 by John Wiley & Sons, Inc.

maxillary bone. A panoramic radiograph plus selective periapical and/or bitewing films should be available for dental assessment previous to radiotherapy. Consultation with the patient's physician on the timing, nature (external beam radiotherapy or radioactive implant), and features (location and size of treatment fields, radiotherapy fractionation and total dose) of the radiotherapy is essential for overall risk assessment and scheduling of any required dental intervention. (White and Pharoah, 2009)

Gag reflexes

Gag reflexes occur in most patients as a natural reaction to tactile stimulation of the soft palate, base of the tongue and parts of the pharynx. In some patients, these reflexes are so predominant that dental procedures such as impression making, dry field maintenance, and placement of dental X-ray films intraorally are made difficult. In extreme cases, adequate examination and dental treatment of these patients may be impossible (Bassi et al., 2004).

The gag reflex is a normal defense mechanism, in preventing foreign bodies from entering the trachea. During the reflex, the shape of the pharynx and its openings are altered by spasmodic muscle contractions.

Characteristic elements of the gagging behavior have been described as follows: (1) puckering the lips or attempting to close the jaws, (2) elevating and furrowing the tongue, (3) elevation of the soft palate, (4) contraction of the anterior and posterior pillars of the fauces, (5) elevation, contraction, and retraction of the larynx and closure of the glottis, (6) forcing air through the closed glottis, producing the characteristic retching sound, (7) excessive salivation, lacrimation, and sweating, (8) respiratory muscle spasm, and (9) vomiting (Kumar et al., 2011).

The regions most sensitive to stimuli that produce the gag reflex are the fauces, base of the tongue, palate, uvula, and posterior pharyngeal wall. Sensory nerves forming afferent pathways for impulses to the reflex center in the medulla oblongata are the trigeminal, glossopharyngeal, and vagus (cranial nerves V, IX, and X). At the release of the complex muscular and secretory elements of

the gag reflex, a number of cranial nerves as well as sympathetic and parasympathetic nerves participate. Gag reflexes may be initiated by psychological factors as well as by tactile stimulation. Anxiety and awareness of a previous gagging problem may heavily influence the severity of the condition.

Recommendations for suppressing and reducing gag reflexes during intraoral radiographic examination

1. Gain confidence of the patient by demonstrating a professional and confident behavior and by demonstrating technical competence.
2. The operator explains the procedure.
3. The patient rinses the mouth with ice-cold water.
4. Salt is placed on the patient's tongue.
5. The patient is requested to initiate deep and audible respiration.
6. The patient holds his/her breath
7. Film placement is done quickly and in a gentle and nonirritating manner, with exposure follows immediately to film placement
8. The attention of the patient is distracted by
   a. Biting vigorously on the bite block
   b. Looking fixedly at a point in the room
   c. Concentrating on breathing control (e.g., by counting seconds)
   d. Performing slow muscular activities requiring concentration (e.g., alternately raising legs to a horizontal position)
9. Fingers in the mouth are avoided
10. Film holders are used
11. Tissue edge of the film packet is moistened by holding it in a stream of cold water
12. The patient is asked to swallow immediately prior to film insertion
13. Surface anesthesia

The frequency of gagging during full-mouth radiography was evaluated in 478 patients. Gagging was observed in 13% of the patients. The frequency of gagging differed significantly in groups radiographed by trained radiologists and by students (9% and 26%, respectively). Gagging occurred in all regions but most frequently in the maxillary molar area. The technical skill, authority, and self-confidence of the operator were major factors of importance in preventing and suppressing gag reflexes in dental radiography (Sewerin, 1984).

Torus

Mandible torus

Mandible (or mandibularis) Torus is a bony growth in the mandible along the surface nearest to the tongue. Mandibular torus is usually present near the mandibular premolars and above the location of the mylohyoid muscle's attachment to the mandible. The prevalence of mandibular torus ranges from 5% to 40%. In 90% of cases, there is a torus on both the left and right sides, making this finding a bilateral condition.

Mandibular torus is more common in Asian and Inuit populations, and slightly more common in males. In the United States, the prevalence is 7–10% of the population. It is believed that mandibular torus is caused by several factors. They are more common in early adult life and are associated with bruxism. The size of the torus may fluctuate throughout life, and in some cases the torus can be large enough to touch each other in the midline of mouth. Consequently, it is believed that mandible torus is the result of local stresses and is not solely due to genetic influences. Mandibular torus is usually found during a clinical examination and no treatment is necessary. Ulcers may form on the torus due to trauma. The torus may also complicate the fabrication of dentures. If removal of the torus is needed, surgery can be done to reduce the amount of bone, but the torus may return in cases where nearby teeth still receive local stresses. (Neville et al., 2002)

Palatal torus

Palatal torus or Torus palatinus is a bony protrusion on the palate. Palatal torus is usually present on the midline of the hard palate. Most palatal tori are less than 2 cm in diameter, but their size can change throughout life. Prevalence of palatal tori ranges from 9% to 60%. Palatal tori are more common in Asian and Inuit populations, and twice more common in females. In the United States, the prevalence is 20–35% of the population. They are more common in early adult life and can increase in size. In some older people, the size of the tori may decrease due to bone resorption. Palatal tori are usually a clinical finding with no treatment necessary. It is possible for ulcers to form on the area of the tori due to repeated trauma. Also, the tori may complicate the fabrication of dentures. If removal of the tori is needed, surgery can be done to reduce the amount of bone present (Neville et al., 2002)

Radiographic examination

Radiographically, mandibular and palatal torus appears as radiopaque masses, often obliterating details of the teeth and the maxillary sinus. For a large palatal torus, the spongy layer appears as a less dense radiopaque mass compared with the compact layer. (Seah, 1995)

Patients with physical disabilities

Patients with physical disabilities may require special handling during a radiographic examination. These patients usually are cooperative and eager to assist. Members of the patient family often help in holding the films (White and Pharoah, 2009).

Patients with trismus

Trismus is defined in Taber's *Cyclopedic Medical Dictionary* as a tonic contraction of the muscles of mastication. In the past, this word was often used to describe the effects of tetanus, also called "lockjaw." More recently, the term "trismus" has been used to describe any restriction to mouth opening, including restrictions caused by trauma, surgery or radiation. This limitation in the ability to open the mouth can have serious health implications, including reduced nutrition due to impaired mastication, difficulty in speaking, and compromised oral hygiene. In persons who have received radiation to the head and neck, the condition is often observed in conjunction with difficulty in swallowing (Garnett et al., 2008). Causes of limited mouth opening can be temporary or permanent. The most obvious effect of trismus is difficulty in opening the mouth.

If the trismus is temporary, the dental treatment and intraoral radiographs need to be postponed until the condition will improve.

A technique to place the radiograph in the mouth of the patient with limited mouth opening is the following (White and Pharoah, 2009):

1. Place the film in haemostatic pliers.
2. Place the film in the mouth of the patient in an horizontal position.
3. Turn the film in the vertical position.
4. Use smaller size films.
5. Take occlusal films.

Patients where the floor of the mouth is nondepressible

These patients have a high insertion of the mylohyoid muscle. Both muscles mylohioides uniting constitute the muscular substance of the floor of the mouth. This is a muscle plane with parallel fibers, which beginning in the mylohyoid line of mandible medially directed raphe ending in a tendon that extends from the inner surface of the chin to the body of the hyoid bone, through a midline along the boundaries between the two mylohyoid. The back of the muscle attaches to the hyoid body.

Placing a periapical radiograph in the area of the lower premolars or canine when the floor of the mouth is high can be impossible. Occlusal, panorex, or Cone Beam Computed tomography (CBCT) radiographs should be considered instead of periapical films (White and Pharoah, 2009).

Narrow palatal

Palatal width is measured as the distance between the maxillary first permanent molar on the right and left sides, at the palatal cervical line, using a specific device. Palate width is typically assessed subjectively in routine clinical practice. Narrowing is often associated with a high palate, but this should be assessed separately. Gingival over-

growth can give the impression of a narrow palate but should be distinguished separately. The term "gothic palate" is used to indicate that the roof of the palate is not round but rather has an inverted V-shape, and therefore, only the upper part of the palate is narrow.

Taking peripaical radiographs in patients with a narrow palate can be a challenge. Cotton rolls can to be used to try to make the film parallel to the X-ray tube as possible. Or occlusal films can be used (White and Pharoah, 2009).

References

Bassi, G.S., Humphris, G.M., and Longman, L.P. (2004) The etiology and management of gagging: a review of the literature. *J Prosthet Dent* 91(5), 459–467.

Carlton, R.R., Adler, A.M., and Burns, B. (2000) *Principles of Radiographic Imaging*, 3rd ed. Thompson Delmar Learning, Clifton Park, NY.

Freeman, J.P. and Brand, J.W. (1994) Radiation doses of commonly used dental radiographic surveys. *Oral Surg Oral Med Oral Pathol*, 77(3), 285–289.

Garnett, M.J., Nohl, F.S., Barclay, S.C. (2008) Management of patients with reduced oral aperture and mandibular hypomobility (trismus) and implications for operative dentistry. *Br Dent J*, 204(3), 125–131.

Kumar, S., Satheesh, P., Savadi, R.C. (2011) Gagging. *N Y State Dent J*, 77(4), 22–27.

Seah, Y.H. (1995) Torus palatinus and torus mandibularis: a review of the literature. *Aust Dent J*, 40(5), 318–321.

Michalowicz, B.S., DiAngelis, A.J., Novak, M.J., Buchanan, W.P., Apapanou, P.N., and Mitchel, D.A. (2008) Examining the safety of dental treatment in pregnant women. *J Am Dent Assoc*, 139(6), 685–695.

National Council on Radiation Protection and Measurements (2003) Recommendations on limits for exposure to ionizing radiation. Bethesda, Md. NCRP, 1987. NCRP report no. 91., Katz VL. Prenatal care. In: J.R. Scott, R.S. Gibbs, B.Y. Karlan, and A.F. Haney, eds., *Danforth's Obstetrics and Gynecology*, 9th ed. Lippincott, Williams and Wilkins, Philadelphia, pp. 1–20.

Neville, B.W., Damm, D., Allen, C., and Bouquot, J. (2002) *Oral & Maxillofacial Pathology*, 2nd ed. Saunders, Medical University of South Carolina, Charleston.

Sewerin, I. (1984) Gagging in dental radiography I. *Oral Surg Oral Med Oral Pathol*, 58(6), 725–728.

White, S.C. and Pharoah, M.J. (2009) *Oral Radiology, 6th Edition Principles and Interpretation*. Mosby Elsevier, St. Louis.

4 Intraoral Digital Imaging

Ernest W. N. Lam

Intraoral radiography with digital sensors should be considered the primary radiographic technique in endodontics. Should digital intraoral radiography not provide adequate diagnostic information for the clinician, occlusal radiography and small field, high-resolution cone beam computed tomography (CT) may be used to supplement periapical images. The purpose of this chapter will be to review intraoral digital imaging sensor technology as it applies to endodontics.

Intraoral digital imaging

Intraoral imaging is performed using an alternating current (AC) or direct current (DC) X-ray unit with a focal spot size of between 0.4 mm and 0.7 mm, operating between 60 kVp and 70 kVp using a filament current of between 4 mA and 7 mA, and an X-ray target-to-exit distance of at least 12 in.

Contemporary X-ray systems use either an AC or DC generator in the X-ray housing to produce X-rays. The AC waveform can be visualized as being sinusoidal in nature with regular peaks and troughs (Figure 4.1), and a periodicity of 1/60th of a second or 60 Hz. This means that the waveform repeats itself between successive peaks or troughs, every 1/60th of a second. When the waveform reaches its peak, electrons flow from the tungsten filament inside the X-ray tube to the tungsten target where the X-rays are generated. X-rays are generated throughout the entire positive cycle of the waveform, every 1/120th of a second; during the trough, no X-rays are generated.

There are inherent inconsistencies or errors in the timing systems of X-ray machines, and these may be more pronounced with shorter exposure times. For less sensitive film-based image receptors that in the past relied on longer exposure times, the pulsed nature of the X-ray beam was not significantly impacted by inconsistencies in the timing or generation of each waveform. For more sensitive film-based or digital sensors that use very short exposure times, inconsistencies may be more noticeable. For example, for very short exposure times of say 0.1 or 0.2 second, an inconsistency of the waveform that disrupts X-ray production for 0.02 or 0.03 second may substantially reduce image density. In an attempt to lessen this problem, manufacturers have developed DC or constant potential systems that incorporate technology that

Endodontic Radiology, Second Edition. Edited by Bettina Basrani.
© 2012 John Wiley & Sons, Inc. Published 2012 by John Wiley & Sons, Inc.

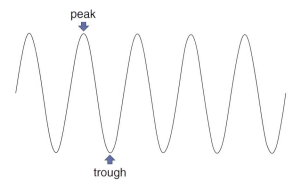

Figure 4.1   Active current (AC) waveform. This trace demonstrates the peaks and troughs of the AC waveform. The duration of one cycle of the waveform (peak-to-peak or trough-to-trough time) is 1/60th of a second. The frequency of the waveform is therefore 60 Hz.

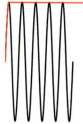

Figure 4.2   Constant or direct current (DC) X-ray tube heads increase the frequency to some 70,000 Hz (70 kHz) (black trace). As a result of the ultra-high frequency of the waveform, the output of radiation attains an almost steady-state peak.

increases the frequency of the AC waveform from 60 Hz to near 70,000 Hz (i.e., 70 kHz) (Figure 4.2, black line). Consequently, X-ray generation becomes almost steady state (Figure 4.2, red line). DC systems also theoretically contribute to lower effective radiation doses. Because the voltage generated is always at or near its peak, less lower energy, less-penetrating, or "soft" radiation is produced, and consequently, less radiation is absorbed by superficial tissues such as skin. The practical decrease in patient dose has not, however, been well documented.

The size of the focal spot or tungsten target may also impact the quality of the image. A smaller focal spot diameter (0.4 mm vs. 0.7 mm) theoretically produces less divergence of the X-ray beam from focal spot to receptor. A less divergent X-ray

beam produces less penumbra or edge unsharpness around an object, creating an image that is theoretically sharper with better defined edges. Other factors that affect X-ray beam divergence include the distance between the focal spot and the exit point of the X-ray beam from the X-ray collimator and collimator shape. Some intraoral X-ray systems employ distances as short as 8 in. Shorter focal spot-to-exit point distances also create a more divergent X-ray beam in comparison to those that use longer collimation, for example, 12 or 16 in. Although 16-in. collimators may be difficult to find, most intraoral X-ray machine manufacturers have, as an option, collimators that result in a 12-in. focal spot-to-exit point distance.

Rectangular collimation in which the exit field of the X-ray beam is not substantially larger than the size of an American National Standards Institute (ANSI) number 2 size sensor limits the size of the X-ray field on the patient. The use of rectangular collimation limits not only reduces the skin entrance dose of the X-ray beam by as much as two-thirds, which is substantial, but the amount of X-ray scatter as well (Velders et al., 1991).

Both operating peak kilovoltage (kVp) and filament current (milliamperage [mA]) affect the quality and/or quantity of the X-ray photons produced. While increasing both peak kilovoltage and milliamperage increases the total bolus of X-ray photons produced, only peak kilovoltage affects the quality of the photons; that is, the distribution of lower energy, less penetrating photons and higher energy, more penetrating photons. As well, higher peak kilovoltage X-ray beams impact on image contrast by affecting the number of gray values that are visible. For viewing subtle changes in tooth or bone mineralization, lower peak kilovoltage settings that produce greater short scale (high image) contrast are preferable. X-ray filament current affects only the number of X-ray photons produced. Therefore, lowering either or both peak kilovoltage and milliamperage will necessitate a concomitant increase in exposure time to maintain image density within the diagnostic range.

Digital sensors

There are three competing intraoral digital receptor technologies: solid-state charge-coupled device

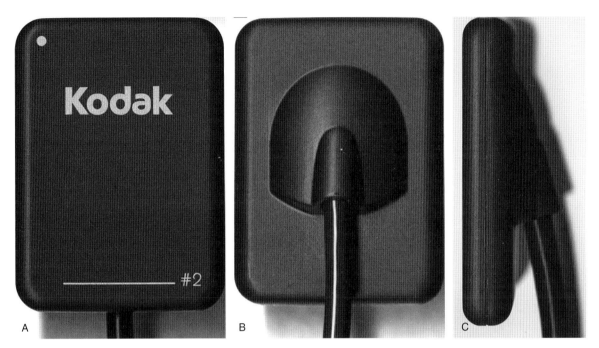

Figure 4.3 Intraoral charge-coupled device (CCD) size 2 sensor (Kodak 6100, Carestream, Rochester, NY). A. Sensitive surface; B. Back surface with wire connection; C. Side profile.

(CCD), complementary metal-oxide semiconductor (CMOS), and photostimulatable phosphor (PSP). The different technologies all capture patient anatomy on a two-dimensional, 2 by 2 matrix of picture elements or pixels.

All sensor types are capable of displaying up to 16,384 shades of gray, from white to black, with each shade of gray represented by a value between 0 and 16,383. Such sensors are referred to as 14-bit sensors (2^{14} = 16,384). Interestingly, most computer monitors that display black and white images are only capable of displaying 256 shades of gray or 2^8, and the human eye is only capable of differentiating between 64 shades of gray or 2^4.

All digital sensors convert X-ray information to electronic information, but they do so in different ways. The components of the CCD (Figure 4.3A–C) and CMOS sensors are encased in a sealed plastic case, typically with an electrical connection to a computer. The thickness of this case may range between 4 mm and 7 mm (Farman and Farman, 2005). For CCD and CMOS sensors, X-ray photons exiting the patient are converted to visible light photons by a scintillator within the sensor. The visible light is then converted into electrons by a fiber optic plate, and finally, the electrons are captured in the CCD or CMOS element of the sensor. The number of electrons captured is directly proportional to the number of X-ray photons that exits the patient and strikes the sensor surface. Although CCD and CMOS sensors differ in the manner in which the electrons are captured and converted to an electronic signal, a discussion of the specific electronic requirements of the two sensors is beyond the scope of this chapter.

In contrast, PSP plates (Figure 4.4A,B) consist of a photoluminescent material consisting of a mixture of different barium fluorohalides containing trace amounts of europium. Europium is incorporated as an activator or luminescence center. This material is mounted on a polyester support. X-rays arriving on the surface of the PSP sensor liberate electrons from europium atoms, and the escaping electrons become entrapped in the halide lattice. Following exposure, the PSP plate is fed into a machine that contains a laser that scans the plate, releases the electrons, converting them to a proportionate number of light photons that are collected

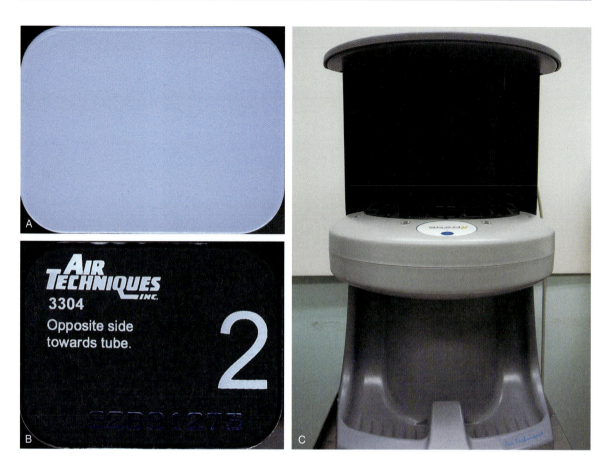

Figure 4.4   Intraoral photostimulatable phosphor (PSP) ANSI size 2 sensor (Air Techniques, Melville, NY) and plate reader. A. Sensitive surface; B. Nonsensitive back surface; C. Plate reader.

and assigned a numerical value like the CCD or CMOS sensor (Figure 4.4C).

CCD and CMOS receptors are substantially more costly than PSP receptors, costing in the range of thousands of dollars versus the hundred dollar range or less for each PSP receptor. Despite the lower cost of PSP receptors, regular replacement is necessary as the active surface of the plate may be damaged by scratches or abrasions generating images that may be nondiagnostic (Bedard et al., 2004).

Like conventional film, PSP receptors are available in ANSI sizes 0, 1, 2, and 4, and the entire surface of the receptor is active. In contrast, less than 80% of the CCD or CMOS sensor surface is active due to the electronics contained within the sensor. A CCD or CMOS sensor the size of the

ANSI 4 receptor is not available. One resultant effect of the smaller active surface area of CCD and CMOS sensors is that compared with PSP sensors and conventional film, more images may be required to cover a particular area within the jaws (Berkhout et al., 2003). The thickness and rigidity of CCD and CMOS sensors make them more difficult to position in children and adults with small mouths, in particular when making bisecting-the-angle images (Wenzel and Møystad, 2001b). And indeed, the CCD and CMOS wire sensors may confound this all the more. One manufacturer does, however, have a wireless CCD sensor, but it is comparatively bulky (Figure 4.3C).

With regard to radiation effective dose to the patient, it has been reported that the mean dose reduction when using digital sensors is between

55% compared with ANSI D speed film (Wenzel and Møystad, 2001a). Indeed, the reduction may also be less than expected if more images are required to adequately cover a particular region of the jaws (Bahrami et al., 2003), or remaking of images is required due to the constraints already alluded to for CCD and CMOS sensors.

Finally, image resolution and display may be considerations for clinicians. The median resolution of CCD and CMOS sensors has been reported in in vitro studies to be approximately 11 line pairs per millimeter (lp/mm). This compares with approximately 8 lp/mm for PSP sensors. The newest generation of CCD and PSP sensors have recently achieved tested resolutions of greater than 20 lp/mm and 13 lp/mm, respectively, rivaling conventional film (>22 lp/mm) (Farman and Farman, 2005). By comparison, the human eye is capable of resolving 8 lp/mm, unaided. It has also been reported that the PSP sensor has greater receptor latitude, allowing it to capture a greater number of gray shades compared with CCD/CMOS sensors.

In general, digital images are more easily managed after exposure compared with film, and the time-savings that dentists who use digital systems experience is significant; 36 min/day for CCD/CMOS users (range, 10–120 minutes) and 25 min/day for PSP users (5–120 minutes). The decrease in savings from PSP users is likely due, in part, to the scanning process required of the sensor plates (Figure 4.4C) (Berkhout et al., 2002).

After an image is captured, software enhancement of the images can be performed, although changes to image contrast and density appear to the most widely used applications. It should, however, be noted, that there is little published evidence that suggests modifying an image using software has a biological correlate.

Bisecting-the-angle and occlusal radiography

Bisecting-the-angle radiography is performed when a position-indicating device (PID) is not used or cannot be used to make intraoral images using the paralleling technique. Typically, the receptor is held in place by a device that can be stabilized by the patient. Such devices have included a simple hemostat or the commercially available Snap-R-Ray. The use of the patient's own fingers is not considered an acceptable alternative to the use of a film-holding device if the patient's finger(s) fall within the X-ray beam.

Unlike the paralleling technique where the receptor is placed parallel or nearly parallel to the long axis of a tooth, the receptor is placed at an angle relative to the long axis of the tooth. Should the incident X-ray beam strike the tooth at 90 degrees to its buccal surface, the projected image of the tooth on the receptor will appear elongated. Alternatively, should the incident X-ray beam strike the receptor plane at 90 degrees, the tooth will appear foreshortened. In both cases, one can expect errors should measurements be required. In practice, errors associated with misjudgments in tooth or X-ray beam angulation may be more pronounced in the anterior regions of the jaws where the incisors are more prominently proclined compared with the more posterior parts of the jaws where the teeth appear more upright in their alveolar processes.

In addition to periapical radiography, some occlusal radiographic techniques may also rely on the use of bisecting-the-angle radiography. Classically, occlusal radiography has relied primarily on the use of large, ANSI 4-sized receptors although ANSI 2 receptors have been used as well. Due to the larger sized receptors, larger regions of the jaws can be captured on a single image, rather than on two or more smaller individual images. More importantly, however, by placing the receptor on the occlusal surfaces of the teeth and using oblique X-ray beam angulations, it may be possible to examine different aspects of the jaws not possible with periapical radiography.

Cross-sectional occlusal radiography is commonly used in the mandible for demonstrating the effects of space-occupying pathoses on the contour of the mandible, including effects on the buccal and lingual cortices. In the anterior maxillae and mandible, an ANSI 4 receptor used with a bite block mounted on a wooden tongue depressor can also demonstrate buccal cortical expansion. This novel technique permits the user to demonstrate changes to the anterior buccal contour of the maxillae or mandible in an extraoral examination that uses the higher resolution capabilities of an intraoral sensor (Figure 4.5).

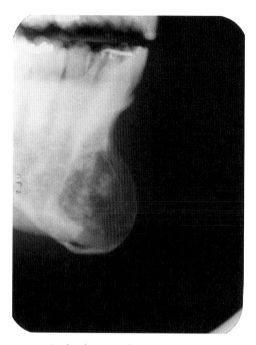

Figure 4.5   Occlusal-on-a-stick image of a simple bone cyst associated with a region of osseous dysplasia. The image shows a mixed radiolucent/radiopaque abnormality in the anterior mandible that has not only expanded the anterior mandible, but has also produced a thinning of the anterior and inferior cortices of the mandible.

References

Bahrami, G., Hagstrøm, C., and Wenzel, A. (2003) Bitewing examination with four digital receptors. *Dentomaxillofac Radiol*, 32, 317–321.

Bedard, A., Davis, T.D., and Angelopoulos, C. (2004) Storage phosphor plates: how durable are they as a digital dental radiographic system? *J Contemp Dent Pract*, 5, 57–69.

Berkhout, W.E., Sanderlink, G.C., and Van Der Stelt, P.F. (2002) A comparison of digital and film radiography in Dutch dental practices assessed by questionnaire. *Dentomaxillofac Radiol*, 31, 93–99.

Berkhout, W.E., Sanderlink, G.C., and Van Der Stelt, P.F. (2003) Does digital radiography increase the number of intraoral radiographs? A questionnaire of Dutch dental practices. *Dentomaxillofac Radiol*, 32, 124–127.

Farman, A.G. and Farman, T.T. (2005) A comparison of 18 different x-ray detectors currently used in dentistry. *Oral Surg Oral Med Oral Pathol Oral Radiol Endod*, 99, 485–489.

Velders, X.L., van Aken, J., and van der Stelt, P.F. (1991) Absorbed dose to organs in the head and neck from bitewing radiography. *Dentomaxillofac Radiol*, 20, 161–165.

Wenzel, A. and Møystad, A. (2001a) Experience of Norwegian general dental practitioners with solid state and phosphor detectors. *Dentomaxillofac Radiol*, 30, 203–208.

Wenzel, A. and Møystad, A. (2001b) Decision criteria and characteristics of Norwegian general dental practitioners seeking digital radiography. *Dentomaxillofac Radiol*, 30, 197–202.

5 Radiographic Considerations Before the Endodontic Treatment Is Initiated

Calvin D. Torneck

Introduction

A correct diagnosis is the foundation of an effective treatment plan, and in endodontics, the dental radiograph is an indispensable diagnostic tool. Interpreting images on a radiograph requires an understanding of anatomy, tissue physiology and pathophysiology, and radiographic physics. It is for this reason that these topics will be briefly reviewed in this chapter dealing with the radiographic expression of endodontic disease. Furthermore, they will be discussed as they relate to two-dimensional or standard radiography. While three-dimensional radiography, as generated by cone beam tomography, has been shown to be more effective in imaging endodontic disease than standard radiography (Patel et al., 2009; Scarfe et al., 2009), it has yet to achieve wide acceptance in everyday clinical practice. This is not to imply that it is not in use in some dental practices, only that the current expense associated with its purchase and the special knowledge associated with the interpretation of its images has limited its use. At present, it is found primarily in dental specialty offices and teaching institutions.

Anatomy of dental tissues

Teeth are composed primarily of dentin, with an enamel cap over the coronal portion and a thin layer of cementum over the root surface. Tooth enamel is the hardest and most highly mineralized substance of the body and with dentin, cementum, and dental pulp is one of the four major parts of the tooth.

Enamel

Enamel appears more radio-opaque than other tissues because of its 90% mineral component that causes greater attenuation of X-ray photons.

Dentine

The dentine will have 70% mineral content. It is less radio-opaque than enamel; its radio-opacity is similar to bone, and the enamel–dentinal junction appears as a distinct interface separating these two structures (Torneck, 1998).

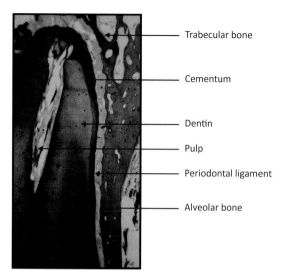

Figure 5.1   Anatomy of the tooth and supporting tissues. (Reprinted from Torneck and Torabinejad, 2002, with permission from Elsevier Ltd.)

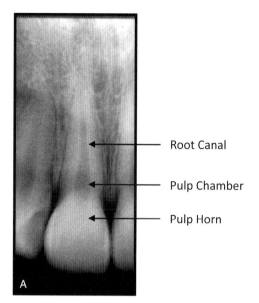

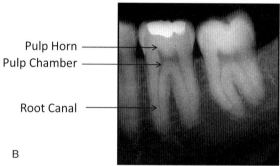

Figure 5.2   A. Divisions of the pulp space of maxillary incisor. B. Divisions of the pulp space of mandibular molar.

Dentine-pulp complex

The dentin–pulp complex, the periodontium and the bone of the maxilla and mandible constitute the endodontic tissues (Figure 5.1). The dentin–pulp complex is a specialized connective tissue with dentin-forming capabilities that define what is referred to radiographically as the pulp space (Figure 5.2A,B). The pulp space, in turn, is divided into the pulp chamber or coronal pulp space, and the root canal, or radicular pulp space. The dentin–pulp complex receives its blood supply via channels that extend through the dentin wall of the tooth root from the periodontium (Torneck, 1998). The major channel is called the apical foramen and is located at or near the anatomical end of the root or apex. It is usually, but not exclusively, the largest of the vascular channels. However, despite its relatively large size when compared to the other vascular channels, it is difficult to image on a radiograph for most adult teeth. The other vascular channels present in the dentin are referred to as accessory and lateral canals. These are found at different sites along the root surface, as well as in the furcation area of multirooted teeth. Channels in close proximity to the apical foramen are often called accessory canals while those located more coronally are called lateral canals. Lateral canals vary in size from very small (0.1 mm) to sizes that approach that of the apical foramen (0.4 mm). Varying methods in identifying the presence of lateral canals in anatomical studies have led to varying reports in their incidence. Suffice it to say that most teeth have one or more canals of this type and that they can play a significant role in the spread of endodontic infection from the root canal to the surrounding tissues. There are rare occasions when large lateral canals can be detected in pre-treatment radiographs, but in most of cases, they are only detected after endodontic treatment, when they become filled with radio-opaque root canal cement or a core material (Figure 5.3A,B).

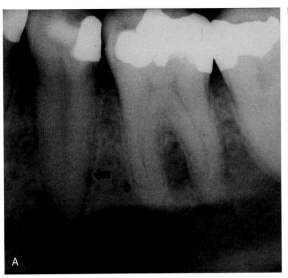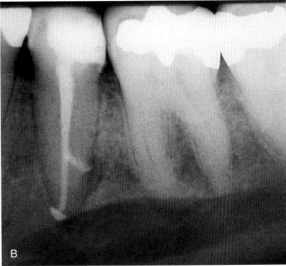

Figure 5.3   A. Lateral lesion associated with lateral canal (arrow) imaged in diagnostic radiograph. B. Lateral canal filled with root canal filling material as seen immediately post treatment.

Periodontium

The periodontium is a complex of hard and soft tissue that supports the tooth in the jaw during function. The soft tissue is a combination of specialized collagen fibers and a loose connective tissue containing progenitor cells, fibroblasts, blood vessels, and nerves. Alternatively called the periodontal ligament, this appears as a radiolucent space that extends around the periphery of the root when the tooth is imaged radiographically (Figure 5.4). The collagen fibers of the ligament are embedded in mineralized tissue on both sides of the space. On the tooth side the anchorage is by cementum, a bone-like mineralized tissue that normally covers the entire root surface, and on the opposite side by the alveolar bone (bundle bone) that lines the bone socket in the jaw. Because alveolar bone is denser than the trabecular bone that comprises the inner structure of the jaw, it appears more radio-opaque than trabecular bone when imaged. This relative opacity is highlighted by the radiolucent appearance of the soft tissue ligament. The name given to alveolar bone radiographically is lamina dura. Although not always detectable in the radiograph due to variances in the way the tooth may be imaged, its continuity in mature teeth is interpreted as a sign of periodontal health, and its

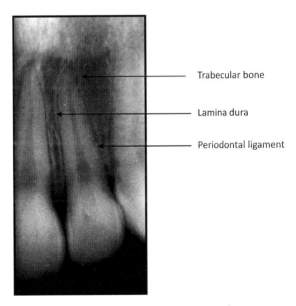

Trabecular bone

Lamina dura

Periodontal ligament

Figure 5.4   Dental supporting tissues as imaged radiographically.

absence, a sign of disease. In partially developed (newly erupted) teeth where apex formation and periodontal development are incomplete, the apical region still contains residual soft tissue elements of the dental papilla and the dental follicle (Figure 5.5). In the radiograph, this combination of

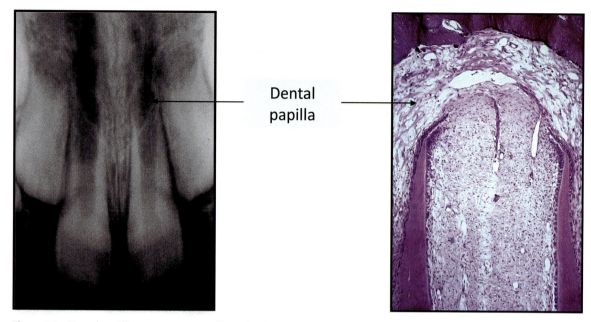

Dental papilla

Figure 5.5   Dental papilla as seen anatomically and radiographically at apex of developing incisor. (Histology reprinted from Torneck and Torabinejad, 2002, with permission from Elsevier Ltd.)

soft tissues is imaged as a circumscribed apical radiolucency without the presence of a of lamina dura. This radiolucency gradually diminishes as root development progresses and disappears when development of the periodontium is complete. The presence of the radiolucency at the apex of a developing tooth can easily be misinterpreted as an area of apical inflammation so it is prudent to support a clinical diagnosis with additional tests before treatment is undertaken. It also makes the early detection of apical inflammation when present, difficult in teeth where root development is incomplete (Torneck 1986).

Cementum

The cementum present on the root surface has a mineral content similar to that of dentin and bone and is therefore difficult to differentiate radiographically from these two other tissues. An exception may be times when the periodontium is healthy and excessive cementum has been formed on one or more of the root surfaces. This produces a benign condition called hypercementosis (Figure 5.6). Its endodontic significance lies in the fact that

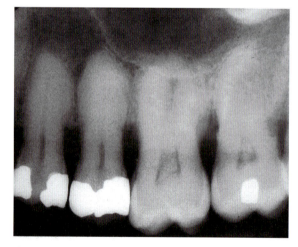

Figure 5.6   Maxillary premolars and molars demonstrating hypercementosis of the roots. Note interproximal bone loss, areas of calculus deposition, and pulp stones in pulp chamber of molar teeth.

it can result in bizarre anatomical changes at the root apex that can make endodontic management of a root canal infection difficult. Generalized hypercementosis is also seen in association with fibro-osseous disease, but in such cases, there is also a change in the architecture of the bone surrounding the teeth that facilitates interpretation of the image.

As previously mentioned, the presence of the periodontal ligament creates a continuous periradicular radiolucent space about the tooth root when the tooth is properly imaged. The space normally averages 0.15–0.38 mm in width in young adults, with the smallest diameter usually present at mid root. It does, however, vary in accordance with age and averages 0.21 mm in 11- to 16-year-olds and 0.15 mm in 51- to 67-year-olds (Nanci, 2008). When lamina dura is not clearly discernable in the dental radiograph, the presence of a periodontal space of uniform and normal width also can be used as a determinant of periodontal health, and conversely, its attenuation as a sign of disease. As in all aspects of interpretive radiology, the use of magnification and multiple views usually proves helpful in properly interpreting information present in the radiograph.

References

Nanci, A. (2008) Periodontium. In: A. Nanci, ed., pp. 239–267. *Ten Cate's Oral Histology*. Mosby, St. Louis.

Patel, S. et al. (2009) Detecting periapical bone defects in human jaws. *Int Endod J*, 42, 506–515.

Scarfe, W.C. et al. (2009) Use of cone beam computed tomography in endodontics. *Int J Dent*, 2009, 1–20. Online article ID 634567, 20 pgs. doi:10.1155/2009/634567

Torneck, C.D. (1986) Endodontic management of partially developed teeth. In: N. Levine, ed., *Current Treatmment in Dental Practice*. Saunders, Philadelphia.

Torneck, C.D. (1998) Dentin–pulp complex. In: A.R. Ten Cate, ed., *Oral Histology*, 5th ed., pp. 150–196. Mosby, St. Louis.

Torneck, C.D. and Torabinejad, M. (2002) Biology of the dental pulp and periradicular tissues. In: R. Walton and M. Torabinejad, eds., *Principles and Practice of Endodontics*, 3rd ed., pp. 4–26. Mosby, St. Louis.

Radiographic Analysis of Anomalous Tooth Forms and Morphological Variations Related to Endodontics

6

Jeffrey M. Coil

An anomaly is a marked deviation from normalcy, especially as a result of congenital or hereditary defects. Recognition and endodontic treatment of dental abnormalities can present a challenge to every practitioner. Radiographic evaluation during a consultation visit is a key element in the pretreatment assessment of a patient's "degree of difficulty" (CAE, 1998). Determination of the complexity of treatment and assessment of the physical nature and condition of a tooth to be treated allows the practitioner to better prepare before treatment commences.

Dens evaginatus

The dens evaginatus is a developmental anomaly that manifests clinically as an extra cusp appearing on the occlusal surface of premolar teeth between the buccal and lingual cusps (Figure 6.1). This projection of enamel can interfere with tooth eruption and occlusion. This tubercle is usually worn down or broken off, which can result in pulp exposure, and subsequent pulp necrosis and periradicular periodontitis (Figure 6.2A). Radiographically, this condition may be recognized by examining the

radiodensity stemming from the cusp of the premolar crown tip before eruption (Figure 6.2B–D), which can influence orthodontic treatment planning (McCulloch et al., 1997). As a tooth is erupting, this extra cusp can also be seen radiographically as well as clinically (Figure 6.2E)

Dens invaginatus

This malformation of teeth usually affects maxillary lateral incisors, and is considered to be an invagination of the dental papilla during development. Although the etiology remains unclear, this tooth abnormality has been described for hundreds of years (Hulsmann, 1997). Various types of this invaginated tooth anomaly were characterized by Oehlers (1957). He categorized this malformation to occur in three different forms as shown in Figure 6.3.

The first type of dens invaginatus, Class I, is a minor form of an invagination that occurs within the crown of the tooth, and does not extend beyond the cementalenamel junction (CEJ). It can be seen radiographically as an invagination in the vicinity of the cingulum (Figure 6.4).

Endodontic Radiology, Second Edition. Edited by Bettina Basrani.
© 2012 John Wiley & Sons, Inc. Published 2012 by John Wiley & Sons, Inc.

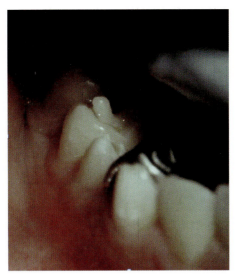

Figure 6.1 Projection of the extra cusp on the occlusal surface of the lower bicuspid tooth is seen clinically. (Image courtesy of Dr. Raymond Greenfeld.)

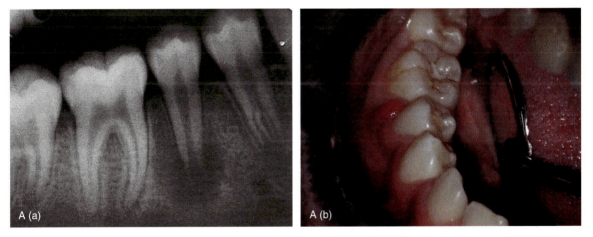

Figure 6.2 A. (a) Periapical lesion associated with the mandibular right premolar tooth. A slight thickening of enamel is seen in the center of the crown near the occlusal surface in the vicinity of the evagination. (b) Clinical view of lower right posterior teeth. The dens evaginatus tubercle has been either broken off or worn down on this second premolar tooth.

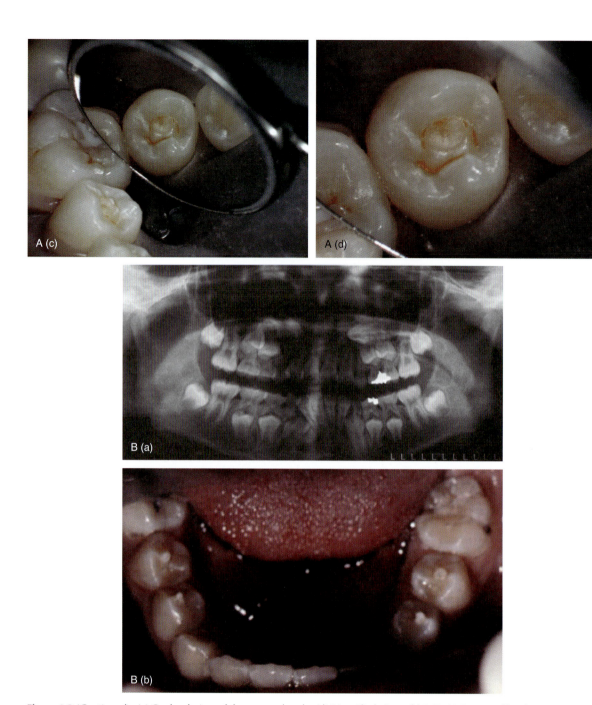

Figure 6.2 (*Continued*) (c) Occlusal view of the worn tubercle. (d) Magnified view of (c). B. (a) Panorex film showing multiple dens evaginatii of unerupted mandibular premolar teeth. Note the thin radiodensity of enamel near the center of the crown near the occlusal surface. All four unerupted mandibular premolar teeth show this radiolucency stemming from their cusps. Such radiodensities exhibiting this condition are not easily seen on the maxillary premolar teeth. (b) Clinical photo after mandibular premolar teeth have erupted, showing dens evaginatus occurring in all four lower premolar teeth (Images courtesy of Dr. Angelina Loo).

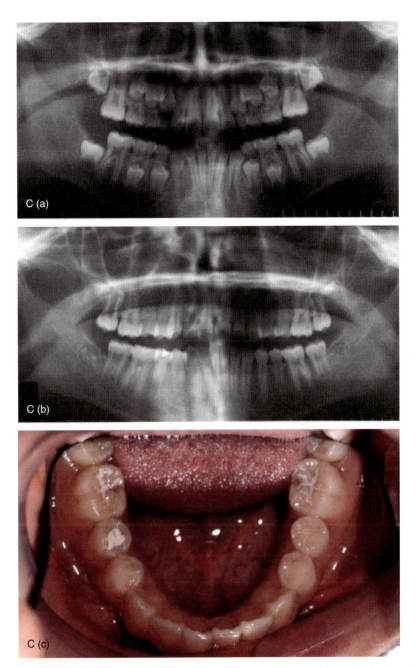

Figure 6.2 (*Continued*) C. Panorex films showing (a) pre- and (b) posteruption states of this patient's dentition. (c) Breakage of the tubercle on the lower right second premolar tooth necessitated a pulp cap and restoration of this tooth (Images courtesy of Dr. Angelina Loo).

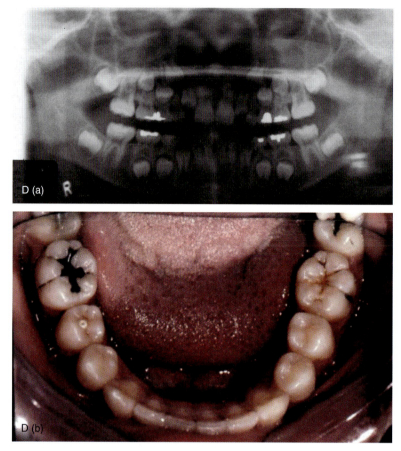

Figure 6.2 (*Continued*) D. (a) Panorex film exhibiting dens evaginatus on both unerupted lower second premolar teeth. (b) Clinical view of erupted teeth exhibits the protruding dens evaginatus along the lingual ridge of the buccal cusp of the lower right second premolar tooth. Note the "target-like" appearance of this worn tubercle indicative of enamel (outer) and dentin (inner) components. The occlusal surface of the left second premolar has a worn tubercle also, but it does not have this same appearance indicating only an enamel involvement (Images courtesy of Dr. Angelina Loo).

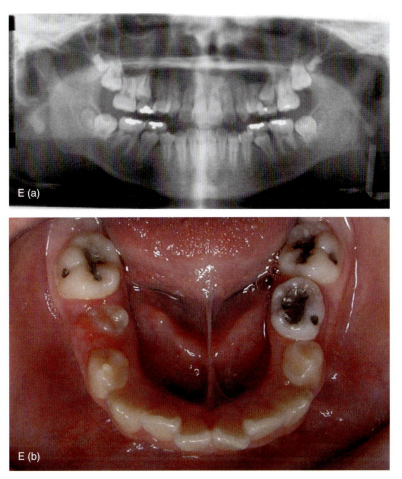

E (a)

E (b)

Figure 6.2 (*Continued*) E. (a) Panorex film showing an erupting lower right first premolar tooth. A typical dens evaginatus seen as a radiodensity stemming from the clinical crown is evident. (b) Clinical view of this partially erupted tooth shows an obvious tubercle associated with the clinical crown (Images courtesy of Dr. Angelina Loo).

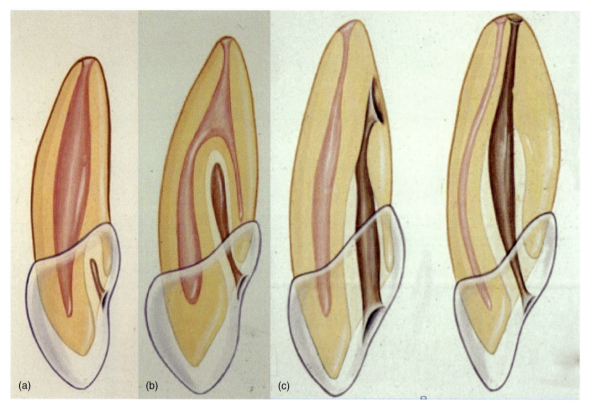

Figure 6.3 Categories of dens invaginatus as characterized by Oehlers (Oehlers, 1957). (a) Class I is an invagination that is limited to the crown of the tooth. (b) Class II invaginations extend beyond the CEJ into the root, but end as a blind sac. (c) Class III invaginations extend deeper into the root and communicate with the external root surface and may extend to the apical root third. Note that none of these invaginations directly communicate with the pulp. (Images courtesy of Dr. Raymond Greenfeld.)

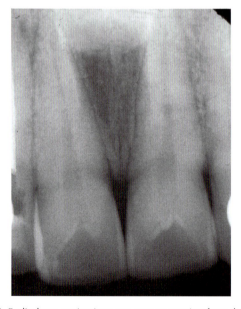

Figure 6.4 Dens invaginatus Class I. Radiodense projections are seen emanating from the cingulum of these maxillary central incisor teeth. (Images courtesy of Dr. Raymond Greenfeld.)

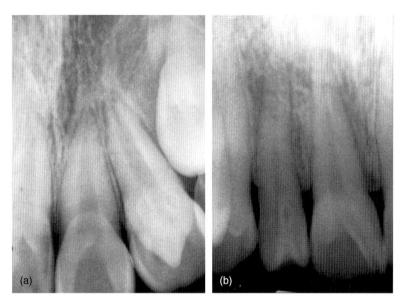

Figure 6.5   Dens invaginatus Class II. (a) Double invagination of the upper left maxillary incisor tooth extending below the CEJ. (b) Invagination near the incisal edge of the upper right maxillary lateral incisor extends below the CEJ and appears directly adjacent to the root canal space. (Images courtesy of Dr. Raymond Greenfeld.)

Deeper forms of invagination that cross the CEJ and invade the root, yet still end in a blind sac, are categorized as Class II. Such invaginations are shown in Figure 6.5. These invaginations may or may not communicate with the pulp. Radiographically, these may appear as a "dens in dente" (tooth within a tooth), although this is a misnomer. It is recognized as a pear-shaped invagination emanating from the crown of the tooth (Figure 6.6). There is a constriction at the beginning of the invagination on the surface of the tooth, before it expands deeper into the root. It may appear that the invagination goes into the pulp because of the superimposition of the invagination over the root canal (Figure 6.7a). Food, bacteria, and debris may get packed into the opening of the invagination, resulting in caries and communication with the pulp. Sealing off the invagination with a bonded resin is shown in Figure 6.7b,c.

Still more severe forms on the invagination, penetrating to communicate with the external root surface and extending to the apical root third, can have quite a malformed appearance (Figure 6.8A). Although this Class III invagination is extensive, there is usually no immediate communication with the pulp. Figure 6.8Ba shows a maxillary lateral incisor tooth with apical periodontitis resulting from infection originating from an invagination. The pulp responded normally to thermal testing. A recall radiograph shows healing of the apical periodontitis, and clinical examination revealed that the pulp continued to respond normally to pulp testing procedures.

Fusion

Fusion is the result of the union of two separate tooth germs. If contact occurs early in development, before calcification begins, two teeth may be united to form one large tooth (Figures 6.9 and 6.10). Radiographically, this can be seen as one large root and root canal system, while having a malformed crown (Figure 6.11). Such clinical presentations have significant orthodontic implications.

Contact of teeth after calcification begins can result in incomplete fusion, where there may be a union of the roots only (Figure 6.12A). The

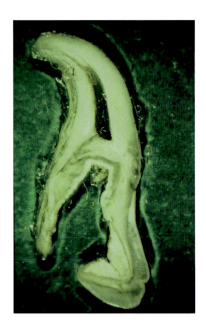

Figure 6.6 Ground section of a tooth exhibiting dens invaginatus Class II. This image shows how this malformation appears like a tooth within a tooth, "dens in dente" (Image courtesy of Dr. Ravindra Shah).

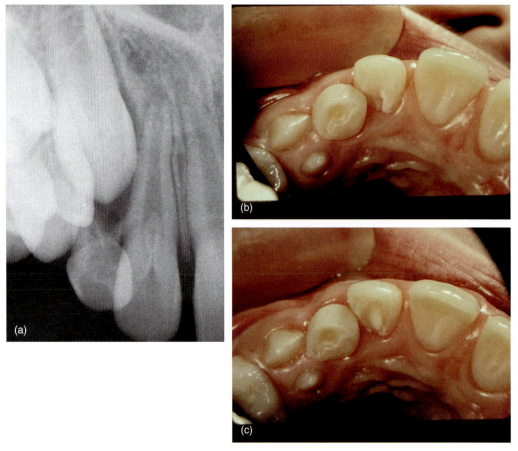

Figure 6.7 (a) Dens invaginatus Class II. Radiographically, the invagination is superimposed over the root canal in this upper right lateral incisor tooth. The pulp in this tooth responds normally to thermal testing. (b) Pre- and (c) posttreatment using an acid etched and bonded resin to seal off the invagination.

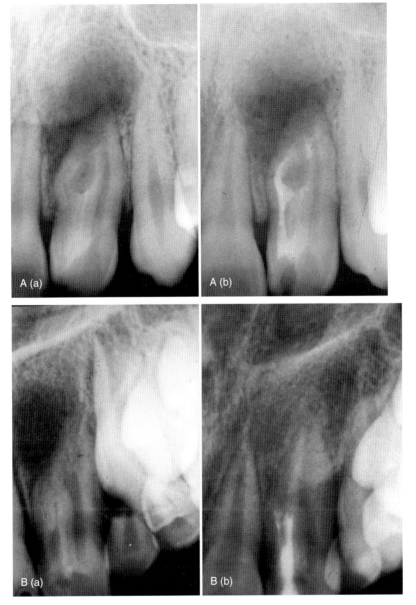

Figure 6.8 A. Dens invaginatus Class III. (a) Pre- and (b) posttreatment radiographs showing an upper left lateral incisor tooth with associated periradicular radiolucency. This tooth responded normally to pulp testing procedures before and after treatment of this invagination (images courtesy of Dr. Raymond Greenfeld). B. A complex anomaly involving dens invaginatus Class III and either fusion or gemination. Notice that the preoperative radiolucency of the upper left lateral incisor (a), resolved after treatment of the invagination (b). This tooth responded normally to pulp testing procedures before and after treatment of this invagination. (Images courtesy of Dr. Raymond Greenfeld.)

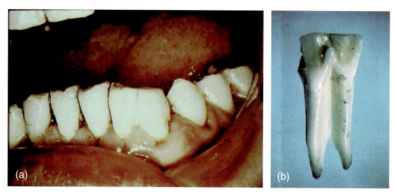

Figure 6.9 (a) Clinical view of fused mandibular anterior teeth. (b) Fusion involves both the crown and root, as seen here. (Images courtesy of Dr. Ravindra Shah.)

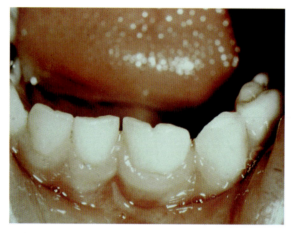

Figure 6.10 Fused teeth are seen clinically here. (Image courtesy of Dr. Ravindra Shah.)

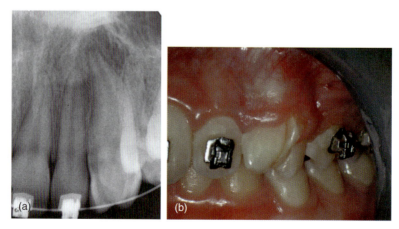

Figure 6.11 Fusion. Radiographically evident are one large root and one large root canal system. Malformation of the crown has significant orthodontic considerations.

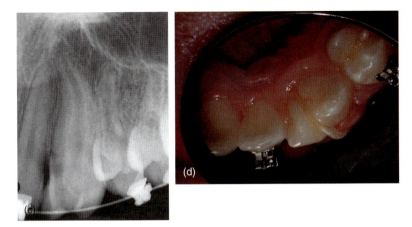

Figure 6.11 (*Continued*)

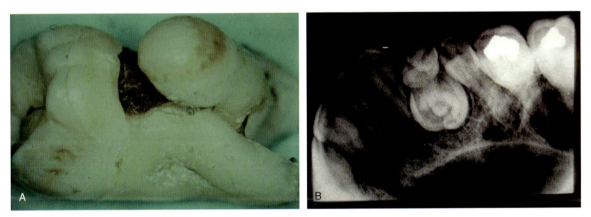

Figure 6.12   A. to D.Fusion of the roots only of this extracted tooth seen here. (Image courtesy of Dr. Ravindra Shah.) B. Fusion of erupted tooth seen radiographically, and possible fusion of unerupted tooth. Note the radiographic appearance of malformed crowns for both the erupted and unerupted teeth. (Image courtesy of Dr. Ravindra Shah.)

radiograph shown in Figure 6.12B shows fusion of teeth in both the deciduous and permanent dentitions. Note the malformed crowns in both the erupted and nonerupted teeth.

The appearance of infections and radiolucent bone in the region of fused teeth can increase the level of diagnostic difficulty. Figure 6.13a,b shows a sinus tract opening over tooth #21 which was traced using a gutta percha point. The radiolucency associated with the fused tooth #1-1 could be mistaken for the origin of this chronic abscess (Figure 6.13c,d). However, pulp testing of the anterior teeth in this region revealed that tooth #1-2 did

not respond to pulp testing procedures. Root canal treatment was initiated and completed for tooth #1-2, and osseous healing is seen after 4 months (Figure 6.13e–g), in addition to the sinus tract healing.

C-shaped canals

C-shaped canals are a result of fusion of roots within a given tooth germ. C-shaped canal systems most commonly occur in mandibular second molar teeth. Mandibular second molars having

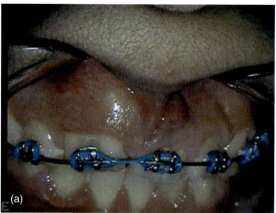

Figure 6.13 Fused tooth, sinus tract, and nonvital adjacent tooth made this endodontic diagnosis difficult. (a) Clinical view of sinus tract opening adjacent to malformed upper right central incisor tooth. (b) Sinus tract exploration with gutta percha point appeared to suggest that the malformed tooth was endodontically involved. (c) Periapical radiolucency extended between upper right lateral and central incisor teeth. (d) Normal bone was present in periapical region of upper left central and lateral incisor teeth. (e) Thermal pulp testing of maxillary anterior teeth revealed that the upper right lateral incisor tooth had a necrotic pulp. (f) Root canal treatment was completed for this tooth. (g) Three months following root canal treatment, the sinus tract had healed, and there was some evidence of osseous healing of the associated periapical lesion also (images courtesy of Dr. Ronald Corber).

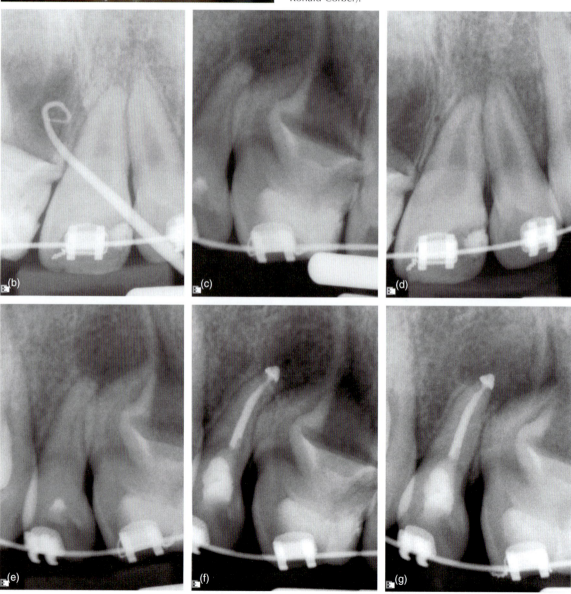

convergent mesial and distal roots should be considered suspicious for having a C-shaped canal configuration. Inadequate cleaning and shaping of this C-shaped lower second molar tooth necessitates endodontic retreatment.

During canal instrumentation, it may appear that one has perforated into the furcation region, but the apex locator should not fire as if the file is in the periodontal ligament space (Figure 6.14A). Clinical views of the access cavity show the joining of discrete canals via an isthmus, hence the term "C-shaped canals." Cone beam computed tomography (CBCT) images showing sagittal and axial views of a C-shaped mandibular second molar tooth are shown in Figure 6.14B. Notice the C-shaped root form throughout the axial slicing of the root. Using CBCT imaging systems will help to visualize three-dimensionally such anomalous root and root canal forms. Obturation of a C-shaped lower second molar tooth is shown in Figure 6.14C (Cooke and Cox, 1979; Melton et al., 1991).

Radicular groove

Lingual radicular groove is most commonly seen on maxillary lateral incisors. This condition is not readily seen on conventional two-dimensional radiographic images. When it does appear, it can be mistaken for a vertical root fracture. However, vertical root fracture can usually be ruled out as this is unusual to occur in non-root canal-treated teeth. Figure 6.15 shows a clinical view of such a lingual groove on tooth #1-2 and the lingual surface of the same extracted tooth (Everett and Kramer, 1972; Greenfeld and Cambruzzi, 1986; Kerezoudis et al., 2003; Lee et al., 1968; Pecora and da Cruz Filho, 1992; Peikoff and Trott, 1977; Peikoff et al., 1985).

Radix entomolaris

Mandibular first molars may have an additional distal root that can be discerned radiographically. When such a root is oriented toward the lingual, it is called the radix entomolaris. This condition can affect both the primary and secondary dentitions as shown in Figure 6.16. Endodontic treatment images of a calcified radix entomolaris tooth are

shown in Figure 6.17. Notice that this "extra" root appears less radiodense than the other two roots. A first molar tooth having radix entomolaris and associated, but unrelated, bony exostosis is shown in Figure 6.18A. Note that both the lingual position of this third root, and the extent and location of this exostosis, would make apical surgery difficult.

Taurodontism

The term taurodontism was introduced by Keith to describe an anomaly where the body of the tooth was enlarged and elongated, leaving short roots (Keith, 1913). Taurodontism means "bull-like teeth." It is a morphological change occurring in multirooted teeth characterized by an elongated pulp chamber in the apico-occlusal dimension resulting in bifurcation or trifurcation of the roots in the apical root third. The challenge for endodontic treatment of such teeth is locating the canal orifi, as they are found in the apical region of the root (Figure 6.18B) (Bernick, 1970; Sert and Bayrili, 2004; Shifman and Buchner, 1976).

Dilaceration

Dilaceration refers to an abrupt change in the root angulation, or a sharp curve or bend in the root of a formed tooth. Usually, abrupt changes in root angulation are also inseparable from abrupt changes in the root canal angulation. One possible etiology is trauma to the developing permanent tooth. Pre- and postoperative endodontic treatment films of a lower left molar tooth are shown in Figure 6.19A. Canal negation to the apical foramen is difficult in severely dilacerated teeth.

Figure 6.19B shows another dilacerated mandibular first molar tooth. Root canal treatment of this tooth is made difficult because of the second and third curvatures in the root, as well as the abrupt change in root canal curvature.

Microdontia

This anomaly describes teeth that are smaller than normal. There are two types of microdontia: (1) generalized microdontia and (2) specific

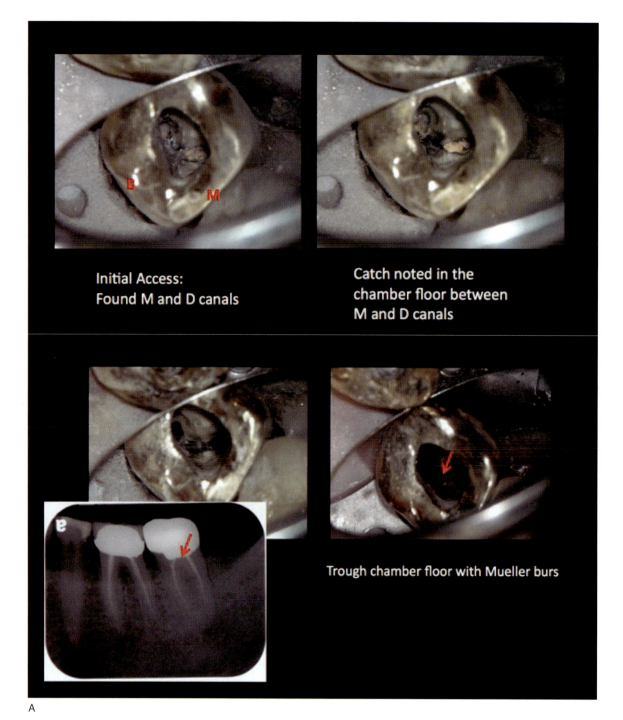

Initial Access:
Found M and D canals

Catch noted in the
chamber floor between
M and D canals

Trough chamber floor with Mueller burs

A

Figure 6.14   A. C-shaped canal. Radiographic images and access cavity photos. (Images courtesy of Dr. James Lin.)

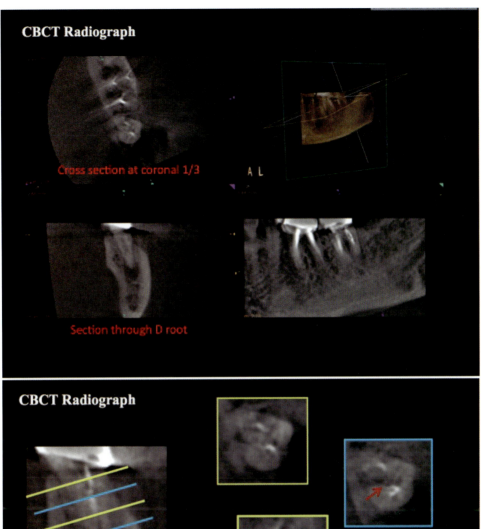

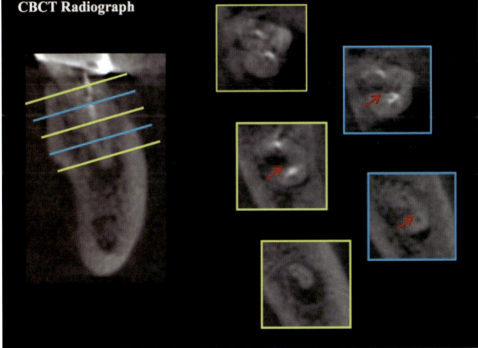

B

Figure 6.14 (*Continued*) B. Cone beam computed tomograhpy (CBCT) images showing sagittal and coronal views of the C-shaped mandibular molar seen in Figure 6.14A. Note the C-shaped root configuration of the (yellow) and (blue) axial slicing seen in the coronal, middle, and apical root thirds. (Images courtesy of Dr. James Lin.)

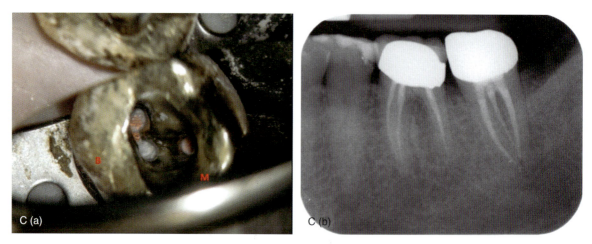

Figure 6.14 (*Continued*) C. Obturation of a C-shaped lower second molar tooth. (a) View of the floor of the pulp chamber shows the canal orifi are joined by a C-shaped isthmus. (b) Final film following root canal retreatment of this lower second molar tooth. It appears that root filling is present in the furcation region in this two-dimensional film. (Images courtesy of Dr. James Lin.)

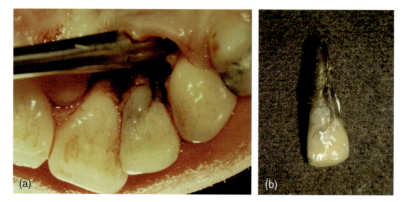

Figure 6.15 Clinical photos of palatal groove on this upper lateral incisor tooth (a) pre-extraction and (b) postextraction. Note that his palatal groove extends to the apical root third of this tooth. (Images courtesy of Dr. Raymond Greenfeld.)

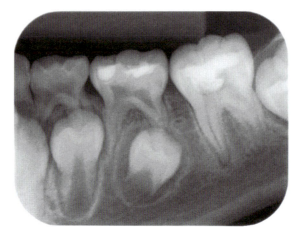

Figure 6.16 Radix entomolaris: Note this condition for both the lower left primary first molar tooth and also for the lower left permanent first molar tooth. (Image courtesy of Dr. Les Campbell.)

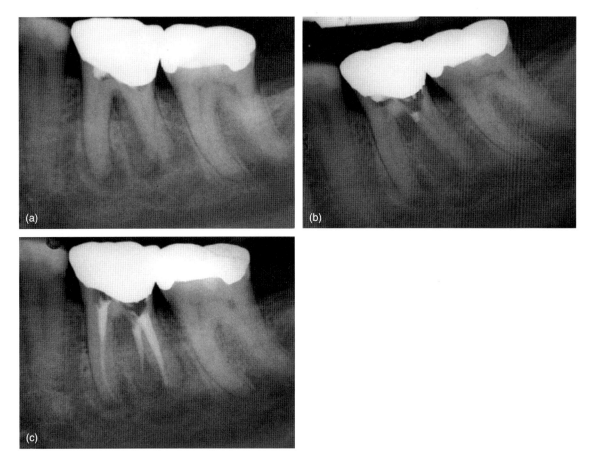

Figure 6.17 Radix entomolaris: (a) Patient was referred because the calcified canals could not be negotiated in this lower left first molar tooth. (b) Film of gutta percha placed in the trough created in the region of the disto-lingual root helps orientate the direction of progression during uncovering the orifice to this calcified disto-lingual canal. (c) Postretreatment film showing obturation of all three roots.

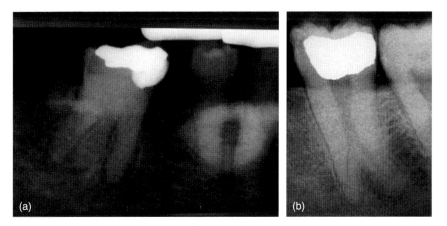

Figure 6.18 (a) Radix entomolaris with bony exostosis; associated but unrelated finding. (b) Taurodontism occurring in this lower molar tooth. Note the elongation of the pulp chamber toward the apical region. (Image courtesy of Visual Endodontics, 2011.)

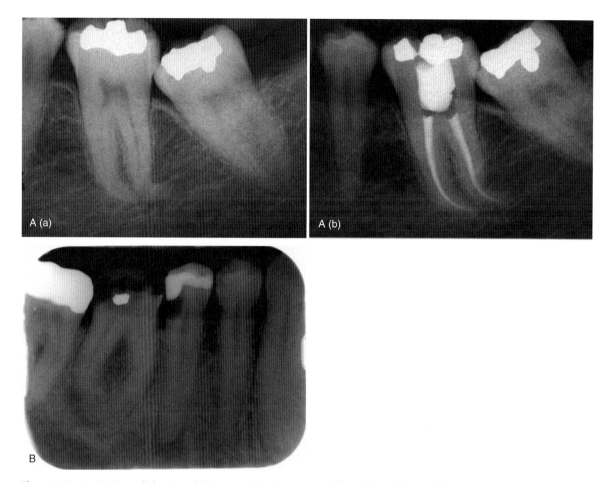

Figure 6.19   A. (a) Pre-endodontic and (b) postendodontic treatment films of this dilacerated lower left first molar tooth. The root canals were instrumented with rotary NiTi files to the beginning of these abrupt curvatures, but then canal shaping was completed using .02 tapered files. B. Dilaceration of this mandibular first molar tooth. Note the abrupt double curvatures of the root canal system in the distal root. (Image courtesy of Dr. Les Campbell.)

microdontia. In generalized microdontia, all the teeth are smaller than normal. This could happen in cases of dwarfism. Specific microdontia involving a single tooth typically affects the third molar tooth and the maxillary lateral incisor. Figure 6.20A shows an unrestored tooth #1-8 adjacent to tooth #1-6, and this tooth appears even smaller than the maxillary first premolar tooth. A "peg lateral" tooth is shown in Figure 6.20B. In both the panorex and periapical films, one can see that tooth #1-2 has a shorter and narrower root than one would expect for the size of the adjacent teeth. Apical periodontitis is also associated with this tooth.

Amelogenesis imperfecta

Amelogenesis imperfecta is a hereditary defect of enamel involving a disturbance in the ectodermal layer. Three types of defect have been classified according to the stage of development in which they occur (Witkop and Sauk, 1976): hypoplastic, a

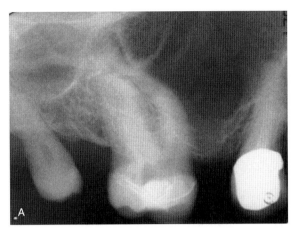

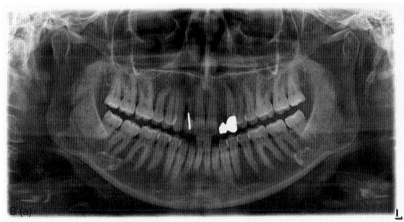

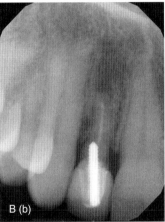

Figure 6.20   A. Microdontia. A microdont is shown in the posterior region of this film of the upper right sextant. B. Microdontia. (a) Panorex and (b) periapical films of this maxillary right lateral incisor tooth. Due to the patient presenting with symptomatic apical periodontitis, and having a large post in this small tooth with a well fitting crown, the treatment decision was to perform periapical surgery. (Courtesy of Dr. Sigrid Coil.)

disruption of the deposition of organic matrix during the formative stage, hypocalcifed, a disruption during the calcification stage, and hypomaturation, where the enamel crystals remain immature.

The clinical appearance can vary greatly among the different forms of amelogenesis imperfecta. The color of affected regions can vary in color from yellow to gray, and the texture can be soft or relatively hard.

Depending on the amount of enamel present on the tooth, the morphology of the crown may appear normal or abnormal. Figure 6.21 shows the thinning of the enamel both radiographically and clinically, toward the incisal edges of the mandibular incisor teeth. Note that the pulp canal space appears to be of normal width.

Dentinogenesis imperfecta

Dentinogenesis imperfecta is a hereditary condition affecting dentin due to a mesodermal defect. Several forms of this disease exist, and the clinical presentation can vary greatly. Clinically, the teeth may appear in color from gray to yellow-brown,

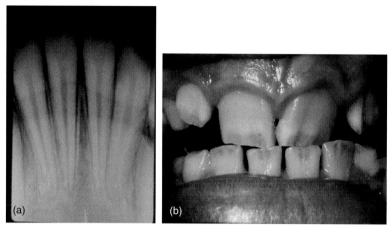

Figure 6.21   Amelogenesis imperfecta. Note the decalcified regions below the incisal edges of the mandibular incisor teeth, evident both (a) radiographically and (b) clinically. (Images courtesy of Dr. Ravindra Shah.)

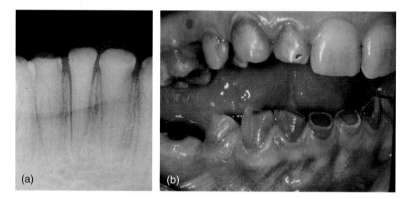

Figure 6.22   Dentinogeneis imperfecta. (a) The typical obliteration of the pulp canal space is seen radiographically. (b) Clinical view showing extensive wear of these lower incisor teeth. (Images courtesy of Dr. Ravindra Shah.)

but all exhibit an opalescent hue. The most profound feature is the partial or complete obliteration of the pulp chamber and root canal space seen radiographically. Figure 6.22 shows a radiographic and a clinical view of this condition. Note that although the root canal space is obliterated, the periodontal membrane space and surrounding bone appear normal.

Dentine dysplasia

Dentin dysplasia is a condition affecting dentin formation. This anomaly was reported by

Ballschmiede who reported observed premature exfoliation of multiple teeth and called it "rootless teeth" (Steidler et al., 1984). The radiographic features of this condition include roots that are short, blunt, and conically shaped. The pulp chambers and root canal spaces are typically obliterated (Figure 6.23). This obliteration occurs pre-eruptively in permanent teeth.

Talon cusp

The talon cusp is an anomalous projection of tooth structure, projecting from the cingulum region of

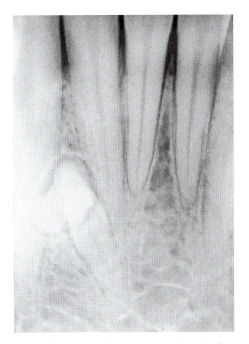

Figure 6.23 Dentine dysplasia is seen in the apical region of these anterior teeth. (Image courtesy of Dr. Ravindra Shah.)

permanent incisor teeth. This structure resembling an eagle's talon, may interfere with occlusion and can be an esthetic problem. A deep development groove is present where the cusp joins the lingual portion of the tooth. Figure 6.24A shows the radiographic appearance of the Talon cusp for a lower incisor teeth, and the clinical view of extracted tooth with a Talon cusp. A rare combination of dens invaginatus exhibiting a talon cusp on the facial aspect of a maxillary incisor tooth is presented in Figure 6.24B.

Congenital syphilis (Hutchinson incisor and Mulberry molars)

The Hutchinson incisor has a characteristic notch in the incisal edge, particularly evident for the maxillary incisor teeth (Figure 6.25). Radiographically, the undulations of the incisal edges would mimic the clinical view.

Morphological variations

A common complexity for endodontic treatment is the treatment of multiple canals in a given root. Although there are guidelines as to expected

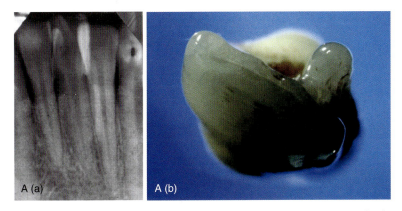

A (a)   A (b)

Figure 6.24 A. (a) Talon cusp is seen radiographically as a discrete cusp on this lower incisor tooth. The incisal view of this talon cusp is shown in (b) (Images courtesy of Dr. Raymond Greenfeld).

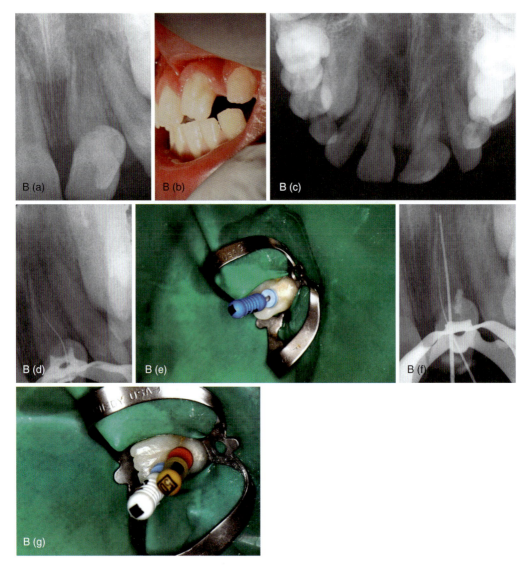

Figure 6.24 (*Continued*) B. Dens invaginatus exhibiting a talon cusp on the facial aspect of the upper left maxillary central incisor tooth. (a) Periapical film showing the invagination and the talon cusp. (b) Clinical image showing the talon cusp on the buccal surface of this tooth. (c) Occlusal film showing the maxillary anterior teeth. (d) Working length film with a file placed in the buccal access cavity. (e) Clinical view of instrument in buccal access cavity. (f) Root canal instruments in two separate canals for this working length film. Note the perforation repair material in the coronal root third just apical to the CEJ. (g) Clinical view of two instruments placed in the buccal access cavity. (Images courtesy of Dr. George Bogen.)

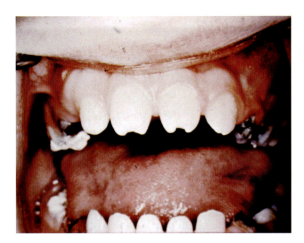

Figure 6.25   Hutchinson's incisor shown clinically are easily identifiable and are easily seen radiographically as well. (Image courtesy of Dr. Ravindra Shah.)

frequencies for the number of canals, and configuration of what to expect in a given tooth type, the true configuration is usually observed following treatment. With the increased use of CBCT, three-dimensional evaluations of teeth and supporting structures are now possible. However, most initial impressions are fettered by careful assessment of two-dimensional periapical radiographs.

References

Bernick, S.M. (1970) Taurodontia. *Oral Surg Oral Med Oral Pathol*, 29, 549.

Canadian Academy of Endodontists. Standards of Practice, August 1998, pp. 4–5.

Cooke, H.G., 3rd. and Cox, F.L. (1979) C-shaped canal configurations in mandibular molars. *J Am Dent Assoc*, 99, 836–839.

Everett, F.G. and Kramer, G.M. (1972) The disto-lingual groove in the maxillary lateral incisor: a periodontal hazard. *J Periodontol*, 443, 352.

Greenfeld, R.S. and Cambruzzi, J.V. (1986) Complexities of endodontic treatment of maxillary lateral incisors with anomalous root formation. *Oral Surg Oral Med Oral Pathol*, 62, 82–88.

Hulsmann, M. (1997) Dens invaginatus: aetiology, classification, prevalence, diagnosis, and treatment considerations. *Int Endo J*, 30, 79–90.

Keith, A. (1913) Problems relating to the teeth of the earlier forms of prehistoric man. *Proc R Soc Med*, 6(Odontol Sect), 103–124.

Kerezoudis, N.P., Sisko, G.J., and Tsatsas, V. (2003) Bilateral buccal radicular groove in maxillary incisors: a case report. *Int Endood J*, 36(12), 898.

Lee, K.W., Lee, E.C., and Poon, K.Y. (1968) Palato-gingival grooves in maxillary incisors. *Br Dent J*, 124, 14.

McCulloch, K.J. et al. (1997) Dens evaginatus from an orthodontic perspective: report of several clinical cases and review of the literature. *Am J Orthodont Dentofac Orthopedics*, 112(6), 670–675.

Melton, D.C., et al. (1991) Anatomical and histological features of C-shaped canals in mandibular second molars. *J Endod*, 17, 384–388.

Oehlers, F.A.C. (1957) Dens invaginatus (dilated composite ondontoma). I. Variations of the invagination process and associated anterior crown forms. *Oral Surg Oral Med Oral Pathol*, 10, 1204–1218.

Pecora, J.D. and da Cruz Filho, A.M. (1992) Study of the incidence of radicular grooves in maxillary incisors. *Braz Dent J.*, 3, 11–16.

Peikoff, M.D. and Trott, J.R. (1977) An endodontic failure caused by an unusual anatomical anomaly. *J Endod*, 3, 356–359.

Peikoff, M.D., et al. (1985) Endodontic failure attributable to a complex radicular lingual groove. *J Endod*, 11, 573–577.

Sert, S. and Bayrili, G. (2004) Taurodontism in six molars: a case report. *J Endod*, 30, 601–602.

Shifman, A. and Buchner, A. (1976) Taurodontism. Report of sixteen cases in Israel. *Oral Surg Oral Med Oral Pathol*, 41, 400–405.

Steidler, N.E. et al. (1984) Dentinal dysplasia: a clinicopathological study of eight cases and review of the literature. *Br J Oral Maxillofac Surg*, 22, 274–286.

Witkop, C.J., Jr. and Sauk, J.J., Jr. (1976) Heritable defects of enamel. In: R.E. Stewart and G.H. Prescott, eds., *Oral Facial Genetics*, pp. 151–226. C.V. Mosby Co., St. Louis.

Part 2

Endodontic Disease

Chapter 7   Radiographic Expression of Endodontic Disease

Chapter 8   Image Interpretation of Periapical Abnormalities

Chapter 9   Radiographic Interpretation of Traumatic Injuries

Chapter 10 Radiographic Analysis of Acquired Pathological Dental Conditions

Chapter 11 Radiographic Analysis of Periodontal and Endodontic Lesions

Chapter 12 Radiographic Imaging in Implant Dentistry

7 Radiographic Expression of Endodontic Disease

Calvin D. Torneck

Endodontic disease

Root canal infection occurs when host tissue interacts with pathogenic microorganisms that colonize the pulp space. This can evoke an inflammatory response during which pathophysiological changes occur in the dental supporting tissues (Stashenko et al., 1998). These are first seen in the periodontium and later in the alveolar bone (Figure 7.1). The initial changes are seen adjacent to sites where blood vessels once entered and exited the dental pulp, that is, in juxtaposition to the apical foramen and/or lateral and accessory canals (Figure 7.2). When inflammation only involves soft tissue (periodontal ligament), no radiographic changes are seen although symptoms of a periodontitis may be clinically present. In time, changes also occur in bone, and it is at that time their presence may be detected radiographically. Their detection is dependent upon their size and their location and the nature of the host's reaction to the presence of the bacteria. Host recognition of pathogenic bacteria is prone to many variables, and these can lead to marked differences in the degree and extent of the inflammation-related tissue changes that occur (Wilson, 2008). Variances in the size and location of

vascular channels also impact on how and where the inflammation is manifested. Small lateral canals or a weak host response, for example, may result in a bone change too small to be detected radiographically (Brynolf, 1967), and larger lesions may not be detectable even when present if they occur on the palatal (lingual) or facial (buccal) aspect of the root where they are masked by root superimposition.

Infection-induced inflammation results in the release of signaling molecules from resident and migrant cells that dysregulate bone metabolism (Torneck and Tulananda, 1969) (Figure 7.3A). In the healthy adult, bone appears relatively constant when imaged because as it remodels, the resorption of bone is balanced by its replacement with new bone (homeostasis). In older adults, there is an innate and acquired-based shift that often leads to a greater removal of bone than formation of bone and hence a reduction in bone mass. When the reduction in bone mass surpasses a calculated norm, the bone is referred to as osteopenic, and when more advanced, it is referred to as osteoporotic. Growing pre-adult patients normally display an increase in overall bone formation and resorption in association with their growth. During the

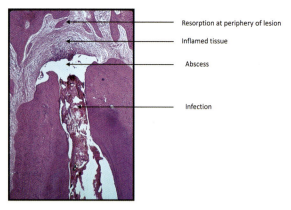

Resorption at periphery of lesion

Inflamed tissue

Abscess

Infection

Figure 7.1   Pathophysiological changes occurring in the apical supporting tissues in association with root canal infection.

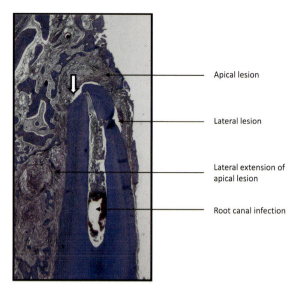

Apical lesion

Lateral lesion

Lateral extension of apical lesion

Root canal infection

Figure 7.2   Lesions of endodontic origin about root of incisor tooth. Note area of resorption at root apex (white arrow).

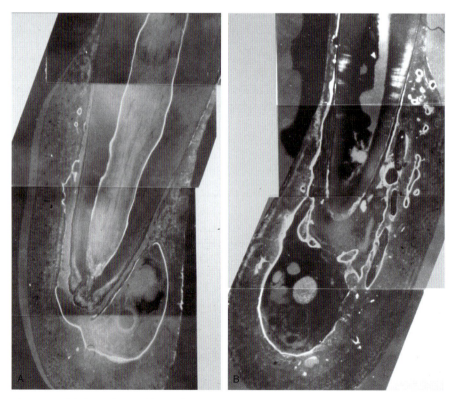

Figure 7.3   A. Fluorescent labeling of normal bone about canine root (dog). White zones indicate bone formed during period of label administration. (Reprinted from Torneck and Tulananda, 1969, with permission from Elsevier Ltd.). B. Dysregulation of bone metabolism about canine root in which there is a root canal infection. Note bone loss (dark area) at apex and new bone deposition (white zones) in supporting tissues. (Reprinted from Torneck and Tulananda, 1969, with permission from Elsevier Ltd.)

growth, bones become altered in size and shape and their density altered by function (an adaptive phenomenon). The rate and degree of alteration seen in bone is mainly under the control of hormonal and locally produced signaling molecules (Boskey and Coleman, 2010).

Myelogenous-derived cells called osteoclasts (OCs) are responsible for bone resorption, and their activity is regulated by hormones and locally produced signaling molecules (Figure 7.4). These molecules are produced not only by resident cells, but also by migrant cells, cells that become attracted to a site when an injury occurs (Cochran, 2008).

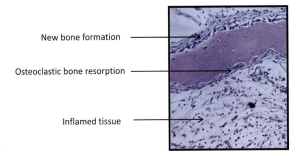

New bone formation

Osteoclastic bone resorption

Inflamed tissue

Figure 7.4 Histological section taken from periphery of apical lesion seen in Figure 7.9B displaying osteoclastic bone resorption in association with tissue inflammation. Deposition of new bone by osteoblasts can be seen in juxtaposition to the resorption site.

Local signaling molecules are called cytokines, and in bone they are normally produced by osteoblasts (OBs) and other cells normal to bone tissue. When infection is present, there is a phenotypic and temporal-related migration of nonresident cells to the site. In the early stages of inflammation, these migrating cells release cytokines that upregulate the production of a signaling ligand called receptor activator of nuclear factor *kappa* B (RANKL) that activates OCs through a surface RANK receptor, to resorb bone (Teng, 2006). While other intra- and extracellular, neurological, and environmental factors also play a role in OC activation, their role appears to be less prominent than that played by RANKL (Tay et al., 2004). With time and control of the infection, OC activation is downregulated by a cytokine called osteopotegrin (OPN) which is a decoy receptor for RANKL and limits its availability for activation of the RANK receptor. OPN upregulation and bone formation are generally seen in the chronic stages of inflammation. The bone formation is initiated locally by cytokines of the transforming growth factor (TGF) super family that, like RANKL, are produced by both resident cells and different subsets of migrant cells attracted to the site (Katagin and Takahashi, 2002). This leads not only to the healing of bone (return to homeostasis) when infection is controlled through treatment (Figure 7.5A–C), but also to the deposition of bone during disease when the intensity of

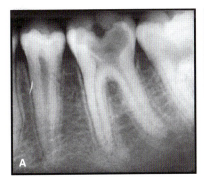
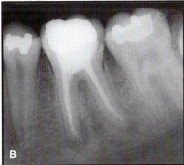
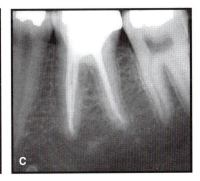

Figure 7.5 A. Changing pattern in bone associated with endodontic infection. In pre-op radiograph, a small diffuse radiolucency in association with increased radio-opacity is seen at apex of mesial roots of mandibular molar. Apex of distal root displays small defined apical radiolucency in association with a slight radio-opacity. B. At completion of endodontic treatment, lesion at apex of mesial roots displays an increase in size of radiolucency. Lesion at apex of distal root displays little change. C. Return to normal bone architecture at apex of mesial and distal root is seen 1 year after completion of endodontic treatment.

the host response is moderated sufficiently to upregulate the release of anti-inflammatory cytokines and downregulate those that are proinflammatory. Another factor that influences bone formation during inflammation is the environmental pH. Mineralization of bone matrix ideally occurs at a slightly alkaline pH. During the early phase of inflammation, the environmental pH becomes acidic, and this tends to locally suppress OB activity and promote OC activity. This too is moderated when proinflammatory cytokines are downregulated. Inflammation is most intense at sites closest to where bacteria and host interact, and it is at those sites that resorption of bone is most apt to persist. At more distant sites where the host response is more moderate, OC activity is usually less intense and OB activity is more prevalent. In low-grade infection, therefore, it is not unusual to see some areas of reactive bone formation at sites peripheral to the root when bone resorption is occurring at the root apex, or bone reactive formation as the most prevalent dysregulative change present. The architecture of this bone, however, is different than that of the bone that is normal to the anatomical site. A local decrease in bone density within the bone is seen as a radiolucency in the radiograph. In endodontic infections, these are initially seen extending out from the periodontal space at sites where a vascular channel is present. When infection leads to an increase in bone formation, a radio-opacity may also be seen

in the radiograph, and again, this occurs in juxtaposition to those sites. Bone changes associated with inflammation are designated with the suffix "itis," hence a radiolucent lesion of endodontic origin is referred to as rarefying osteitis (Figure 7.6A,B), and one that is opaque, condensing (sclerosing) osteitis (Figure 7.7A,B). Condensing osteitis is usually accompanied by some degree of rarefying osteitis (Figures 7.8 and 7.9A–C),

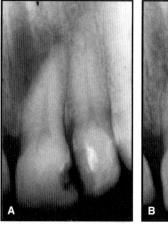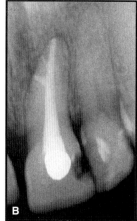

Figure 7.6   A. Apical and lateral endodontic rarefying osteitis associated with root of maxillary incisor. B. Lesion displays healing 8 months post-op. Note presence of two large lateral canals on mesial aspect of root.

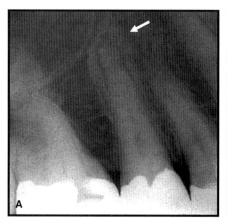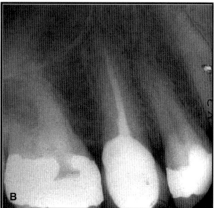

Figure 7.7   A. Widened periodontal space and loss of lamina dura in association with condensing osteitis (arrow) at apex of nonvital maxillary premolar. B. Reestablishment of normal bone 1 year after completion of endodontic treatment.

unlike rarefying osteitis, which can occur without an accompanying radio-opacity. As previously mentioned, because lesions of endodontic origin initially develop in the periodontal ligament, a widening of the periodontal space and an accompanying loss of lamina dura is usually present in a well-exposed radiograph. Several factors, in addition to those that have been already mentioned, influence the ability of the clinician to detect the

lesion radiographically even when it is histologically present. These range from physical factors necessary to generate a good readable image, to the size and location of the lesion in the bone (Brynolf, 1967). Bone imaging of diagnostic quality requires proper alignment of the tooth manifesting endodontic disease with the central ray, as well as sufficient density and contrast to record all the nuances of bone architecture (Figure 7.10). These factors separate tooth from bone and help differentiate normal from bone altered by disease. However, even with properly exposed images, lesions may not be radiographically detectable in standard imaging methods if they are masked by superimposition of roots, as has already been discussed, or when they occur and are restricted to trabecular bone. Studies have shown that extension of the lesion to include junctional bone, bone at the interface of the trabecular and cortical bone, is necessary if it is to be seen radiographically (Bender and Seltzer, 1961a, 1961b). This apparently applies primarily to teeth whose roots are centrally situated in the jaw and less to teeth whose roots approximate the bone surface. It also has been shown that lesion size is usually underrepresented when imaged radiographically (Figure 7.11A,B).

Lesions of endodontic origin can be large or small, concentrically disposed at their site of origin, or highly eccentric. Large eccentric lesions can result in the inclusion of the roots of neighboring healthy teeth within the perimeter of its radiographic presence (Figure 7.12A,B). This can lead to misdiagnosis and unnecessary treatment of

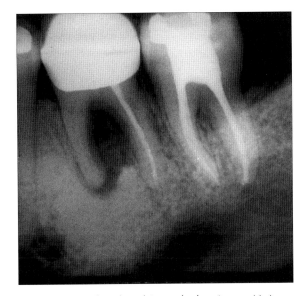

Figure 7.8 Combined rarefying and sclerosing osteitis in mandible associated with endodontic infection of molar tooth.

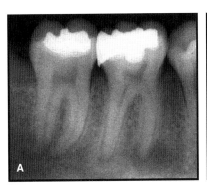
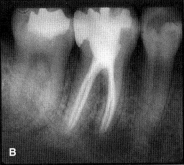
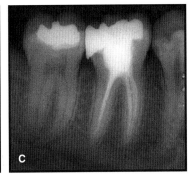

Figure 7.9 A. Mandibular first molar demonstrating condensing and rarefying osteitis at apex of mesial and distal roots. B. Lesions are still present at completion of endodontic treatment. C. Return to normal bone architecture 1 year after completion of endodontic treatment.

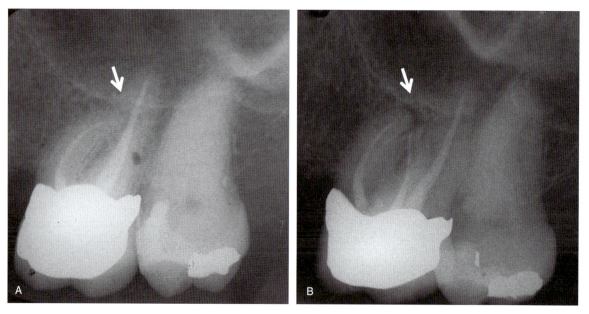

Figure 7.10 A. Underexposure and superimposition of root leaves lesion at apex of mesiobuccal root of maxillary molar undetectable in radiograph. B. Change in angle of central ray (CR) and proper exposure reveals presence of rarefying osteitis at mesiobuccal root apex.

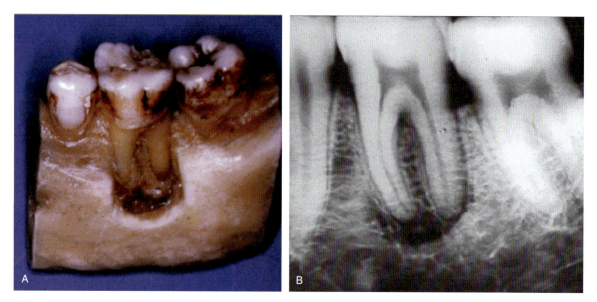

Figure 7.11 A. Experimental removal of bone over roots and around apices of mandibular molar. B. Radiographic appearance of bone removal shown in Figure 7.11A.

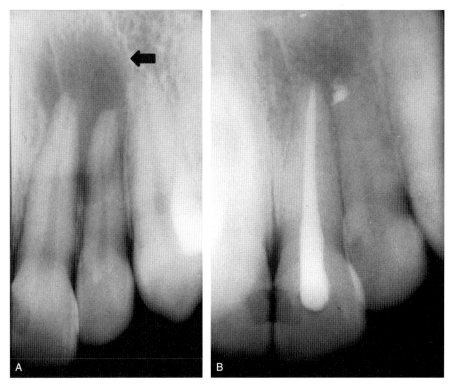

Figure 7.12   A. Lesion of endodontic origin at apex of maxillary central incisor (note deep coronal restoration) extending over apex of lateral incisor (unrestored). Lateral incisor responds positively to thermal and electrical testing. B Radiograph taken 1 year after endodontic treatment of central incisor, indicating healing of lesion. Some extruded root canal cement (opacity over lateral incisor) persists in tissue.

otherwise healthy teeth unless precautions are undertaken to confirm which tooth is responsible for the changes that are seen. This again emphasizes a need to take multiple views of the teeth in question and to utilize additional diagnostic tests, before a working diagnosis is established and treatment is begun. More often than not, only one tooth is responsible for the lesion, hence only one tooth needs to be treated for healing to occur. The challenge lies in identifying that tooth by properly assessing the pulp status of all the teeth present in the area (Figure 7.13A,B).

As stated previously, lesions of endodontic origin can assume a variety of shapes in the radiograph depending upon their location and the nature of the bone changes. One of clinical concern is the extension of a radiolucent lesion from the apex of the root to the crest of the bone (Figures 7.14A,B and 7.15A,B). Another is the presence of a

lesion in the furcation area of a multirooted tooth (Figure 7.16A–C). Both of these patterns are typical of the type of bone loss associated more with lesions of periodontal origin than they are with those of endodontic origin. Care must be exercised to differentiate which disease is responsible for the change if a successful conclusion to the treatment rendered is to be expected.

Radiolucent lesions of endodontic origin can also manifest diffuse or well-demarcated borders. The difference appears to be related to the "acuteness" of the lesion. Acute lesions tend to enlarge rapidly and as such promote more rapid and more aggressive peripheral bone resorption. The presence of this inflammation-activated resorption at the periphery of the lesion appears to be the factor responsible for the poorly demarcated border of the radiolucency seen in the radiographic image. Chronic lesions, on the other hand, tend to have

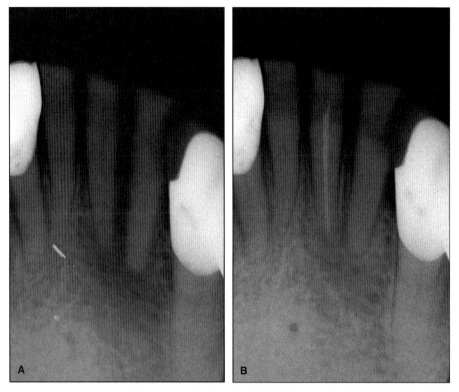

Figure 7.13   A. Rarefying osteitis at apex of mandibular central and lateral incisors. Only central incisor failed to respond to vitality tests. B. Healing is evident about both incisors 1 year after completion of endodontic treatment of central incisor.

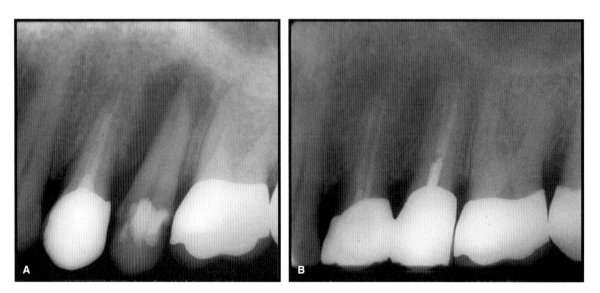

Figure 7.14   A. Rarefying osteitis that extends from apex to crestal region of bone along mesial aspect of root of maxillary premolar. B. Lesion appears healed 1 year after endodontic treatment.

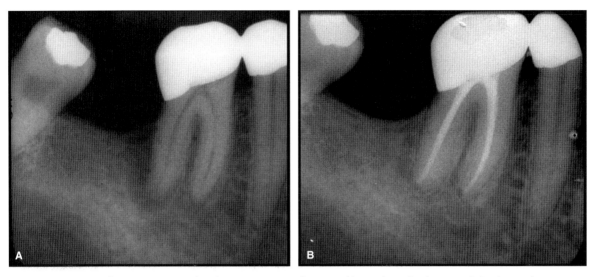

Figure 7.15 A. Rarefying osteitis extending from apex to crestal region of bone along distal aspect of distal root of mandibular molar. B. Lesion appears healed 1 year after endodontic treatment.

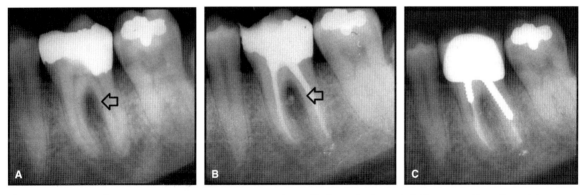

Figure 7.16 A. Rarefying osteitis present in furcation area of mandibular molar (arrow). B. Presence of lateral canal from middle third of mesial root appears to be source of rarefying osteitis as indicated in immediate po radiograph. C. Restoration of normal bone in furcation 1 year after completion of endodontic treatment.

much less resorption present at the periphery, especially those that develop a connective tissue capsule. This results in their having a well-demarcated sharp border separating the lesion from the surrounding bone in the radiographic image (Figure 7.17A,B). Some lesions even become corticated due to the formation of new bone at the periphery. This gives them a cyst-like appearance (to be discussed later in this chapter). This cortication is a reactive response in surrounding bone to a slow or nonexpanding lesion and is not pathognomonic of a cyst.

External resorption of the root apex is a common side effect of endodontic-induced apical inflammation. It occurs histologically in 80–90% of teeth with apical inflammation (Laux et al., 2000; Vier and Figueiredo, 2002) but can be detected in the radiograph in only 10–15%, and usually only when it is relatively severe (Figure 7.18A,B). As seen in the radiographic imaging of bone lesions, the histological extent of the resorption is generally more severe than that seen in the radiographic image. When present it can, and usually does, alter the normal anatomical configuration of the apical

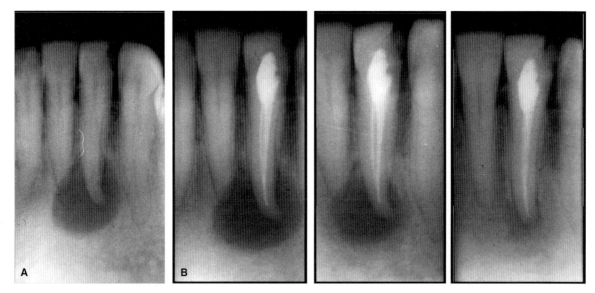

Figure 7.17   A. Well-demarcated radiolucent lesion of endodontic origin at apex of mandibular lateral incisor. B. Series of radiographs taken immed, 6 months, and 18 months, after completion of treatment. On nonsurgical endodontic treatment, note change in angle of CR results in superimposition of root over dilacerated apex. Bone trabeculae are relatively uniform at healed site. Nutrient canal is present near mesial aspect of root apex.

foramen, and this can lead to problems in preparation and filling of the root canal, unless precautions are taken to account for its presence. Only repair of cementum, periodontal ligament, and bone can be expected to occur at the site of resorption when endodontic treatment is successfully undertaken (Figure 7.19A,B). Dentin lost to external resorption is not replaced.

Endodontic-induced periostitis of the nasal cavity and antrum

As lesions of endodontic origin enlarge in size, they can, in accordance with their position in the jaws, induce activity in the periosteum that lines the wall of an osseous cavity or that is present on the surface of the jaw. After resorption has reached the surface of a bone, continued growth of the lesion can raise and stimulate the periosteum to produce new bone about the periphery of the lesion as it slowly expands. This results in a localized alteration in the contour of the bone surface. The term used to describe this effect is "periostitis."

Periostitis that involves the walls of the nasal cavity or antrum can be caused by endodontic infection at the roots of any of the teeth that approximate these structures (Figures 7.20 and 7.21). Unlike the original bone wall that appears smooth and uniform, bone formed in response to an inflammatory stimulus appears irregular and at times discontinuous when imaged radiographically. The change in contour in the cavity wall induced by the lesion may appear as a minor elevation of the cavity floor or as occurs in more severe cases, as a prominent corticated extension of the apical radiolucent lesion into the cavity. It is important to differentiate endodontic-induced periostitis from periostitis that can occur in response to nonodontogenic lesions before treatment is initiated. Because respiratory epithelium overlies periosteum in both of these cavities, endodontic infection may also lead to a localized mucositis (Figure 7.22A–C). This appears as a homogenous grayish radio-opacity that extends outward from the wall of the cavity into the more radiolucent respiratory space. Its association with an endodontic infection and its localized distribution makes it easy to differentiate from the more generalized type of muco-

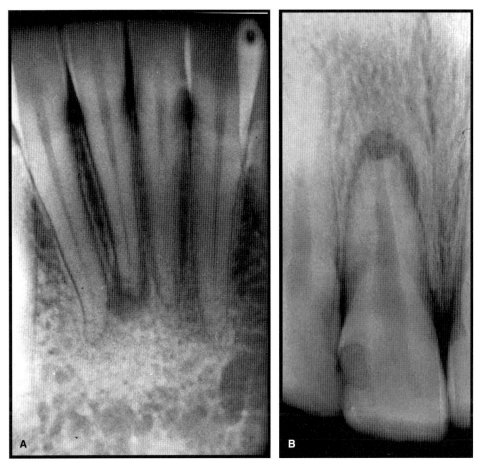

Figure 7.18 A. Mandibular incisor demonstrating rarefying and condensing osteitis accompanied by apical external resorption. B. Maxillary incisor demonstrating rarefying osteitis accompanied by more severe apical external resorption.

sitis associated with primary sinus and nasal infection or allergy. Periostitis and mucositis associated with endodontic infections are reactionary occurrences and as such, resolve over time when the root canal infection is properly managed (Figure 7.22A–C).

Endodontic-induced periostitis of the jaws

Periostitis of the jaws is more common in the mandible than in the maxilla, and is more common in preadolescents and adolescents than it is in adults. It can occur on the buccal and lingual aspect of the jaw and is seen more frequently in the association with posterior teeth than with anterior teeth. As with the periostitis seen in the respiratory cavities, it is caused by the inflammation-related stimulation of the periosteum that leads to a change in the contour of the bone surface. This change may be minor and barely visible when viewed in the radiograph, or be quite pronounced in size to a point where its presence is not only noticed radiographically but clinically as well (Figure 7.23). To properly image periostitis of the jaws, views other than those considered standard for endodontic diagnosis usually have to be taken (Figure 7.24A–C). Because stimuli associated with inflammation are episodic in nature, periosteal activity induced by the inflammation is also episodic in nature. This can give the periosteal new bone a striated or

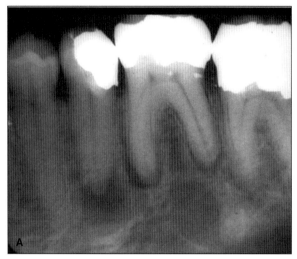 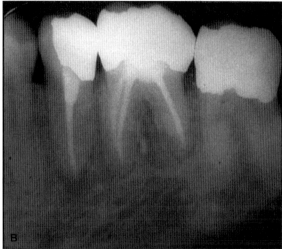

Figure 7.19   A. Mandibular premolar and molar displaying rarefying osteitis and apical root resorption in association with an endodontic infection. B. Repair of resorbed apicies and apical lesions 1 year after completion of endodontic treatment.

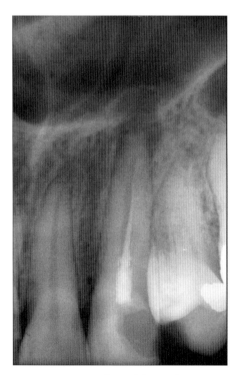

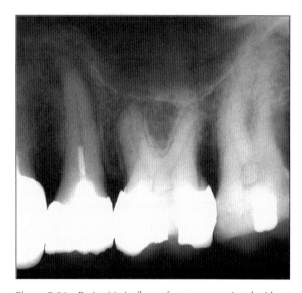

Figure 7.21   Periostitis in floor of antrum associated with lesion of endodontic origin at apex of 2nd premolar.

Figure 7.20   Periostitis in floor of the nasal cavity associated with lesion of endodontic origin at apex of cuspid.

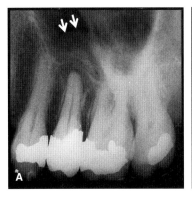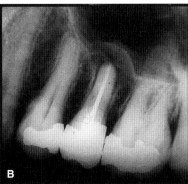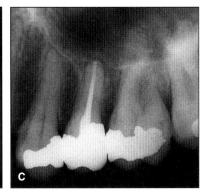

Figure 7.22   A. Periostitis and localized mucositis (arrows) in floor of antrum in association with lesion of endodontic origin at apex of 2nd premolar. B. Resolution of mucositis, but not periostitis, 2 weeks after nonsurgical endodontic treatment. C. Resolution of periostitis 1 year later.

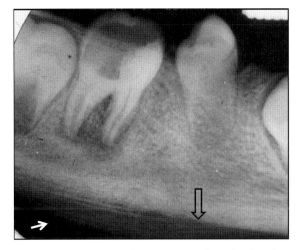

Figure 7.23   Periostitis (white arrow) at inferior border of mandible associated with endodontic infection at the apex of mandibular 1st molar of preadolescent patient. Note striated appearance of periosteal response. Open black arrow denotes original position of inferior border of mandible.

onion-like appearance. Periostitis is usually seen in an area of the jaw that approximates the site of endodontic infection. In many cases, a radiolucent path of communication can be seen between the site of the periostitis and the periapical lesion. Periostitis of the jaws caused by endodontic infection, like periostitis seen in association with bony cavities, is reversible when the infection responsible for its induction is adequately controlled. In the jaws,

however, a longer time is required for the change in surface contour to be fully resolved. It is important to relate this information to the patient when a clinically apparent periostitis is present, as they may think its clinical presentation is one of soft tissue origin and therefore reversible shortly after treatment has been rendered.

Cysts of endodontic origin

Residual epithelial cells called epithelial cell rests of Malassez, derived from Hertwig's epithelial root sheath, are normal cellular inclusions of the periodontium. These cells, once thought to be vestigial cells, have now been shown to play a role in periodontal maintenance and repair (Nanci, 2008). During inflammation of the periodontium, these cells can be stimulated to form sheets or clumps of epithelium within the inflammatory lesion (Figure 7.25). This, in turn, can lead to the development of a radicular cyst. Some cysts have a potential to enlarge at the expense of the bone and the inflammatory tissue within a lesion of endodontic origin and grow to an appreciable size. Cysts can develop in contact with the tooth root (bay cyst) or distant from it (true cyst). As they enlarge, they tend to do so symmetrically and hence produce a smooth peripheral contour when the lesion is imaged ragiographically. If expansion is slow, a bony cortex can develop along the periphery of the lesion (Figure 7.26A–C). As stated earlier, this is as a reactive response and is not of diagnostic significance.

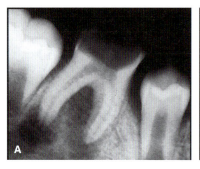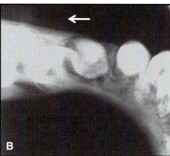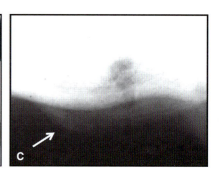

Figure 7.24   A. Lesion of endodontic origin present at apices of mandibular molar in preadolescent patient. B. Occlusal view showing periostitis on buccal aspect of mandible (arrow) of patient in Figure 7.24A. C. Lateral view showing periostitis on inferior border of mandible of patient in Figure 7.24A (arrow). Radiolucent area seen in middle of jaw was continuous with lesion present at root apices.

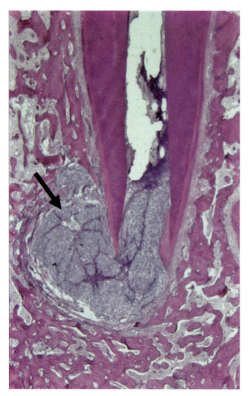

Figure 7.25   Lesion of endodontic origin demonstrating proliferating epithelium (Blue lines) and micro-cyst formation (arrow).

As seen radiographically, cysts can be corticated or noncorticated and are either large or small (Figure 7.27A,B). On average, however, they tend to be larger than noncystic inflammatory lesions of endodontic origin. Like large simple inflammatory lesions of endodontic origin, large cysts also have a potential to induce periostitis when they encroach upon the periosteum of a bone cavity or the surface of the jaw. Large cysts can predispose the jaw to pathological fracture especially if the patient is exposed to a traumatic event (Figure 7.28A,B). This places an onus on the clinician to ensure that the healing of a lesion by nonsurgical endodontic treatment is progressing favorably, before the patient is discharged from care. Cysts can also become infected (as depicted in Figure 7.28B). When this occurs, they lose their well-defined border and assume the clinical and radiographic characteristics of an acute inflammatory lesion. While most radicular cysts occur in association with the root apex, they have also been reported to occur in association with lateral canals. Though such reports are relatively rare in the literature, their presence at such sites would have to be accounted for when a treatment plan for the management of a lateral lesion is presented. Statistics appears to support the premise that some cysts can heal spontaneously after nonsurgical endodontic treatment. Others are known to persist until they are surgically removed. To date, no convincing evidence is available to explain this behavior although several theories have been offered. Subjectively, radiographic evidence appears to suggest that cysts that do resolve nonsurgically do so at a much slower rate than do noncystic inflammatory lesions (Figure 7.29A,B) and that the bone formed when they do heal is more irregular in appearance than the bone formed in the healing of noncystic inflammatory lesions (Figure 7.30A,B).

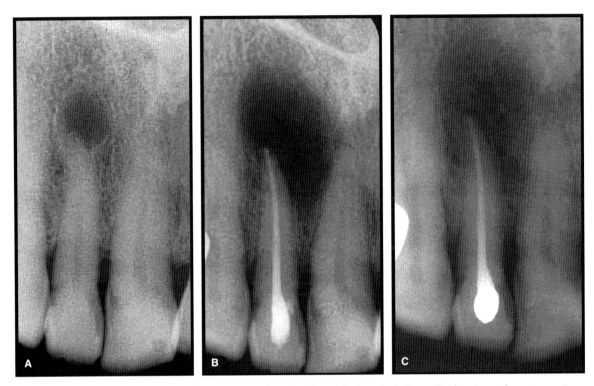

Figure 7.26   A. Corticated radiolucent lesion at apex of nonvital lateral incisor. B. Radiograph taken 6 months postoperative. Lesion was symptomatic and appears to have increased in size. Periphery of lesion is no longer corticated and appears diffuse in some areas. Apical curettage performed shortly afterward (cyst confirmed at biopsy). C. Radiograph taken 6 months after surgery.

Odontogenic keratocyst is a cyst that develops in the jaws from retained dental lamina. It can at times, mimic the appearance of a radicular cyst. While not initiated by endodontic disease, it has been found occasionally in association with teeth that manifest endodontic disease. Unlike a radicular cyst, a keratocyst tends to enlarge aggressively and can, on occasion, cause resorption on the roots of approximating teeth. They are not known to resolve spontaneously and have a high recurrence rate when they are not completely removed surgically.

Internal root resorption

Infection of the dental pulp can, on occasion, lead to the differentiation of monocytic cells, present in the inflammatory lesion into odontoclasts in much the same way that OC differentiate in a periapical endodontic lesion. Odontoclasts are identical to the OCs and behave in much the same manner when in contact with mineralized tissue. In normal pulp, there is a zone of unmineralized dentin, called predentin, at the pulp space periphery that is resistant to resorption. However, during pulp inflammation, some odontoblasts may be irreversibly injured, and this leads to localized unregulated mineralization of predentin at that site. This leaves this area of dentin vulnerable to resorption if monocytic cells and the signaling molecules that trigger their differentiation and activation into odontoclasts are present. In its early stages, internal resorption of the dentin may not be detectable in the radiograph (Vier and Figueiredo, 2002). Advanced internal resorption of dentin is, and appears as a progressive and localized radiolucent enlargement of the pulp space. If left unaddressed, it can quickly lead to a perforation of the root or crown surface (Figure 7.31). In the radiograph, the borders of the

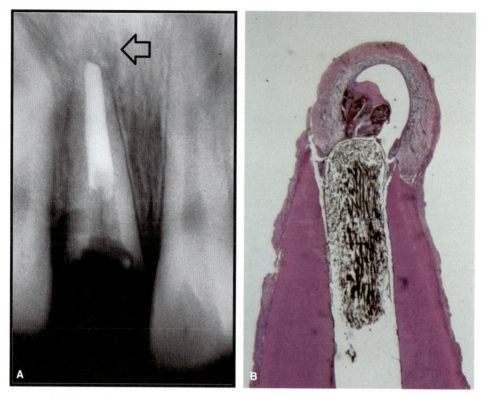

Figure 7.27 A. Small diffuse radiolucent lesion noted at apex of maxillary incisor traumatically fractured 4 years after endodontic treatment. Opacity present in lesion is unresorbed root canal cement. B. Small bay cyst noted at root apex after tooth in Figure 7.34A extracted and examined histologically.

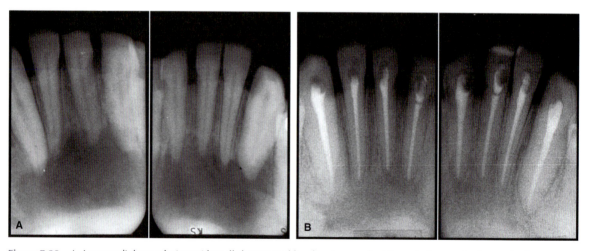

Figure 7.28 A. Large radiolucent lesion with well-demarcated borders (proven by biopsy to be a radicular cyst) of endodontic origin in anterior mandible. B. Healing in anterior mandible 1 year after endodontic treatment of mandiblar anterior teeth and surgical removal of cyst.

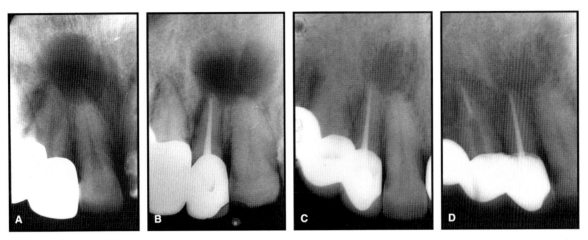

Figure 7.29 A. Corticated radiolucent lesion of endodontic origin associated with apex of lateral incisor and superimposed over apex of central incisor. B. Radiograph taken immediately after nonsurgical endodontic treatment of lateral incisor. C. Radiographs taken 2 years after nonsurgical endodontic treatment. Note irregular trabecular architecture as lesion heals from periphery to center. D. Radiograph taken 11 years after nonsurgical endodontic treatment. Note lesion has healed, but trabecular pattern is irregular as compared to normal bone of maxilla.

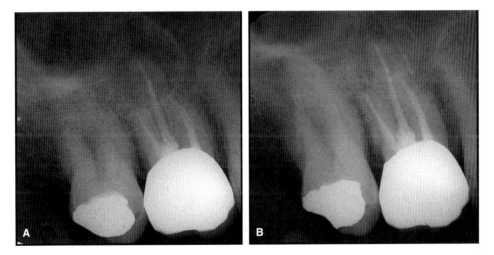

Figure 7.30 A. Radiograph of corticated radiolucent lesion of endodontic origin associated with maxillary 1st molar taken immediately after nonsurgical endodontic treatment. Lesion has induced a periostitis in floor of antrum. B. Radiograph taken 12 years after treatment. Time of healing was prolonged and healed site exhibits irregular trabecular pattern. Floor of antrum still appears elevated despite apparent resolution of cause.

resorbing dentin tend to appear relatively smooth, but histologically, they are highly irregular. Internal resorption can appear symmetrical or asymmetrical relative to its relationship with the pulp space, and can occur anywhere within its length. When internal resorption perforates the tooth surface at a site where there is periodontium, periodontitis can develop in much the same way as it does when a lateral canal is present (Figure 7.32A–C). Internal root resorption can be differentiated histologically from external root resorption (resorption initiated in the periodontium) by a persistence

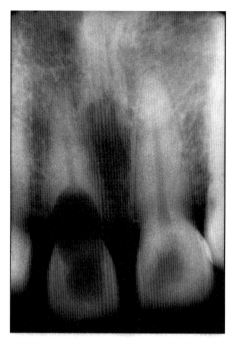

Figure 7.31 Internal resorption in pulp chamber of maxillary incisor. The prognosis for retaining this tooth by endodontic treatment was poor.

of predentin at the periphery of the pulp space when the pulp of the tooth is normal. In the radiograph, the preserved predentin appears as a thin radio-opaque line (relative to the more radiolucent pulp space) outlining the normal pulp space (Figure 7.33). The presence of this outline and the knowledge that internal resorption does not occur in the pulp of normal adult teeth is one means of differentiating between the two. Conversely, it can be assumed that when internal resorption is seen, the pulp is or has been inflamed. Endodontic treatment of teeth manifesting active internal resorption, that is, resorption detected prior to the development of pulp necrosis, should be initiated as soon as possible. This minimizes the degree of dentin loss and reduces the risk of root fracture. Once the pulp is necrotic, as evidenced by the presence of an apical lesion, resorption of dentin ceases, and the need for immediate treatment lessens. Resolution of periodontitis associated with perforating internal resorption can be expected to occur when the root canal infection is effectively controlled and the perforated site is adequately sealed.

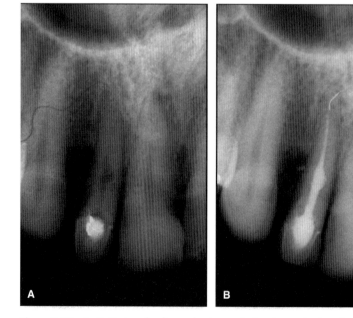
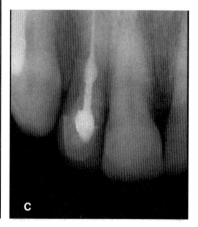

Figure 7.32 A.–C. Series of radiographs demonstrating internal resorption and attending lateral radiolucency associated with endodontic infection in maxillary lateral incisor. Lateral was treated endodontically. Note site of perforation as designated by extrusion of root canal sealer. Healing of lateral lesion 1 year after treatment.

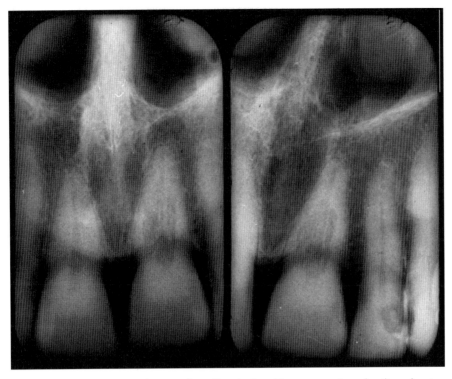

Figure 7.33 External resorption present on the root of maxillary incisor. Note preservation of outline of root canal in central part of radiolucency.

Summary

In the preceding sections of this chapter I have attempted to briefly relate the events and mechanisms that lead to the development of inflammatory lesions caused by infection of the dental pulp. How, why, and where they develop requires an understanding of dental anatomy, head and neck anatomy, and the alterations in normal bone physiology that develop in response to the presence of infection. Needless to say, a detailed discussion of all of these factors goes far beyond my ability and the intent of this chapter. However, by highlighting some of the major aspects of bacteria/host interaction, it has been possible to offer some insight into the radiographic changes that are seen in the jaws when endodontic infection is present. There was a time when only the presence of bone loss about the root of a tooth with an endodontic infection was defined as being an "endodontic lesion." Today, it is apparent the "endodontic lesion" is in actuality a product of all the infection-related changes that occur in the jaws. As such, it is reasonable to define the "endodontic lesion" in the radiograph as one that has both productive and destructive features, features that can be reversed when the infection responsible for their presence has been adequately controlled. This makes the radiograph an important tool not only in identifying and monitoring all the progressive changes that occur in the jaws when an endodontic infection is present, but also in monitoring their reversibility, to assure that a favorable outcome to treatment of the infection responsible for the changes has been realized.

The chapter would be incomplete without mention of the fact that the radiographic expression of endodontic disease can be mimicked by a variety of other odontogenic and nonodontogenic conditions that occur in the jaw and that the radiograph is just one of the diagnostic tools available to a clinician in search of a diagnosis. That is not said to minimize its value, but rather to emphasize that like all such tools, it has limitations that must be recognized by all who are to use it wisely. Finally, there has been hesitation by some clinicians to use the radiograph to its full potential in identifying disease. Radiography is, and will continue to be, one of the most important and widely used diagnostic tools in health care in the foreseeable future. Like most tools, it is potentially harmful to the patient when overused and equally harmful to the patient when underused. Its usefulness in identifying disease and in evaluating the outcome of treatment rendered in endodontics and in many other health-related conditions cannot be overstressed.

References

Bender, I.B. and Seltzer, S. (1961a) Roentgenographic and direct observation of experimental lesions in bone. *J Am Dent Assoc*, 62, 152–160.

Bender, I.B. and Seltzer, S. (1961b) Roentgenographic and direct observation of experimental lesions in bone. *J Am Dent Assoc*, 62, 708–716.

Boskey, A.L. and Coleman, R. (2010) Aging and bone. *J Dent Res*, 89, 1333–1348.

Brynolf, I. (1967) A histologic and roentgenographic study of the periapical region of human incisors. (Thesis). *Odont Revy*, 18(Suppl 2), 1–176.

Cochran, D.L. (2008) Inflammation and bone loss in periodontal disease. *J Periodontol*, 79(Suppl), 1569–1576.

Katagin, T. and Takahashi, N. (2002) Regulatory mechanisms of osteoblast and osteoclast differentiation. *Oral Dis*, 8, 147–159.

Laux, M. et al. (2000) Apical inflammatory root resorption: a correlative radiographic and histological study. *Int Endod J*, 33, 483–493.

Nanci, A. (2008) Periodontium. In: A. Nanci, ed., *Ten Cate's Oral Histology*, pp. 239–267. Mosby, St. Louis.

Stashenko, P., Teles, R.D., and D'Souza, R. (1998) Periapical inflammatory responses and their modulation. *Crit Rev Oral Biol Med*, 9, 498–521.

Tay, J.Y.Y. et al. (2004) Identification of RANKL in osteolytic lesions of the facial skeleton. *J Dent Res*, 83, 349–353.

Teng, Y.-T.A. (2006) Protective and destructive immunity in the periodontium: Part 2. T cell-mediated immunity in the periodontium. *J Dent Res*, 85, 209–219.

Torneck, C.D. and Tulananda, N. (1969) Reaction of bone and cementum to experimental abscess formation in the dog. *Oral Surg Oral Med Oral Pathol Oral Radiol Endod*, 25, 404–416.

Vier, F.V. and Figueiredo, J.A.P. (2002) Prevalence of different periapical lesions associated with human teeth and their correlation with the presence and extension of apical external root resorption. *Int Endod J*, 35, 710–719.

Wilson, A.G. (2008) Epigenetic regulation of gene expression in the inflammatory response and relevance to common diseases. *J Periodontol*, 79(Suppl), 1514–1519.

8 Image Interpretation of Periapical Abnormalities

Ernest W. N. Lam

General principles

Still more of an art than a science, image interpretation relies on both visual and cognitive skills that enable the clinician to make sense of a series of discrete observations.

After an image series and/or image volume is acquired, the images should be viewed under dimly lit conditions without interference from extraneous or ambient light, even when viewing on a computer monitor. The first step in this process is to determine if the region of interest represents an area of normal anatomy or pathosis. Indeed, the identification of normal radiographic appearances is the most elementary step in the interpretive process, requiring the clinician to have an appreciation for a broad range of normal appearances; the so-called range of normal.

Once an entity has been deemed not to be within this range of normal, the following features or characteristics should be assessed:

1. Number
2. Location(s)
3. Attenuation (radiolucent, radiopaque, mixed radiolucent/radiopaque)
4. Border Characteristics
5. Internal Structure
6. Effects on Surrounding Structures and
7. Associations and Effects on/with Adjacent Teeth.

It should be noted that feature identification is largely, but not always, imaging modality-independent. While one modality may be able to produce images that depict certain features better than another, should the clinician be incapable of either identifying the feature or understanding its biological context, the usefulness of even the most sophisticated image becomes questionable.

The use of a structured interpretation algorithm such as the one provided above may serve as a useful prompt, ensuring that radiographic features are systematically evaluated, and none are missed. The systematic evaluation of features may result in a more focused interpretation or diagnosis that "makes sense," in light of what is seen (Baghdady et al., 2009).

Endodontic Radiology, Second Edition. Edited by Bettina Basrani.
© 2012 John Wiley & Sons, Inc. Published 2012 by John Wiley & Sons, Inc.

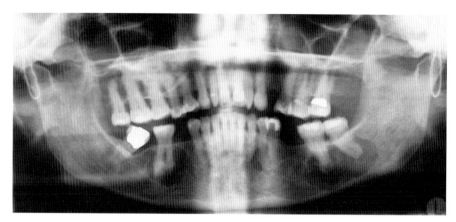

Figure 8.1 Florid osseous dysplasia with simple bone cysts. The panoramic image shows multiple, well-defined, delicately corticated, mixed radiolucent/radiopaque areas in the mandible and right maxilla. Note the central location of the areas of radiopacity within the larger radiolucent simple bone cysts in the mandibular right and left first molar areas.

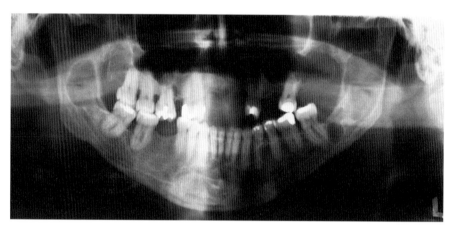

Figure 8.2 Keratocystic odontogenic tumors in nevoid basal cell carcinoma syndrome. The panoramic image shows four, well-defined, corticated, radiolucent entities in the mandibular rami, and left premolar and molar areas. The mandibular left ramus lesion demonstrates little anterior–posterior expansion.

Number

There are relatively few abnormalities that arise within the jaws with multiple areas of involvement. Unfortunately, endodontists, who may see only a small region of the jaws during their work, may be at a disadvantage, not being able to examine the jaws in their entirety. The appearances of multiple entities within the same image may reflect a bone dysplasia involving the jaws (Figure 8.1) or a disease with underlying systemic involvement that may require further investigation (Figure 8.2).

Location(s)

The geometric center of an abnormality may provide information about biological origin. Abnormalities that arise in positions coronal or pericoronal to the crowns of the teeth generally arise from odontogenic sources, as are abnormalities that arise along tooth root surfaces. Abnormalities with centers located at or minimally apical to the root apex may be odontogenic in origin (Figure 8.3), as well as nonodontogenic (Figure 8.4). And should an abnormality develop with location well-apical

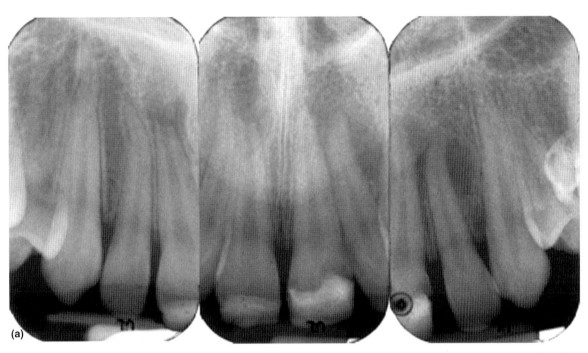

Figure 8.3   Rarefying osteitis, anterior maxillae. (a) Periapical images and small field cone beam CT reconstructions through the (b) (on next page) maxillary right and (c) (on next page) left permanent central incisors show well-defined, corticated, "hydraulic" radiolucent/low-attenuation abnormalities. On the right side, the abnormality is associated with the root apex of the externally resorbed central incisor. On the left side, the abnormality encompasses the roots of the central and lateral incisors. The reconstruction through the maxillary left lateral incisor (lower right) shows the abnormality to overlay the buccal root of the tooth with a portion of the buccal periodontal ligament space intact.

to the tooth root, these are generally nonodontogenic in origin.

Attenuation (radiolucent, radiopaque, mixed radiolucent/radiopaque)

The terms radiolucent and radiopaque are relative terms that describe the attenuation or absorption characteristics of a tissue to radiation. Radiolucent entities have not attenuated radiation to any significant degree, whereas radiopaque entities have.

The terms radiolucent and radiopaque are said to be relative because object radiolucency or radiopacity are dependent on what other tissues are located adjacent to the object or area/volume of interest. Among the tissues or materials that may appear on dental images (Figure 8.5), metal, whether in the form of a dental material or foreign body, is always the most radiopaque entity on any image. This is followed by radiopaque restorative

materials and cements, and then by tooth-related tissues, enamel, dentin, and cementum. Cortical bone and trabeculae within the cancellous bone are next on this hierarchy, followed by calculus. Nearest the bottom of the list are the soft tissues, including mucosa and cartilage, body fluids, and radiolucent composite restorative materials and cements. At the very bottom of this hierarchy are fat and air. Both are radiolucent, relative to other tissue.

Border characteristics

Definition of border periphery reflects the growth behavior of an abnormality: slow or fast growing, indolent or aggressive. The terms well-defined, moderately well-defined, poorly or ill-defined are used to describe these peripheries. Imagine trying to outline the periphery of an abnormality with a pencil or pen. If the majority of an abnormality's

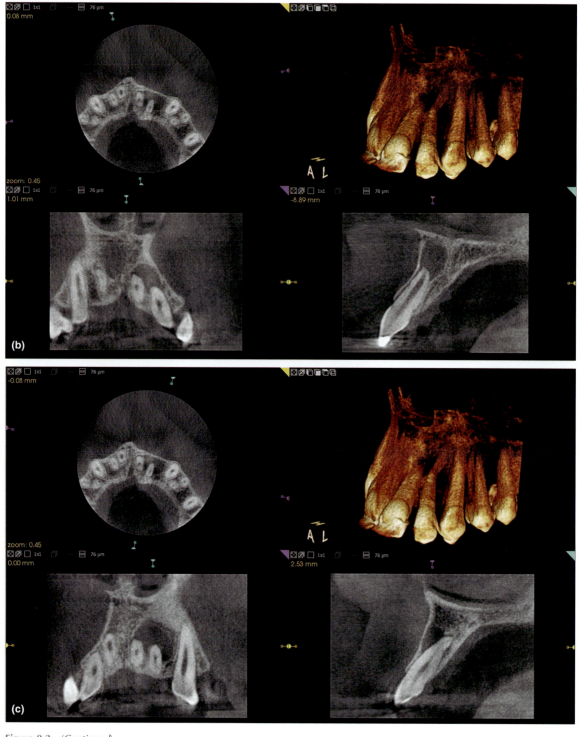

Figure 8.3 *(Continued)*

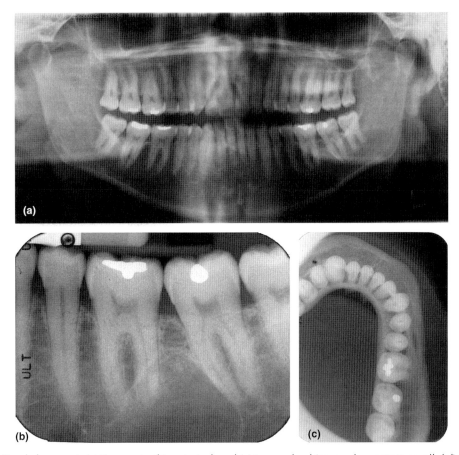

Figure 8.4 Simple bone cyst. (a) Panoramic, (b) periapical, and (c) true occlusal images demonstrate a well-defined, delicately corticated, "hydraulic," unilocular radiolucency situated in the mandibular left molar area extending from the mid-root levels of the molar teeth to the inferior cortex. The abnormality encroaches on the inferior and buccal cortices of the mandible in this area, but the periodontal ligament space and lamina dura of the first molar roots are undisturbed.

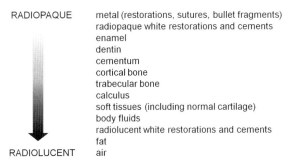

RADIOPAQUE	metal (restorations, sutures, bullet fragments)
	radiopaque white restorations and cements
	enamel
	dentin
	cementum
	cortical bone
	trabecular bone
	calculus
	soft tissues (including normal cartilage)
	body fluids
	radiolucent white restorations and cements
	fat
RADIOLUCENT	air

Figure 8.5 Relative radiopacities and radiolucencies of materials and tissues appearing on dental radiographs.

periphery is easily traced and definable, the abnormality likely has a well-defined periphery (Figure 8.6). For abnormalities where a substantial portion or majority of the periphery is easily definable, this periphery is likely moderately well-defined. For entities where the abnormality's edge is difficult to ascertain in a majority of locations, the abnormality likely has a poorly defined periphery (Figure 8.7). Lesions that have well-defined or moderately well-defined borders tend to show a slower, more indolent, or controlled pattern of growth. As such, the surrounding bone is better able to contain the abnormality as it grows. Abnormalities with more poorly defined peripheries tend to have a faster, more uncontrolled pattern of growth. These abnormalities may also be more aggressive in nature.

The presence or absence of a bone cortex encircling an abnormality may also indicate biological indolence or aggression. A cortex is a discrete radiopaque line that scribes the edge or border of an abnormality (Figure 8.6). Some have used the word "sclerotic" to describe this feature; however, the term sclerosis from which the term sclerotic is derived, refers to a diffuse area of radiopacity in bone (Figure 8.8), commonly associated with inflammation. The transition between a cortex and an adjacent area of cancellous bone is both sharp and discrete. In contrast, the transition between an area of sclerosis and adjacent cancellous bone is more gradual, with the periphery of the sclerotic reaction blending into the surrounding adjacent cancellous bone. Therefore, peripheral cortication and peripheral sclerosis are terms that should not be used synonymously as both reflect different biological processes. Like a well-defined border, the presence of a cortex infers that an abnormality is growing slowly, indolently, and at a more controlled rate.

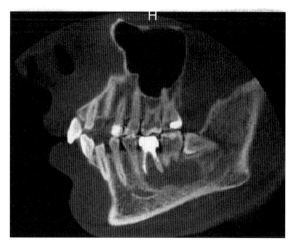

Figure 8.8   Secondarily infected keratocystic odontogenic tumor. The oblique sagittal reconstruction of the mandibular left body derived from a cone beam CT volume shows a moderately well-defined, elliptical low-attenuation area extending from the first molar roots to the region of the impacted third molar. Note the loss of definition of the trabecular bone pattern around the abnormality, and the presence of diffuse radiopaque area extending primarily mesially and inferiorly from the edge of the abnormality.

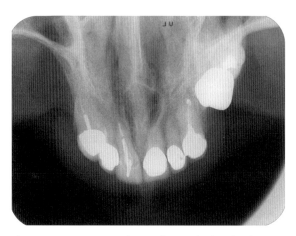

Figure 8.6   Incisive canal cyst. The standard occlusal image shows a well-defined, corticated, "hydraulic," radiolucent abnormality located in the anterior maxillae. The periodontal ligament space and the lamina dura of the maxillary left central incisor are undisturbed.

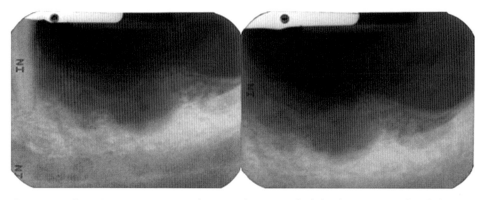

Figure 8.7   Squamous cell carcinoma. Two periapical images show a poorly defined, noncorticated, radiolucent surface abnormality that has produced nonuniform destruction of the crest of the alveolar process of the mandible.

The periphery of an abnormality can also take on other features, depending on the local effects the abnormality has on adjacent soft tissues such as periosteum. Should an abnormality have the capacity to stimulate the proliferation of the adjacent periosteum overlying a nearby bone cortex, lamellar, or more exuberant hair-on-end, starburst or sunray appearances can also be generated at bone peripheries. For example, when an intrabony inflammatory reaction reaches a cortical boundary, the overlying surface periosteum may be mechani-cally stripped, and then elevated from the surface of the bone cortex. Osteoprogenitor cells located on the endosteal surface of the periosteum may be stimulated to differentiate and deposit new bone matrix on the deep surface of the displaced periosteum. Should there be no resolution of the inflammatory reaction, and it is permitted to continue, additional layers of new bone may develop. Such a response is often referred to as a lamellar or "onion skin" type of response (Figure 8.9). More intense stimulation of the periosteum may occur

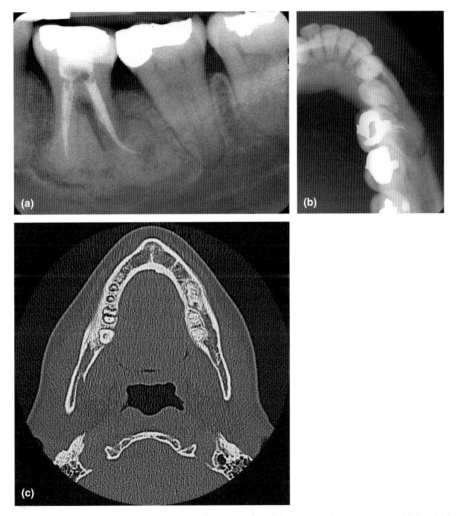

Figure 8.9 Florid osseous dysplasia and osteomyelitis. (a) Periapical and (b) true occlusal images and (c) axial bone window medical CT image show moderately well-defined, mixed radiolucent/radiopaque areas located at the apices of the mandibular left first molar teeth. Surrounding the central areas of radiopacity are thin, radiolucent rims, and these, in turn are surrounded by radiopaque lines. The true occlusal and medical CT images show a lamellar bone pattern located adjacent to the buccal cortex of the mandible in this area. At least three radiopaque layers of periosteal new bone are seen on the higher resolution occlusal image.

with other disease processes such as blood dyscrasias or intrabony osteoblastic metastases. In these instances, the appearance of a "hair-on-end" or sunray type of new bone formation may be seen at a bone border (Figure 8.10).

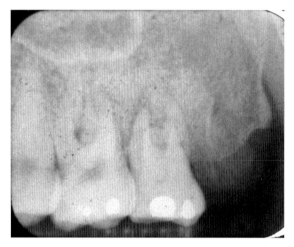

Figure 8.10 Osteosarcoma. The periapical image of the left posterior maxilla shows a poorly defined, primarily radiopaque area of abnormal bone pattern located in the molar and tubersity areas. Note the bone spicules radiating in an occlusal direction, distal to the second molar. As well, the lamina dura of the molars have been lost, and there is widening of the periodontal ligament spaces around the roots; Garrington's sign.

Internal structure

The cells within some abnormalities have the capacity to produce a mineralized matrix of bone, bone-like, tooth, or tooth-like material. The deposition of such material may impart a mixed radiolucent/radiopaque appearance on images. Where the X-ray beam passes through these mineralized deposits, there is attenuation of the beam by these materials such that focal areas of radiopacity may be visualized (Figure 8.11).

For some abnormalities, deposition can be diffuse, dispersed over an initially small area or volume. With time, separate smaller areas may begin to coalesce, forming larger "clumps" of radiopacity (Figure 8.12). For other abnormalities, the mineralization is very discrete and appears to have a high degree of organization. To the extent that enough of the normal bone pattern is removed, disturbed, or replaced, and depending on what other tissues are mixed into the bone matrix, the bone may take on an appearance that is more radiolucent than cortical bone, but more radiopaque than cancellous bone.

Internal structure may also occur in the form of septation or in regions of entrapped remnant bone. Such abnormalities do not, however, have the capacity to lay down a mineralized matrix. Therefore, the presence of septae should not be misinter-

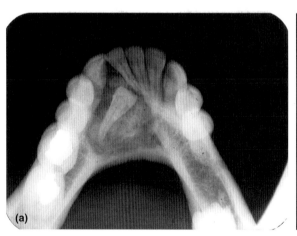
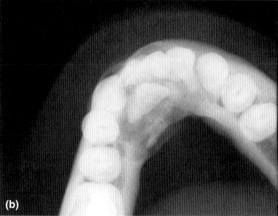

(a)   (b)

Figure 8.11 Ossifying fibroma. (a) The anterior occlusal image of the mandible shows a poorly-to-moderately well-defined, mixed radiolucent/radiopaque area in the anterior mandible associated with the impacted mandibular right permanent lateral incisor. Note the almost cotton wool-like deposition of mineralized matrix centrally within the abnormality, and the broad radiolucent rim more peripherally. The concentric growth pattern of the abnormality (b) is consistent with the interpretation of a benign tumor.

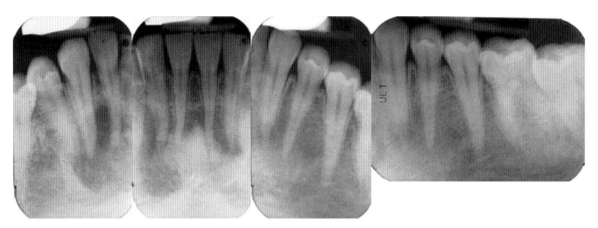

Figure 8.12 Periapical osseous dysplasia. The periapical images of the mandibular anterior and left premolar teeth show a moderately well-defined, mixed radiolucent/radiopaque area located at the periapices of the anterior teeth. The central radiopaque focus is surrounded by a thick, radiolucent boundary, and this in turn, is surrounded by a variably thick radiopaque line. Note that the periodontal ligament spaces around the apices of the central incisor teeth are intact.

preted to convey the mixed radiolucent/radiopaque quality of other abnormalities that have the capacity to lay down a mineralized matrix.

Effects on surrounding structures

Some abnormalities may grow to a size where they begin to impinge on the positions of normal anatomic structures like the teeth and their supporting structures or anatomical boundaries.

When an abnormality arises near a bone boundary, there may be displacement of these cortices (Figure 8.13). In the case of the maxillary sinus or nasal fossa, displacement of these cortices may result in a loss of air volume within these cavities. Lesions that have a faster, more aggressive growth pattern may introduce discontinuities in bone boundaries should the growth of the abnormality overtake the ability of osteoblasts to maintain the integrity of the boundary.

Benign, space-occupying abnormalities have a tendency to displace the teeth as well as the bone boundaries. Where space-occupying abnormalities disturb the positions of the teeth or impact on their supporting structures, there can also be both displacement and directional external resorption of the teeth (Figure 8.14). In this process, clast-like cells located at the expanding front of an abnor-

mality slowly begin to resorb tooth material. While patients may develop gross asymmetries due to the enlarging abnormality, changes may also occur to the dental occlusion, and there may be loss of normal interproximal tooth contacts.

Associations and effects on/with adjacent teeth

The appearance of an abnormality having an association with the apex of a tooth and/or its supporting structures may indicate derivation of the abnormality from an odontogenic source. Unfortunately, such an association may be difficult to ascertain on a single two-dimensional image, such as a periapical image. Additional images (a second periapical image or an occlusal image) and a cone beam computed tomography (CT) volume may be required to demonstrate the association (or nonassociation) (Figure 8.13). Abnormalities that arise within the periodontal ligament space in close association with the root of the tooth or arise with an attachment to a tooth are more likely to be of odontogenic origin. Entities that arise outside of the ligament space are nonodontogenic in origin.

Malignant lesions that invade or metastasize to the bone may grow around the teeth, leaving them

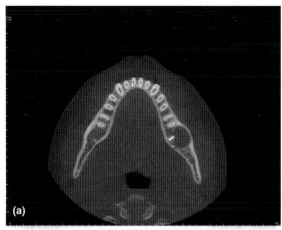

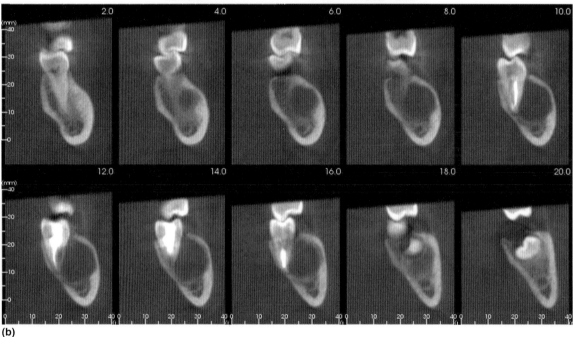

Figure 8.13 Buccal bifurcation cyst. (a) Axial and (b) cross-sectional/buccal-lingual cone beam CT reconstruction through the mandible show a well-defined, corticated, "hydraulic" low-attenuation abnormality associated with the buccal root surface of the endodontically treated mandibular right second molar. Note the expansion of the mandible in this area and the thinning of the buccal cortex. The root apices of the molar tooth have been displaced significantly into the lingual cortex of the mandible.

appearing as if to be "standing in space". Although not a common feature, some sarcomas have the capacity to externally resorb tooth roots. Malignant cells may also infiltrate the periodontal ligament space around a tooth, resulting in a generalized widening of the ligament space (Figure 8.10).

Periapical pathoses

At best, the terms "periapical pathosis" or "periapical radiolucency" are descriptive; they are non-specific and are certainly not diagnostic. Such terms simply identify the existence of a pathologic

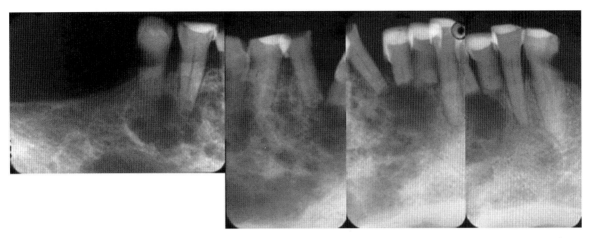

Figure 8.14 Ameloblastoma. Periapical images of the anterior and right premolar area of the mandible show a moderately well-defined, multilocular, radiolucent area associated with the root apices of the incisor and premolar teeth. Note the small, curvilinear septations separating out individual small radiolucent tumor nests and the prominent external resorption of the teeth.

entity at the periapices of one or more teeth. Indeed, there are numerous radiolucent (and radiopaque and mixed radiolucent/radiopaque) pathoses that may occur at the periapices of teeth, the majority of which have nothing whatsoever to do with the status of the dental pulp. Other terms such as "endodontic lesion" or "lesion of endodontic origin" are completely meaningless diagnostically and should not be used at all as radiographic descriptors. In this next section, we will address some of the more common abnormalities that may occur at the apices of teeth that may be of particular importance and concern to the endodontist.

Chronic apical periodontitis/ rarefying osteitis

Chronic apical periodontitis and rarefying osteitis are localized inflammatory responses of bone that may manifest in the apical periodontal ligament space (chronic apical periodontitis) and destroy periapical bone (rarefying osteitis), commonly the result of pulpal necrosis or periodontal disease.

When rarefying osteitis is identified radiographically at the apex of a tooth with a nonvital pulp, the term is used to refer to one of three distinct histopathologic entities that cannot be distinguished radiographically: (peri)radicular abscess,

granuloma, or cyst. Histopathologically, the cavity of the last of these entities, the radicular cyst, is lined with odontogenic epithelium derived from Hertwig's epithelial root sheath (Neville et al., 2009).

The radiographic interpretation of rarefying osteitis relies on the identification of a localized increase in the width of the periodontal ligament space and early loss of bone, typically at the apex of a tooth root, with a geometric center at or apical to the apex of the root. In the earliest stages of this process, periodontal ligament space widening may be subtle and very localized (Figure 8.15). With time, there may be more obvious displacement or loss of definition of the lamina dura away from the root apex (Figure 8.3a). As the entity enlarges, the radiographic appearance becomes that of a moderately well-defined to well-defined, variably corticated, circular radiolucent abnormality, with the lamina dura of the tooth root ultimately becoming the corticated periphery (Figure 8.3b,c). The near-uniform multidirectional pattern of enlargement of this abnormality has been described as being "hydraulic." At the periphery of such inflammatory abnormalities, a sclerotic bone reaction may encircle the borders of the abnormality where there is osteoblastic deposition of additional bone (e.g., sclerosing osteitis). Rarefying osteitis may also be associated with external resorption of the involved

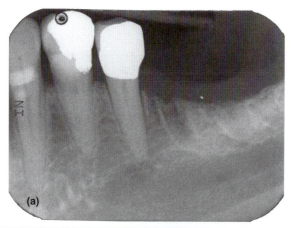

(a)

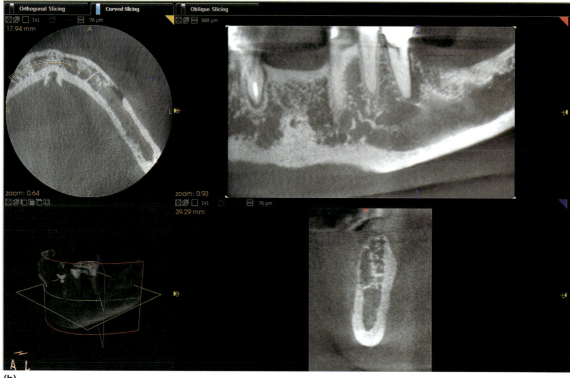

(b)

Figure 8.15 Rarefying osteitis. (a) Periapical image and (b) small field cone beam CT image of the same region of the mandibular left premolar area. The patient presents with a parulis located on the distolingual root surface of the second premolar. Although the periapical image shows a loss of definition to the lamina dura along the distal root surface of the tooth, no discrete radiolucent area is seen. The 1-mm thick cone beam reconstruction through this area shows loss of lamina dura and a pararadicular low-attenuation region extending down the distal surface of the premolar to the apex.

tooth root, or of adjacent tooth roots, depending on the size and extent of the lesion.

Intraoral periapical and occlusal radiography are the best methods of imaging rarefying osteitis, and in some cases, these images may be supplemented with a small field cone beam CT study should the periapical images fail to allow definitive interpretation or when the abnormality grows very large in size or volume.

Simple bone cyst

The simple cyst is known by a myriad of other terms such as hemorrhagic, idiopathic, or traumatic bone cyst or cavity. The simple bone cyst is a pseudocyst and lacks any epithelial lining. In some instances, small amounts of fibrous connective tissue may be found within the bone cavity, and this may be accompanied by a small amount of fluid.

The etiology of the simple bone cyst is unknown. Three etiopathogeneses have been postulated (Harnet et al., 2008; Shimoyama et al., 1999). The first hypothesis relates to local imbalances in osteoblast and osteoclast activities during growth and development. A second hypothesis relates the development of the cavity to a tumor that has undergone liquefactive degeneration. Both these hypotheses infer that the osteoblastic component of the bone has failed to repair the defect produced by the osteoclasts or the tumor. A third hypothesis suggests that the bone cavity develops as a result of a microtraumatic or traumatic event that has failed to induce a fracture but has produced bone ischemia and aseptic necrosis. In the majority of instances, no tumors have been identified, and traumas have not been documented. Interestingly, simple bone cysts may also arise in the long bones (Lokiec and Wientroub, 1998). Here, they can be associated with considerable pain, the result of pathological fracture. In the jaws, simple bone cysts are often found incidentally on images made for other purposes. And unlike the long bones, large simple bone cysts in the jaws are not known to induce fracture or be associated with pain.

Simple bone cysts are unilocular radiolucent entities in bone that have one of the most delicately corticated peripheries of almost any abnormality arising in the jaws (Figure 8.4). They are well

defined, and may occur in almost any location in the jaws. As the simple bone cyst enlarges and encroaches on the dentition, the superior border of the cavity can scallop around the roots of the teeth, leaving the periodontal ligament spaces and lamina dura undisturbed. When simple bone cysts arise near the follicles of developing teeth, the follicular cortices also remain undisturbed. Such features demonstrate the indolent nature of simple bone cysts and help differentiate these entities from other more aggressively growing radiolucent abnormalities in the jaws that can affect the dental and peridental structures more significantly (Chadwick et al., 2011).

Intraoral periapical and occlusal radiography, as well as panoramic imaging, are the recommended imaging modalities for simple bone cysts. Should the cavity be large or if expansion of the bone is seen, small field cone beam CT may be useful to characterize the extent of the cavity.

Buccal bifurcation cyst

The buccal bifurcation cyst is found mostly in young children and adolescents, and is often associated with a partially erupted permanent molar. The development of the cyst impedes eruption of the molar, and displaces the roots of the tooth toward the lingual cortex of bone, a classic feature (Pompura et al., 1997). The lining of the cyst is believed to be derived from the epithelial cell rests of Malassez, and as such, inflammation has been proposed as a possible pathogenesis. There is, however, no evidence to support this hypothesis.

The buccal bifurcation cyst is a well-defined, corticated, unilocular, radiolucent entity with a geometric center located within or at least at the level of the furcation of multirooted teeth. The rather unique position of the cyst in the buccal furcation, and the displacement of the tooth roots toward the lingual cortex are hallmarks of this entity (Figures 8.13 and 8.16).

Intraoral periapical radiography should appropriately demonstrate the location of the cyst relative to the tooth furcation, and a true occlusal image (Figure 8.16b) of the tooth will demonstrate the buccal expansion of the bone as well as the displacement of the roots toward the lingual cortex.

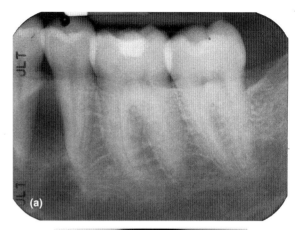

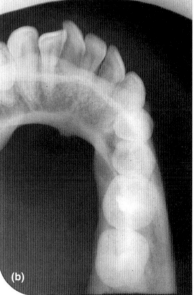

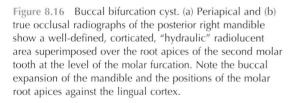

Figure 8.16 Buccal bifurcation cyst. (a) Periapical and (b) true occlusal radiographs of the posterior right mandible show a well-defined, corticated, "hydraulic" radiolucent area superimposed over the root apices of the second molar tooth at the level of the molar furcation. Note the buccal expansion of the mandible and the positions of the molar root apices against the lingual cortex.

Figure 8.17 Lateral periodontal cyst. (a) Periapical and (b) true occlusal images show a bilocular, well-defined, corticated, radiolucent, "hydraulic" abnormality located between the roots of the mandibular premolars. The periodontal ligament spaces along the adjacent root surfaces appear intact, and the lamina dura along the mesial surface of the second premolar is intact. The occlusal image shows encroachment on the lingual cortex.

Lateral periodontal cyst

The epithelial lining of the lateral periodontal cyst is believed to arise from the vepithelial cell rests of Malassez located alongside the lateral aspects of the premolar tooth roots. Indeed, this is the most common place for their occurrence (Suljak et al., 1998).

The lateral periodontal cyst may be unilocular or multilocular (botryoid) (Figure 8.17). The cysts are small, with well-defined, corticated peripheries, and they are radiolucent. Circular in appearance, the lateral periodontal cyst arises along the mesial or lateral root surfaces of teeth. There may be disruption of the lamina dura of the tooth root, and if large enough, may cause tooth displacement.

As these lesions are typically very small in size, a periapical image together with a true occlusal image of the area should suffice.

Incisive canal cyst

The incisive canal cyst arises near the maxillary midline, palatal in a position palatal to the maxillary incisors (Figure 8.6). Although the cavity is continuous with the midline incisive canal, it may sometimes be difficult to demonstrate this association using conventional two-dimensional imaging. The normal incisive canal can attain horizontal widths of up to 10mm, and it is generally accepted that the width becomes abnormal when it attains a horizontal dimension greater than 10mm. Interestingly, the incisive canal cyst epithelium is derived from respiratory epithelium which is a pseudostratified columnar, ciliated epithelium.

Radiographically, the incisive canal cyst is a well-defined, variably corticated, radiolucent, "hydraulic" entity superimposed over the roots of the maxillary central incisors. The periodontal ligament spaces and lamina dura of the incisors should appear intact and undisturbed by the radiolucent cyst.

An anterior or standard occlusal image of the maxillae, supplemented with periapical images, should suffice for imaging and diagnosis. Should significant palatal expansion be noted clinically, or should the cavity not appear in the midline, a limited or small field cone beam CT of the anterior maxillae may be helpful to develop an interpretation (Figure 8.18).

Central giant cell lesion

There is some controversy related to the pathogenesis of the central giant cell lesion. Some believe the lesion to be a benign neoplasm (i.e., central giant cell tumor), while others believe the lesion to be reactive in nature.

Central giant cell lesions occur typically in younger individuals, mesial to the maxillary canines or the mandibular first permanent molars. These abnormalities demonstrate well-defined peripheries with delicate cortices. Internally, they exhibit a delicate, wispy, lace-like network of septation (Figure 8.19), many of which may be straight, extending toward the radiolucent center from the periphery at 90 degrees. Larger lesions may produce considerable expansion of the bone, displace teeth, and induce external resorption of the tooth roots.

Intraoral periapical and occlusal images are useful for visualizing intralesional septation. A panoramic image may also be useful to demonstrate the extent of the lesion, unless the lesion is located in the anterior maxillae or mandible. Given the soft tissue nature of the lesion, cone beam CT is not advised for this lesion. Rather, medical CT should be used to demonstrate involvement of adjacent soft tissues should a fenestration or discontinuity of a bone border be revealed on intraoral images.

Giant cell lesions can arise as solitary entities within the jaws, be associated with hyperparathyroidism (brown tumors) or craniofacial anomalies such as cherubism or Noonan's syndrome. Treatment of these lesions has included direct intralesional injections of corticosteroids or calcitonin (Suárez-Roa Mde et al., 2009).

Keratocystic odontogenic tumor

Recently, the World Health Organization (2005) reclassified the odontogenic keratocyst as an odontogenic tumor because of its aggressive clinical growth, the propensity of the basal cell layer of the epithelial lining to undergo "budding," and the identification of mutations of a tumor suppressor gene, the *PATCH* (*PTCH*) gene (Madras and Lapointe, 2008). The reclassification also resulted in a name change to keratocystic odontogenic tumor.

Keratocystic odontogenic tumors may occur in a variety of locations in and around teeth, or be associated with the crowns of unerupted teeth, mimicking the appearances of a dentigerous cyst. Because of the epithelium's ability to undergo budding, some keratocystic odontogenic tumors may take on a multilocular appearance, mimicking other odontogenic tumors such as ameloblastoma.

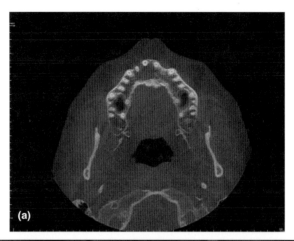

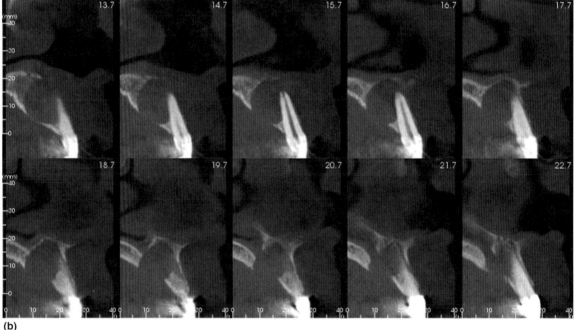

Figure 8.18 Incisive canal cyst. (a) Axial and (b) cross-sectional buccal/palatal reconstructions through the anterior maxilla. The images show a well-defined, variably corticated, low-attenuation, "hydraulic" entity situated in the anterior and anterior right maxilla that is continuous with the incisive canal (cross-sectional images 20.7 to 22.7).

Keratocystic odontogenic tumors are well-defined, variably corticated, radiolucent entities. In the posterior mandible, when they involve the anterior border of the ramus, there may be fenestration or loss of this or other bone cortices. The mandibular canal may be displaced. There is a strong tendency for these abnormalities to tunnel or grow through the bone, producing relatively little buccal/lingual expansion relative to the mesial/distal dimension of the abnormality; this is a hallmark growth pattern of keratocystic odontogenic tumors (Figure 8.20). Those keratocystic odontogenic tumors that develop in the maxilla and encroach on the maxillary sinus may display

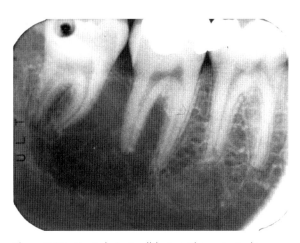

Figure 8.19 Central giant cell lesion. The periapical image shows a moderately well-defined, delicately corticated, radiolucent area superimposed over the roots of the mandibular right second and third molars. Internally, there are several delicate, lace-like septae. Definition of the lamina dura and periodontal ligament space around the distal root of the first molar has been lost, and there has been subtle external resorption of the second molar distal root.

a more classical cyst-like pattern of growth. In these instances, they may take on a more hydraulic shape, displacing the floor of the maxillary sinus superiorly as the abnormality enlarges.

Multiple keratocystic odontogenic tumors may arise in nevoid basal cell carcinoma or Gorlin–Goltz syndrome (Figure 8.2). The syndrome may be accompanied by other stigmata including the development of multiple basal cell carcinomas of the skin, bifid ribs, palmar and plantar pitting, benign dermal cysts, and ectopic falx calcification. Indeed, should a keratocystic odontogenic tumor be identified in a young individual, three-dimensional imaging may be useful for identifying other lesions in the jaws, and a referral should be made to the patient's physician, or to a medical geneticist so that other stigmata of the syndrome and *PTCH* mutations can be identified.

Panoramic and intraoral periapical and occlusal radiography should be used to first characterize the extent of the lesion in the jaws and teeth. Because of the potential involvement that larger lesions may have with the adjacent soft tissues

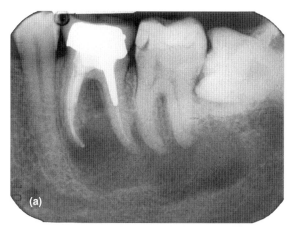

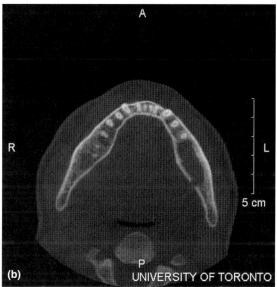

Figure 8.20 Secondarily infected keratocystic odontogenic tumor. (a) Periapical image, (b) axial, and (c) cross-sectional buccal/lingual cone beam CT reconstructions of the mandibular left molar area show a well-defined, variably corticated, radiolucent/low-attenuation area located apical to the molar teeth. Note the elongated growth pattern of the abnormality. While there has been thinning of the buccal and lingual cortices of the mandible, there has been no appreciable buccal/lingual expansion of the bone in spite of the sizable mesial/distal dimension.

should they grow beyond bone borders, cone beam CT should not be used. Rather, medical CT is advised for such lesions. Advanced imaging is also suggested for follow-up of the jaw lesions (Lam et al., 2009).

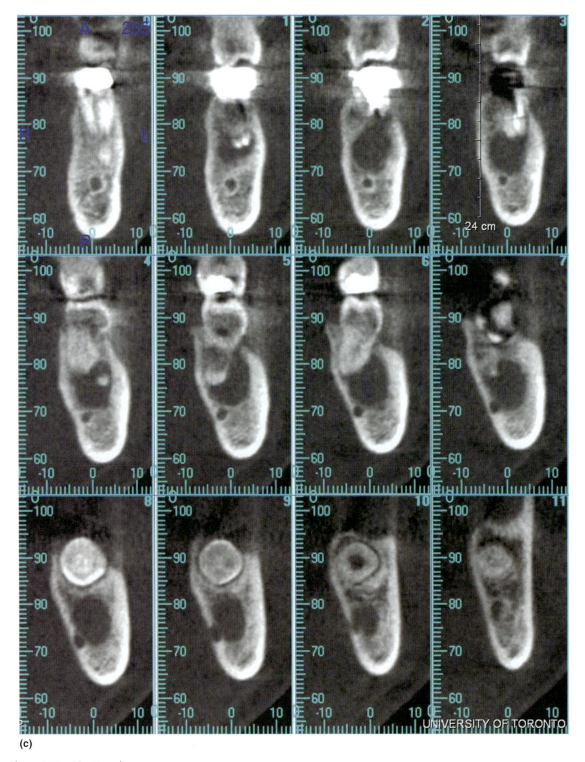

(c)

Figure 8.20   (Continued)

Ameloblastoma

The ameloblastoma is a benign odontogenic tumor arising from the neoplastic proliferation of odontogenic epithelium without ectomesenchyme. In these tumors, the microenvironment may dictate tumor cell phenotypes, and this may be reflected radiographically as differences in regional growth patterns of individual groups or nests of cells within the larger tumor. In general, ameloblastomas have well-defined, but variably corticated peripheries. They are radiolucent and do not have the hydraulic expansile characteristics that are seen in most cysts or cyst-like entities. Ameloblastoma can produce significant expansion of the bone with displacement of adjacent anatomical structures, and significant displacement and directional external resorption of the teeth.

Worth (1963) described four radiographic patterns of ameloblastoma, all of which could potentially be seen within the same lesion: unilocular, unilocular with coarse trabeculae, multilocular, and honeycomb (Figures 8.14 and 8.21). The subdivision of the tumor into smaller, possibly phenotypically distinct cellular subpopulations creates the appearance of remnant bone between these populations (septation). In ameloblastoma, the presence of septation and, in particular, curvilinear septation within a larger cavity to produce partial or complete loculation, greatly adds to the possibility of ameloblastoma. Moreover, where there is more aggressive growth of the lesion, there may be loss of a bone border. This is a particularly important feature to assess in the retromolar alveolar crest area or anterior border of the ramus.

Given the extensive nature of the soft tissue tumor mass and the possible extension of the soft tissue mass into adjacent soft tissues (Figure 8.22), medical CT or magnetic resonance imaging (MRI) are the modalities of choice for characterizing this lesion. Cone beam CT, due to its current limitation of not being able to depict soft tissues, should not be used as any soft tissue extension of the ameloblastoma will not be appreciated. The failure to characterize tumor extension into the adjacent soft tissue planes increases patient morbidity and results in mismanagement.

Hematogenous abnormalities

The hematogenous abnormalities are a group of diseases that arise from blood-forming cells. These include lymphoma, leukemia, Langerhan cell histiocytosis (formerly histiocytosis X), and multiple myeloma.

The first two of these diseases, lymphoma and leukemia, are blood-borne malignancies that are

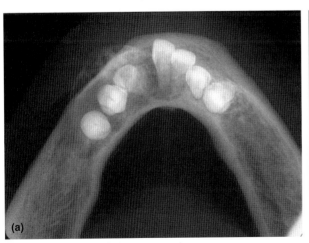
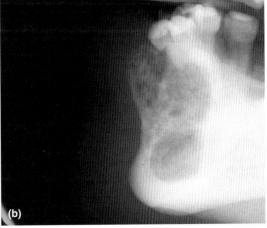

Figure 8.21 Ameloblastoma. (a) True occlusal and (b) occlusal-on-a-stick images of the anterior mandible show a well-defined, multilocular abnormality. Note the pattern of small radiolucencies within the abnormality and the curvilinear septations. Both images also demonstrate the expansile nature of the abnormality.

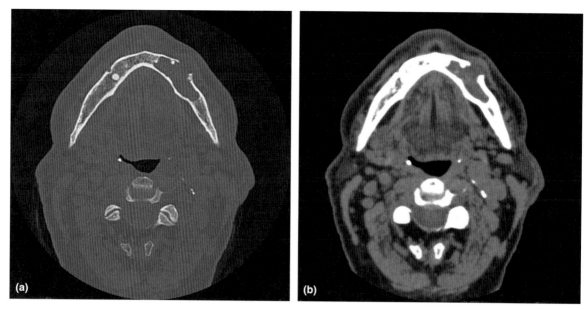

Figure 8.22   Ameloblastoma. (a) Bone and (b) soft tissue window medical CT images show a well-defined, corticated, low-attenuation abnormality in the mandibular left premolar area. The images show spill-through of the soft tissue tumor mass into fat and platysma muscle overlying the buccal surface of the mandible.

characterized by an infiltrative pattern of piece-meal bone destruction as small groups of cells begin populating marrow spaces within the bone. As this population of cells begins to proliferate, there is gradual enlargement of the marrow spaces and a concomitant loss of the normal trabecular bone pattern. With time, the appearance of multiple, poorly defined radiolucencies appear within the bone. In Langerhan cell histiocytosis, a similar pattern of destruction can also be seen. In this disease, cell proliferation may progress to a point where bone support surrounding the teeth is all but lost, and the teeth have the appearance of "floating in space". In reality, though, the teeth are suspended within a large soft tissue mass.

Multiple myeloma, another blood-borne malignancy, is characterized by larger, more well-defined circular radiolucencies within the bone. The circular appearance of individual entities in the bone has been described as "punched out" (Figure 8.23). When these small radiolucencies encroach on an adjacent cortex, they may produce small "cookie bites" out of the cortex.

Intraoral, panoramic, and skull views are easily made of patients with hematogenous abnormalities to achieve a diagnosis in the head and neck.

Advanced imaging of regions of the body and nuclear medicine may be ordered by the patient's physician to characterize involvement beyond the skull and jaws.

Solid malignancies

Solid malignant tumors that involve the jaws may be associated with a significant soft tissue component that may be locally aggressive and destructive, extending into and around normal tissues. Lesions that involve the bone arise late in the course of disease and are generally rare in the jaws.

Squamous cell carcinoma is the most common primary malignancy in the oral cavity. Extension into adjacent soft tissue spaces or into bone increases the stage and therefore severity of disease. Floor of mouth, gingival, or retromolar tumors may be locally infiltrative, producing poorly defined, noncorticated radiolucent areas in the bone (Figure 8.24). When bone destruction involves the crest of the alveolar process, the pattern that may be seen is reminiscent of warm water poured onto snow (Figure 8.7); the slow

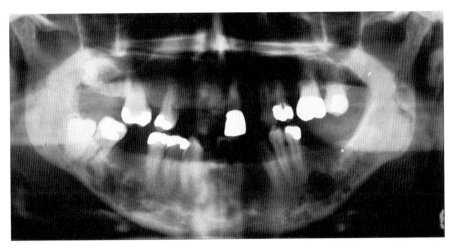

Figure 8.23 Multiple myeloma. Panoramic image shows multiple, variably sized, well-defined, variably corticated, circular, radiolucencies extending throughout the mandible. Some of the smaller areas located near the inferior cortex of the mandible have made "cookie bite" defects here. Image courtesy of Dr. G.E. Lily.

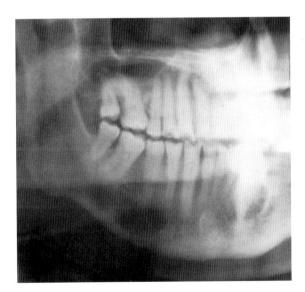

Figure 8.24 Squamous cell carcinoma. Cropped panoramic image shows two moderately well-defined, radiolucent areas located apical to the roots of the mandiublar right premolars and first molar. The abnormalities have encroached minimally on the inferior cortex of the mandible. Image courtesy of Dr. K. Dolan.

melting away of individual flakes as they come into contact with the warm water. Should the lesions involve the mandibular canal, some degree of dysesthesia or paresthesia may reported. With time, a distinct cookie bite loss of bone support

around the teeth may be visualized, and the teeth may appear as if to be floating in space.

Primary sarcomas of the bone, including chondrosarcoma and osteosarcoma of the jaws, are even rarer. When these malignancies develop, there may be considerable expansion of the bone, and dystrophic calcification may be visible within the lesion. An early sign of involvement of the teeth may be uniform widening of the periodontal ligament space (Figure 8.10), the result of tumor cell infiltration (Garrington and Collett, 1988; Garrington et al., 1967). This has been referred to as Garrington's sign and is visible on intraoral periapical images.

While it is important for the clinician to be able to recognize the features of malignancy, should a malignancy involve the jaws, patients should be promptly referred for medical management. Medical CT and MRI, modalities that can characterize the soft tissue components of these lesions and demonstrate the involvement of adjacent soft tissues, are the modalities of choice. Cone beam CT is not indicated for these lesions.

Bone or fibrous scar

Bone healing is difficult to quantify radiographically, particularly in the early stages of the process.

Following intervention, there is an initial hyper-emic response in the bone, and a blood clot is estab-lished that is slowly replaced by granulation tissue. At this time, a slow loss of the cortical outline defect may be seen radiographically. Osteoblasts are recruited from the defect's periphery, and a mineralized matrix is laid down from the defect periphery toward the center. If there is an insuffi-cient number of osteoblasts available, endosteal pluripotential stem cells that differentiate into osteoblasts may be recruited to the site. In the event that the defect fails to completely fill with bone matrix, a "rolled" border of radiopaque bone may be seen at the periphery accompanied by a central circular area of radiolucency. This "doughnut-shaped" appearance is often referred to as a fibrous scar (Figure 8.25).

As with any scar, the healing here in bone is considered sound in spite of the incomplete infill of bone. In some instances, the bone that does infill the defect may have a consistency that is reminis-cent of "ground glass," depending on the amount of fibrous connective tissue admixed into the bone (Figure 8.26). With less connective tissue and more bone matrix, the scar will appear more radiopaque, although some internal detail may still be visible (Figure 8.27).

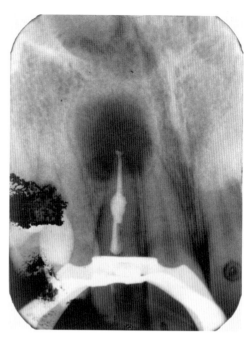

Figure 8.25   Fibrous scar. Periapical radiograph showing a well-defined, variably corticated radiolucent area located at the root apex of the endodontically treated maxillary right lateral incisor. Peripherally, the radiolucent area is bordered by a thick radiopaque border with a pattern of trabeculae radiating from the periphery, centrally.

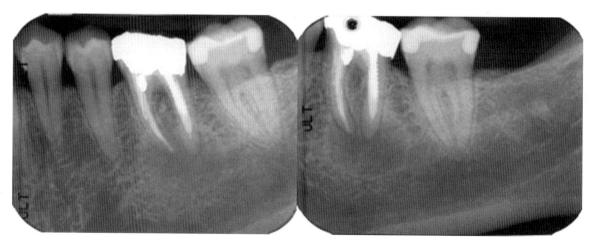

Figure 8.26   Healed bone. Periapical radiographs show a well-defined, delicately corticated, radiolucent area with a subtle, ground-glass type of internal pattern. The periodontal ligament spaces at the apices of the first molar tooth are intact.

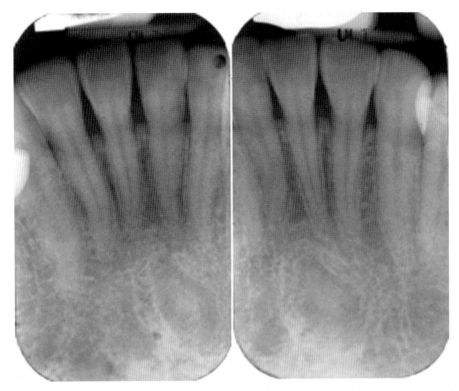

Figure 8.27   Healed bone. Periapical radiographs of the anterior mandible show a well-defined, corticated, radiopaque area located at the apices of the incisor teeth. Note the concentric internal lamellae within the now-healed defect.

Osseous dysplasia

The osseous dysplasias (formerly known as the cemento-osseous dysplasias) are a group of bone abnormalities that result in the deposition of a fibrous connective tissue matrix with a matrix of bone and, in some instances, cementum-like material. Histopathologic interpretation of these lesions is difficult and not definitive due to the overlapping of features of these entities with other bone dysplasias including fibrous dysplasia and benign tumors such as ossifying fibroma (Alsufyani and Lam, 2011a). For such lesions, radiologic examinations are diagnostic (Alsufyani and Lam, 2011b).

Two subtypes of the osseous dysplasias have been defined: periapical and florid. Although arguable, some believe both to be manifestations of the same disease process along a spectrum. Others, however, believe these entities represent different abnormalities due to their different clinical behav-

iors. The etiology of the osseous dysplasias is unknown, although it has been hypothesized that they may reflect a decoupling of normal osteoblastic and osteoclastic activities during normal bone remodeling.

Three stages of the osseous dysplasias have been described based on their radiographic appearances; an early stage radiolucent appearance, a mixed radiolucent/radiopaque stage where a radiopaque focus appears centrally within the radiolucency, and a mature stage in which the entity is almost entirely radiopaque except for perhaps a thin, radiolucent line or rim encircling the radiopacity. In all cases, the pulps of the involved teeth are vital.

The early stage lesion of osseous dysplasia appears, for all intents and purposes, to be radiographically identical to rarefying osteitis. There may be disruption and loss of the apical lamina dura of the involved tooth roots, and a small,

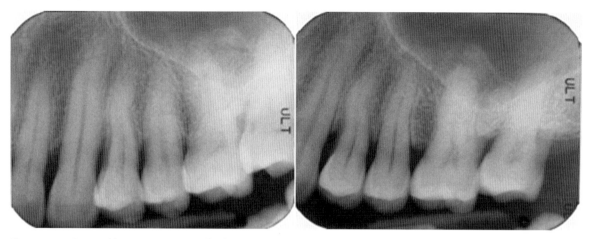

Figure 8.28 Periapical (cemento) osseous dysplasia. The periapical images show a well-defined, corticated, mixed radiolucent/radiopaque area located at the apices of the maxillary left first molar. The radiopaque component appears centrally within the abnormality, and a thin, radiolucent rim surrounds these. The elevated floor of the maxillary sinus forms the superior border of the abnormality.

moderately well-defined, variably corticated radiolucent area may appear. With time, a focal area of increased radiopacity may begin to appear at the apices of the involved teeth within the radiolucent area, and this should serve as a radiographic clue that the entity is an osseous dysplasia and not rarefying osteitis (Figure 8.28). As well, this appearance should be easily distinguishable from sclerosing osteitis as the area of sclerosis in the inflammatory lesion occurs at the lesion peripherally and not centrally as is the case with osseous dysplasia.

Should the mature lesion become large and the radiopaque areas coalesce (Figure 8.12), there can be local expansion of the bone to accommodate the increased size of the radiopacity (Figure 8.29). Furthermore, florid osseous dysplasia can be associated with the development of simple bone cysts in the jaws, and these can produce sizable radiolucencies (Figure 8.1) and substantial expansion (Figure 8.30). Another complication of the florid subtype is the development of osteomyelitis (Figure 8.9). Florid osseous dypslasias are believed to have a

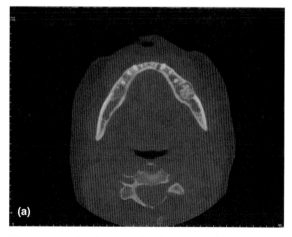

Figure 8.29 Florid osseous dysplasia. (a) Axial and (b) panoramic (upper right) and cross-sectional buccal/lingual (lower panel) cone beam CT reconstructions of the mandible show a multiple well-defined, radiolucent, and mixed radiolucent/radiopaque entities at the apices of the mandibular right first molar and second premolar, and left lateral incisor and first molar teeth. In particular, the entity associated with the apices of the mandibular left first molar shows buccal expansion and thinning of the cortex.

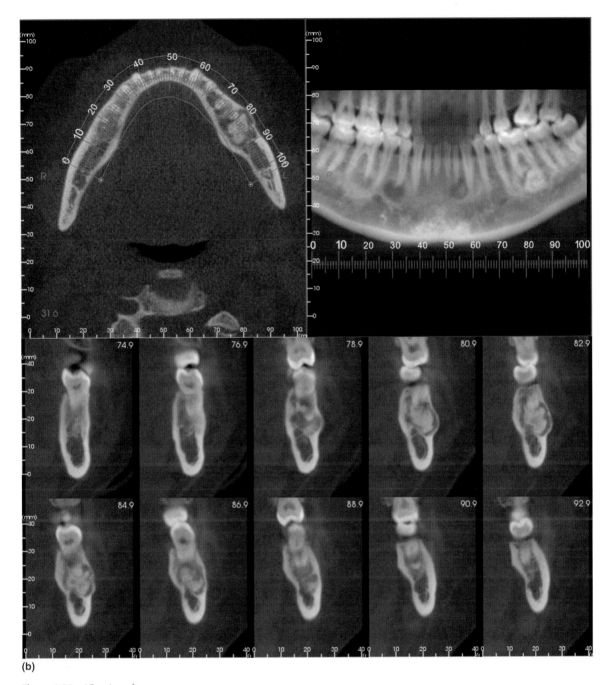

(b)

Figure 8.29   (*Continued*)

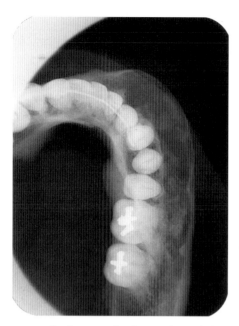

Figure 8.30 Florid osseous dysplasia with simple bone cysts. The true occlusal radiograph of the mandible shows prominent buccal expansion of the mandible, thinning of the buccal cortex, and internal areas of mixed radiolucent and radiopaque entities. The substantially sized simple bone cysts have produced significant expansion of the bone.

compromised blood supply. As such, secondary infection of the lesions can occur should bacteria be introduced either through the tooth or bone. In such cases, this may lead to osteomyelitis in the jaws (Groot et al., 1996).

Intraoral periapical and occlusal radiography should be used to image the associations of individual lesions with the teeth. Should osteomyelitis develop, medical or cone beam CT should be used to rule out sequestration or periosteal new bone formation and to determine the spread of infection (Orpe et al., 1996).

Dense bone island

The dense bone island is an asymptomatic, noninflammatory hamartoma of bone that may or may not have an association with the teeth. Should there be an association, the tooth pulp is vital.

Dense bone islands are well-defined, noncorticated, radiopaque entities situated in and around the teeth. They may have an association with a bone cortex, including the lamina dura (Figure 8.31) or they may arise centrally in the cancellous bone. Should they grow to involve the teeth and

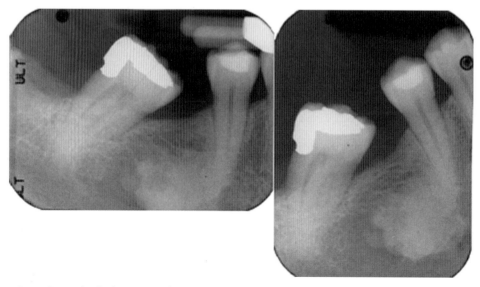

Figure 8.31 Dense bone island. The periapical images show a well-defined, noncorticated, radiopaque area located adjacent to the mandibular right second premolar and the edentulous area, just distal to this. In some areas, the periphery of the dense bone island appears to blend, imperceptibly with the surrounding trabecular bone pattern.

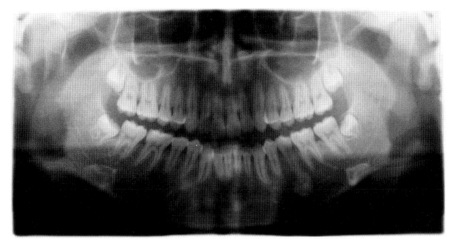

Figure 8.32   Dense bone island. The panoramic image shows a well-defined, non-corticated, radiopaque area associated with the root of the mandibular left second premolar. Note that the apical periodontal ligament space is intact.

peridental structures, the periodontal ligament space is undisturbed and remains intact. In cases where a dense bone island is associated with the root apex of a mandibular molar, the molar root may undergo a finite amount of external root resorption (Figure 8.32). Interestingly, the apical periodontal ligament space remains intact as does the vitality of the pulp.

Intraoral periapical and occlusal radiography is all that is necessary to interpret and diagnose dense bone islands.

References

Alsufyani, N.A. and Lam, E.W. (2011a) Cemento-osseous dysplasia of the jaws: clinical and radiographic analysis. *J Can Dent Assoc (Tor)*, 77, b70.

Alsufyani, N.A. and Lam, E.W. (2011b) Cemento-osseous dysplasia of the jaw bones: key radiographic features. *Dentomaxillofac Radiol*, 40, 141–146.

Baghdady, M.T., Pharoah, M.J., Regehr, G., Lam, E.W., and Woods, N.N. (2009) The role of basic sciences in diagnostic oral radiology. *J Dent Ed*, 73, 1187–1193.

Chadwick, J.W., Alsufyani, N.A., and Lam, E.W. (2011) Clinical and radiographic features of solitary and cemento-osseous dysplasia-associated simple bone cysts. *Dentomaxillofac Radiol*, 40, 230–235.

Garrington, G.E. and Collett, W.K. (1988) Chondrosarcoma: II. Chondrosarcoma of the jaws: analysis of 37 cases. *J Oral Pathol*, 17, 12–20.

Garrington, G.E., Scofield, H.H., Cornyn, J., and Hooker, S.P. (1967) Osteosarcoma of the jaws. Analysis of 56 cases. *Cancer*, 20, 377–391.

Groot, R.H., van Merkesteyn, J.P., and Bras, J. (1996) Diffuse sclerosing osteomyelitis and florid osseous dysplasia. *Oral Surg Oral Med Oral Pathol Oral Radiol Endod*, 81, 333–342.

Harnet, J.-C., Lombardi, T., Klewansky, P., Rieger, J., Tempe, M.-H., and Clavert, J.-M. (2008) Solitary bone cyst of the jaws: a review of the etiopathogenic hypotheses. *J Oral Maxillofac Surg*, 66, 2345–2348.

Lam, E.W., Lee, L., Perschbacher, S.E., and Pharoah, M.J. (2009) The occurrence of keratocystic odontogenic tumours in nevoid basal cell carcinoma syndrome. *Dentomaxillofac Radiol*, 38, 475–479.

Lokiec, F. and Wientroub, S. (1998) Simple bone cyst: etiology, classification, pathology, and treatment modalities. *J Pediatr Orthop B*, 7, 262–273.

Madras, J. and Lapointe, H. (2008) Keratocystic odontogenic tumour: reclassification of the odontogenic keratocyst from cyst to tumour. *J Can Dent Assoc (Tor)*, 74, 165–165.

Neville, B., Damm, D.D., Allen, C.M., and Bouquot, J. (2009) *Oral and Maxillofacial Pathology*, 3rd ed. Saunders, Chicago, IL.

Orpe, E.C., Lee, L., and Pharoah, M.J. (1996) A radiological analysis of chronic sclerosing osteomyelitis of the mandible. *Dentomaxillofac Radiol*, 25, 125–129.

Pompura, J.R., Sandor, G.K., and Stoneman, D.W. (1997) The buccal bifurcation cyst: a prospective study of treatment outcomes in 44 cases. *Oral Surg Oral Med Oral Pathol Oral Radiol Endod*, 83, 215–221.

Shimoyama, T., Horie, N., Nasu, D., Kaneko, T., Kato, T., Tojo, T., Suzuki, T., and Ide, F. (1999) So-called simple bone cyst of the jaw: a family of pseudocysts of diverse nature and etiology. *J Oral Sci*, 41, 93–98.

Suárez-Roa Mde, L., Ruíz-Godoy Rivera, L.M., Asbun-Bojalil, J., Dávilla-Serapio, J.E., Menjívar-Rubio, A.H., and Meneses-García, A. (2009) Interventions for central giant cell granuloma (CGCG) of the jaws. *Cochrane Database Syst Rev*, October 7(4), CD007404.

Suljak, J.P., Bohay, R.N., and Wysocki, G.P. (1998) Lateral periodontal cyst: a case report and review of the literature. *J Can Dent Assoc (Tor)*, 64, 48–51.

World Health Organization (2005) *Pathology and Genetics, Head and Neck Tumours*. L. Barnes, J.W. Eveson, P. Reichart, and D. Sidransky, eds., IARC Press, Lyon.

Worth, H.M. (1963) *Principles and Practice of Oral Radiologic Interpretation*. Year Book Medical Publishers, Chicago, IL.

9 Radiographic Interpretation of Traumatic Injuries

Nestor Cohenca

Introduction

The world of endodontics has witnessed several changes in the past decade. New technologies, instruments, and materials have resulted in better diagnosis and more predictable therapy. The application of computer based-systems and the development of electronic sensors have provided the technical means to apply theoretical principles to diagnostic imaging. Among these innovations, digital radiographic imaging has introduced a new dimension with many potential benefits for endodontic practice and has significantly improved the ability to accurately diagnose in a cost- and dose-efficient manner (Berkhout et al., 2004). Recent improvements in three-dimensional (3D) digital radiographic imaging introduced a new perspective, allowing us to evaluate the anatomic structures, both hard and soft tissue, in three spatial planes (Scarfe, 2005). Comparing with the traditional projection (plain film) radiograph, which is a two-dimensional shadow of a 3D object, 3D imaging overcomes this major limitation by providing a true representation of the anatomy while eliminating superimpositions. Several studies have reported the use of computerized

tomography and digital radiography for differential diagnosis (Shrout et al., 1993; Simon et al., 2006; Trope et al., 1989), assessment of treatment outcomes (Camps et al., 2004; Cotti et al., 1999), endodontics (Cotton et al., 2007), oral and maxillofacial surgery (Danforth et al., 2003a; Eggers et al., 2005; Ziegler et al., 2002), implantology (Hatcher et al., 2003; Sato et al., 2004), and orthodontics with reliable linear measurements for reconstruction and imaging of dental and maxillofacial structures (Baumrind et al., 2003; Danforth et al., 2003b; Maki et al., 2003).

The incidence of dental trauma due to falls, sports, automobile accidents, and violence has increased significantly in recent decades, affecting children's and teenagers' anterior teeth (Andreasen and Andreasen, 1994). In combination with clinical tests and observations such as percussion, palpation, tooth mobility, coronal color changes, pulp sensitivity, and vitality, the first clinical and radiographic examination of the traumatized patient is critical. The information gathered allows the clinician to determine the initial diagnosis, severity of the injury, develop a treatment plan, and create a baseline for follow-up. When correctly performed and adequately interpreted,

Endodontic Radiology, Second Edition. Edited by Bettina Basrani.
© 2012 John Wiley & Sons, Inc. Published 2012 by John Wiley & Sons, Inc.

these tests are reliable in diagnosing pulp necrosis (Andreasen, 1988a).

Following a traumatic injury, we must differentiate between the first radiographic examination of the patient, immediately after the injury, and the follow-up examinations. During the first radiographic examination, our focus should be on diagnosing bone fractures of the mandibular and maxillary processes, alveolar bone fracture(s), root fracture(s), displacement of teeth, and stage of root development/maturation. Follow-up radiographic examination is aimed at diagnosing widening of the periodontal ligament (PDL), disturbance of lamina dura, periapical radiolucencies, root resorptions, repair of root fractures, pulp canal obliteration, and root maturation/development.

Stage of root development

In 1960, Nolla published classification for odontogenic development using radiographic interpretation (Table 9.1) (Nolla, 1960). This classification has been widely used by all specialties throughout the years including current articles (Oliveira et al., 2008; Pioto et al., 2005).

Knowledge of the developmental stages of permanent teeth is essential for clinical practice in several dental specialties, since it may influence diagnosis, treatment planning, and outcomes. This is particularly true in cases of immature and traumatized teeth. In 1976, Fulling and Andreasen demonstrated that the late differentiation of Ad nerve fibers in the dental pulp could explain the lack of a reliable and predictable response of erupt-

Table 9.1 Radiographic classification for odontogenic development.

0	No crypt
1	Presence of crypt
2	Initial calcification
3	One-third crown completed
4	Two-thirds crown completed
5	Crown almost completed
6	Crown completed
7	One-third root completed
8	Two-thirds root completed
9	Root almost open (open apex)
10	Root apex completed

ing and undeveloped teeth to thermal and electrical stimulation (Fulling and Andreasen, 1976). In young patients with immature teeth, carbon dioxide (CO_2) snow and dichlorodifluoromethane are the most reliable sensitivity tests followed by the electric pulp test and ethyl chloride and ice (Fuss et al., 1986). Therefore, in absence of reliable clinical tests, radiographic evidence of root development and dentin maturation during follow-up examination may be critical in providing the clinician with reliable information related to the presence of a vital dental pulp.

Traumatic injuries

Radiographic interpretations of traumatic injuries will be thoroughly described and illustrated using the classification proposed by Andreasen and Andreasen in 1994 (Glendor et al., 2007) and adopted by the World Health Organization (WHO). Feliciano and Franca Caldas evaluated 164 articles and 54 different classifications and they concluded that, according to the literature, the most frequently used classification system was that of Andreasen (32%) (Feliciano and de Franca Caldas, 2006). Treatment recommendations are based on the official guidelines of the International Association of Dental Traumatology (IADT) (Flores et al., 2007a, 2007b, 2007c).

Injuries to the hard dental tissues and the pulp

1. Enamel fracture
   a. Definition: A fracture confined to the enamel with loss of tooth structure.
   b. Clinical features: Crown fracture involving enamel only with no visible sign of exposed dentin (Figure 9.1).
   c. Radiographic features: The enamel loss is visible.
   d. Recommended radiographs: Periapical radiographs at different horizontal angles (Brynolf, 1970a, 1970b; Wilson, 1995). This recommendation is aimed at ruling out the possible presence of a root fracture or a luxation injury (Bender and Freedland, 1983a). In case of lip laceration or swelling,

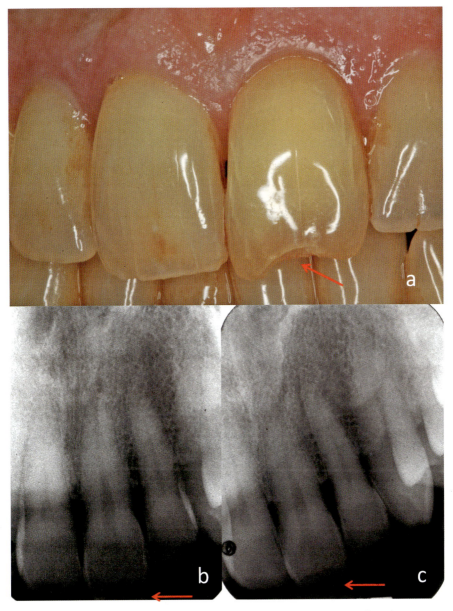

Figure 9.1 Clinical and radiographic diagnosis of enamel fracture of the maxillary left central incisor.

a radiograph of the lip is indicated to search for tooth fragments or foreign material (Figure 9.2).

e. Recommended treatment: The main purpose is to restore esthetics. Etch-bond resin restorations are the treatment of choice.

2. Uncomplicated enamel and dentin fracture

   a. Definition: A fracture confined to enamel and dentin with loss of tooth structure, but without pulpal exposure.

   b. Clinical features: Crown fracture involving enamel and dentin with no visible exposure of the pulp (Figure 9.3a).

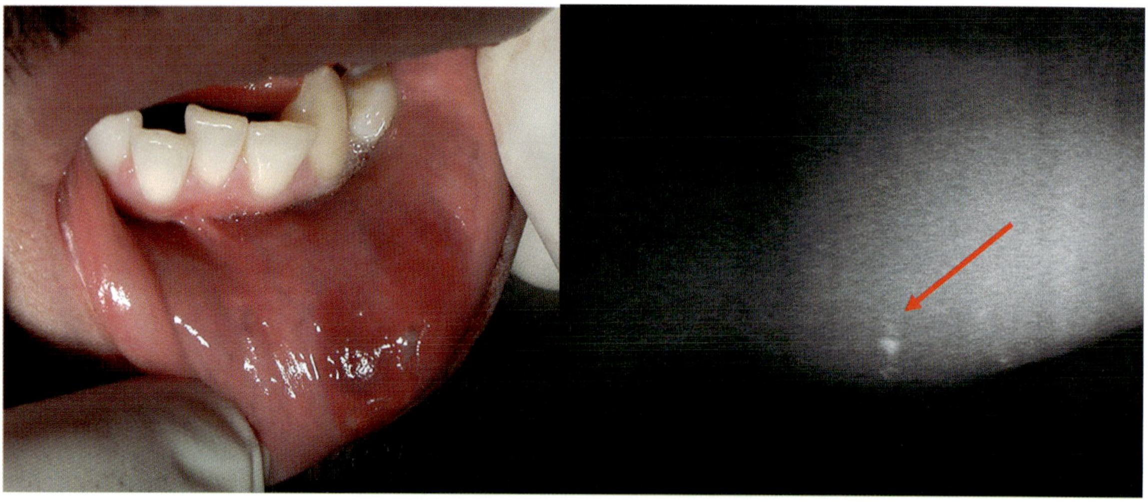

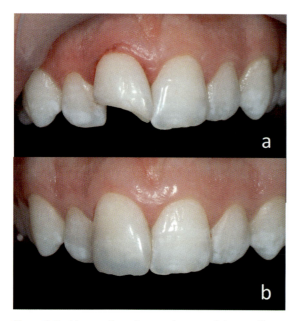

Figure 9.2 Lip laceration and swelling. A radiograph of the lip demonstrated the presence of tooth fragments within soft tissues.

Figure 9.3 Uncomplicated crown fracture of the maxillary right central incisor. (a) Preoperative and (b) postoperative restoration with composite resins. Courtesy of Dr. Gabriela Ibarra.

c. Radiographic features: A visible fracture is observed involving the loss of enamel and dentin, with no evidence of pulpal involvement.

d. Recommended radiographs: Periapical radiographs at different horizontal angles. This recommendation is aimed at ruling out the possible presence of a root fracture or a luxation injury. In case of lip laceration or swelling, a radiograph of the lip is indicated to search for tooth fragments or foreign material. Evaluate size of the pulp chamber and determine the stage of root development.

e. Recommended treatment: Clinical tests and radiographic examination. The exposed dentin should be protected by placing glass ionomer liner over the exposed dentin. A bonding agent and composite restoration is then indicated to restore the esthetics and function (Figure 9.3b). If an intact fragment exists, a bonding procedure may be carried out (Yilmaz et al., 2010). Check the occlusion.

f. Patient instructions: Soft diet and good oral hygiene.

g. Urgency: Subacute (within 24 hours) or delayed (more than 1 day).

h. Follow-up. Clinical and radiographic examination at 6–8 weeks and 1 year.

3. Complicated enamel and dentin fracture

a. Definition: A fracture confined to enamel and dentin with loss of tooth structure and pulpal exposure.

b. Clinical features: Crown fracture involving enamel and dentin with a visible exposure of the pulp (Figure 9.4a).

c. Radiographic features: A visible fracture is observed involving the loss of enamel and dentin reaching the pulp chamber (Figure 9.5).

d. Recommended radiographs: Periapical radiographs at different horizontal angles. In case of lip laceration or swelling, a radiograph of the lip is indicated to search for tooth fragments or foreign material. For moderate to severe trauma, Cohenca et al. recommended the use of cone beam computed tomography (CBCT) for accurate diagnosis and treatment planning

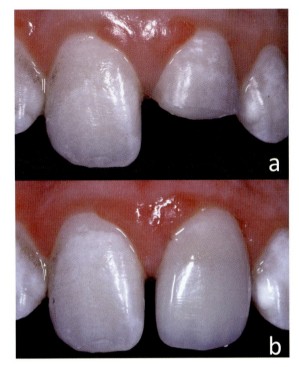

Figure 9.4 Complicated crown fracture of the maxillary left central incisor. (a) Preoperative and (b) postoperative restoration with composite resins. Courtesy of Dr. Gabriela Ibarra.

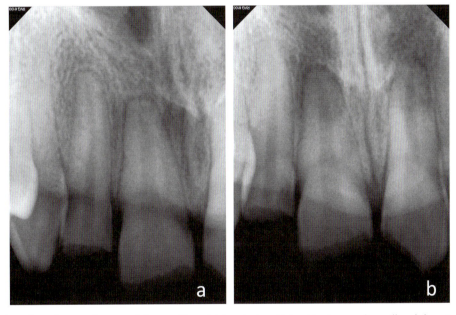

Figure 9.5 Complicated crown fracture of the maxillary right central and lateral incisors and maxillary left central incisor. (a–b) Periapical radiographs at different horizontal angles.

(Cohenca et al., 2007). Periapical radiographs indicated the presence of complicated fractures on the right maxillary lateral incisor and both maxillary central incisors (Figure 9.5). However, further evaluation of the case using CBCT illustrated a clear crown–root facture on the lingual aspect of the right maxillary lateral incisor (Figure 9.6). Evaluate size of pulp chamber and determine the stage of root development.

e.　Recommended treatment: Clinical tests and radiographic examination. Pulp capp-

ing, partial pulpotomy, cervical pulpotomy, or pulpectomy are all alternative treatment options. Cvek et al. (Cvek, 1978) recommended partial pulpotomy using pure calcium hydroxide. A dentinal barrier was radiographically evident at 3–6 months in 96% of the cases. Fuks et al. obtained similar results with no correlation between healing and size of pulp exposure, type of trauma, time frame, and root development (Fuks et al., 1987). Current literature recommends the use of mineral trioxide aggregate (MTA) as the

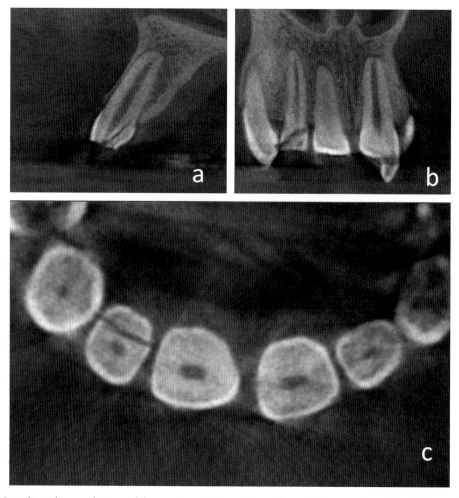

Figure 9.6　Complicated crown fracture of the maxillary right central and lateral incisors and maxillary left central incisor (same case of Figure 9.5). Cone beam computed tomography demonstrating an additional crown–root fracture on the maxillary right lateral incisors that was not visible on the periapical radiographs.

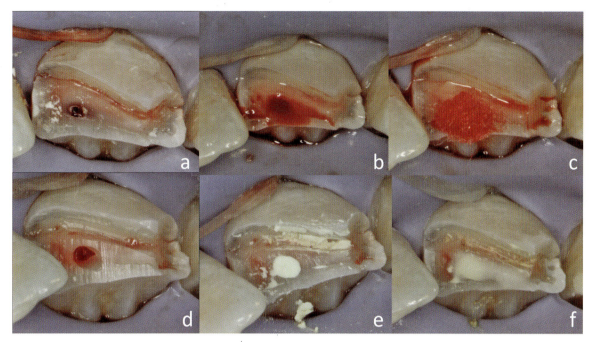

Figure 9.7   Complicated crown fracture of the maxillary right central incisor. Partial pulpotomy procedure clinically illustrated by steps: (a) Pulp exposure, (b) pulpal tissue excised 2 mm below the exposure, (c) bleeding control by pressure only (cotton pellet moisted on saline), (d) hemostasis obtained, (e) white MTA seal, and (f) protection of the MTA using a layer of glass ionomer lining.

material of choice instead of calcium hydroxide (Karabucak et al., 2005). The rational for this recommendation relies on the sealing ability and biocompatibility of MTA. Figure 9.6 illustrates the treatment of a complicated crown fracture with partial pulpotomy and MTA (Figure 9.7). Upon completion of the pulpal treatment, a composite-based restoration is indicated to restore the esthetics and function (Figure 9.4b). Check the occlusion.

   i.   Patient instructions: Soft diet and good oral hygiene.

   ii.   Urgency: Subacute (within 24 hours).

   iii. Follow-up. Clinical and radiographic examination at 6–8 weeks and 1 year.

4.   Crown and root fracture

   a.   Definition: Fracture involves enamel, dentin, and root structure.

   b.   Clinical features: Crown fracture involving enamel and dentin extending into the root structure (Figure 9.8). The pulp may or may not be exposed. Additional findings may include loose, but still attached, segments of the tooth. Sensibility testing is usually positive.

   c.   Radiographic features: Apical extension of fracture may be visible on a regular periapical radiograph (Figures 9.9 and 9.10).

   d.   Recommended radiographs: Periapical and occlusal exposures. A cone beam exposure might be necessary to reveal the extent of the fracture.

   e.   Recommended treatment: Treatment considerations are similar to the ones described for complicated crown fractures. As an emergency treatment, stabilization of the coronal fragment with acid etch/resin splint to the remaining tooth structure and adjacent teeth is recommended (Figure 9.11). If the fracture is subgingival, expose the fracture site by gingivectomy or orthodontic/surgical extrusion. If root formation is completed, endodontic therapy

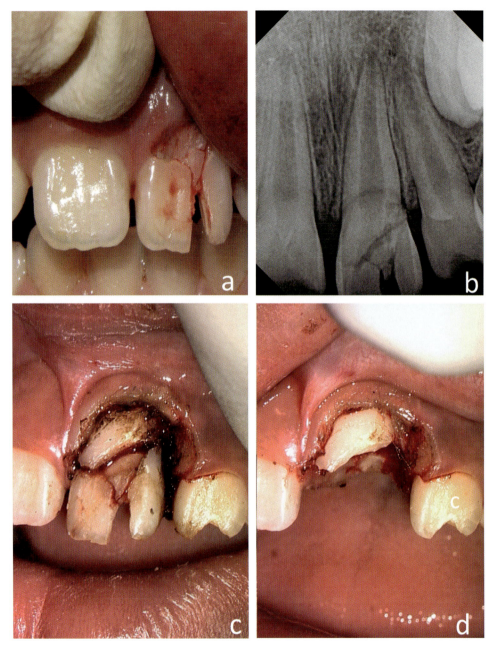

Figure 9.8 Crown–root fracture of the maxillary left central incisor. (a) Clinical view of the fracture immediately after injury, (b) periapical radiograph demonstrating the complicated crown–root fracture, (c) clinical gingivectomy exposing all the fracture's fragments, and (d) remaining tooth structure after removal of the fracture fragments.

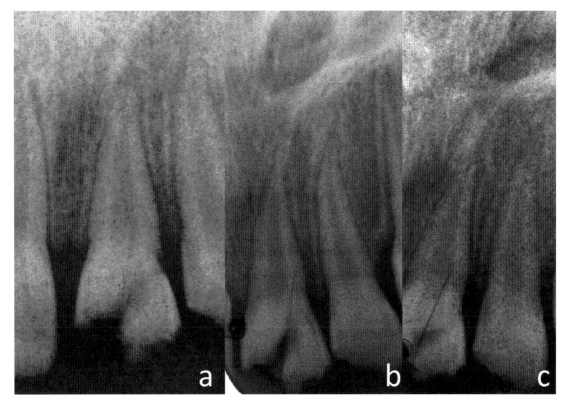

Figure 9.9 Crown–root fracture of the maxillary left central incisor. (a–c) Periapical radiographs at different horizontal angles.

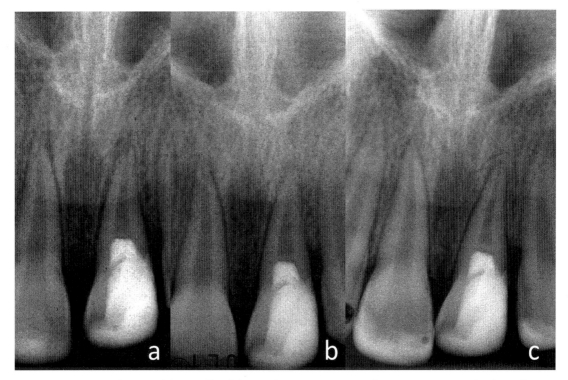

Figure 9.10 Crown–root fracture of the maxillary left central incisor (same case of Figure 9.9). Periapical radiographs. (a) Immediately postoperative, (b) 2 months follow-up, and (c) 6 months follow-up.

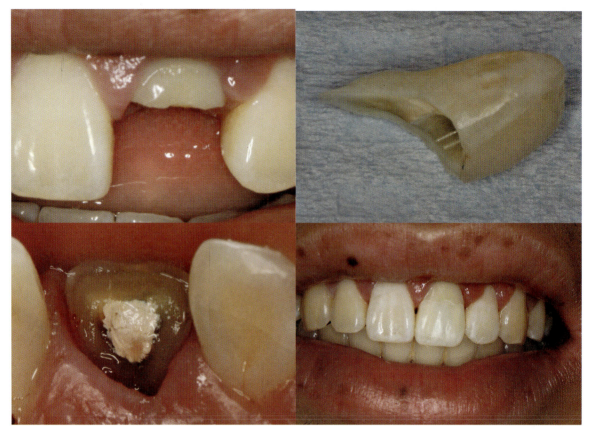

Figure 9.11   Crown–root fracture of the maxillary left central incisor. (a–d) Emergency procedure for stabilization of the coronal fragment with acid etch/resin splint to the remaining tooth structure and adjacent teeth.

is indicated. Otherwise, if the root is immature, partial or cervical pulpotomy is indicated.

f. Patient instructions: Soft diet and good oral hygiene.

g. Urgency: Subacute (within 24 hours).

h. Follow-up. Clinical and radiographic examination at 6–8 weeks and 1 year.

5. Root fracture

a. Definition: A fracture confined to the root of the tooth involving cementum, dentin, and the pulp. Root fractures can be further classified by level in coronal, middle-root, and apical. It can also be classified based on the direction in vertical, horizontal, and oblique planes. Most root fractures related to traumatic injuries are horizontal and are at the middle-root level. The coronal frag-

ment of the tooth is often displaced. Apical segment is usually not displaced.

b. Clinical features: The coronal segment may be mobile and in some cases displaced. Transient crown discoloration might be present.

c. Radiographic features: The root fracture line is usually visible on a periapical radiograph. The fracture involves the root of the tooth and is more often horizontal (Figure 9.12).

d. Recommended radiographs: A multidirectional approach using a conventional periapical exposure and two additional vertical periapical projections that vary ±15–20 degrees from the central beam has been advocated by several authors (Andreasen et al., 2007; Bender and Freedland, 1983a,

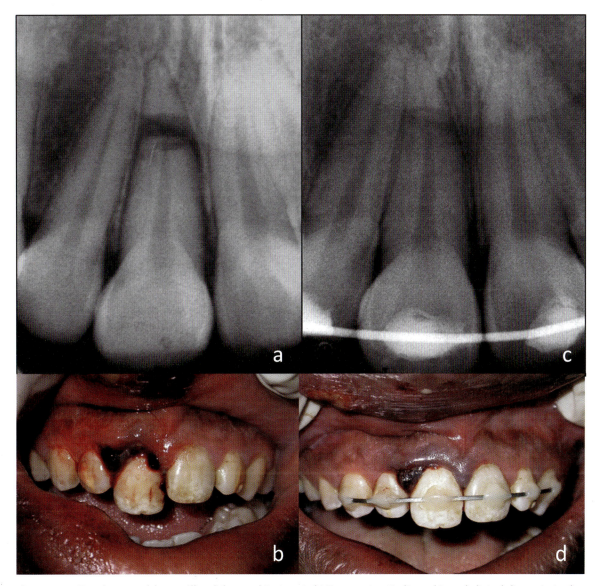

Figure 9.12   Root fracture of the maxillary left central incisor. (a–b) Preoperative. Radiographic and clinical diagnosis. (c–d) Postoperative. Reduction, repositioning, and splinting.

1983b; Degering, 1970; Wilson, 1995). A cone beam exposure might be necessary to reveal the extent and direction of the fracture (Figure 9.13a–c) (Cohenca et al., 2007). Recently, Bornstein et al. compared intraoral occlusal and periapical radiographs versus limited CBCT in diagnosing root-fractured permanent teeth and concluded that the diagnosis of the location and angulation of root fractures based on limited CBCT imaging differs significantly from diagnostic procedures based on intraoral radiographs (PA/OC) alone (Bornstein et al., 2009).

e.   Recommended treatment: Clinical tests and radiographic examination. Cardinal rules of fractures include immediate reduction and immobilization. Reposition

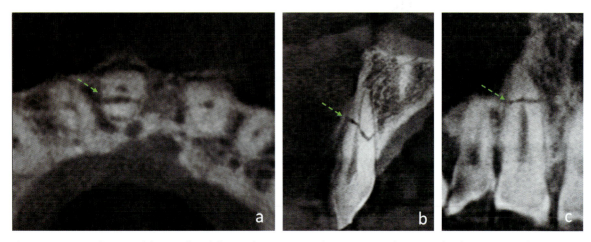

Figure 9.13   Root fracture of the maxillary left central incisor. Cone beam computed tomography demonstrating the fracture on all three planes: (a) axial, (b) sagittal, and (c) coronal.

of the coronal fragment and immobilization with a flexible acid-etch resin splint for 3–4 weeks is recommended. Despite the severity of this injury, the dental pulp is expected to regenerate in 77% of the cases (Cvek et al., 2001; Zachrisson and Jacobsen, 1975). Initially, clinical and radiographic follow-up is recommended. If pulp necrosis is diagnosed, it involves the coronal fragment only and therefore, endodontic therapy should be performed on the coronal segment.

f.   Patient instructions: Soft diet and good oral hygiene. Chlorhexidine mouth rinse (0.12%) twice a day for 7 days.

g.   Urgency: Acute (within a few hours).

h.   Follow-up. Splint removal with clinical and radiographic examination at 3–4 weeks. Clinical and radiographic examination at 6–8 weeks, 6 months, 1 year, and yearly for 5 years.

Injuries to the periodontal tissues

1.   Concussion.

a.   Definition: An injury to the supporting structures without loosening or displacement, but with a marked reaction to percussion.

b.   Clinical features: Tooth is tender to percussion without clinical displacement or mobility. Marginal bleeding may or may not be present at the sulcular level.

c.   Radiographic features: Since there is no displacement of the tooth, no significant changes or abnormalities are expected during the radiographic examination.

d.   Recommended radiographs: Periapical radiographs at different horizontal angles. Since no displacement occurred, no radiographic abnormalities are expected. However, these radiographs will serve as a baseline for further follow-up.

e.   Recommended treatment: Clinical tests and radiographic examination. Recommendations are aimed at preventing further injury to the periodontium and to facilitate periodontal and pulpal regeneration. Mandel and Vidik demonstrated that the PDL achieved 70% of its original strength 14 days after severe traumatic injuries (Mandel and Viidik, 1989). The occlusion should be evaluated and relieved if necessary.

f.   Patient instructions: Soft diet and good oral hygiene. Chlorhexidine mouth rinse (0.12%) twice a day for 7 days.

g.   Urgency: Sub-acute (within 24 hours).

h. Follow-up. Clinical and radiographic examination at up to 3 weeks, 6–8 weeks, 6 months, and 1 year.

2. Subluxation.

   a. Definition: An injury to the supporting structures with loosening, but without clinical or radiographic displacement of the tooth.

   b. Clinical features: Tooth is tender to percussion without clinical displacement. Tooth presents with some degree of clinical mobility. Marginal bleeding may or may not be present at the sulcular level.

   c. Radiographic features: Since there is no displacement of the tooth, no significant changes or abnormalities are expected during the radiographic examination.

   d. Recommended radiographs: Periapical radiographs at different horizontal angles. Since no displacement occurred, no radiographic abnormalities are expected. However, these radiographs will serve as a baseline for further follow-up.

   e. Recommended treatment. Same as for concussion injuries. Splint is indicated only in case of marked loosening or mobility. In such cases, a flexible splint of up to 0.16 mm thick should be applied for 7–14 days. The occlusion should be evaluated and relieved if necessary.

   f. Patient instructions: Soft diet and good oral hygiene. Chlorhexidine mouth rinse (0.12%) twice a day for 7 days.

   g. Urgency: Subacute (within 24 hours).

   h. Follow-up. Splint removal on or before 3 weeks. Clinical and radiographic examination at up to 3 weeks, 6–8 weeks, 6 months, and 1 year.

3. Luxation or displacement.

   a. Definition: An injury to the supporting structures with loosening and clinical or radiographic displacement. Based on the direction of the displacement, luxation injuries are further classified in lateral, extrusive and intrusive.

   b. Clinical features:

      i. Lateral luxation: Lateral displacement of the tooth other than axially. Lateral luxation injuries are characterized by partial or total separation of the PDL. Since most impacts are coming in a buccolingual direction, the crown is generally displaced lingually and the root buccally. Displacement is often accompanied by fracture of either the labial or the palatal/lingual alveolar bone. If both sides of the alveolar socket have been fractured, the injury should be classified as an alveolar fracture (alveolar fractures rarely affect only a single tooth). In most cases of lateral luxation, the apex of the tooth has been forced into the bone by the displacement, and the tooth is frequently nonmobile.

      ii. Extrusive luxation: An injury to the tooth characterized by partial or total separation of the PDL resulting in loosening and displacement of the tooth in an axial direction. The alveolar socket bone is intact in an extrusion injury as opposed to a lateral luxation injury. Depending of the degree of displacement, the tooth might be extremely loose.

      iii. Intrusive luxation: Displacement of the tooth into the alveolar bone. This injury is often accompanied by fracture of the alveolar socket. The tooth is displaced axially into the alveolar bone and immobile. Clinically, the crown might be partially or completely intruded (Figure 9.14a).

   c. Radiographic features: In cases of extrusive and lateral luxations, the tooth appears displaced with increase in the periapical ligament space (Figure 9.15a,b). On the contrary, in cases of intrusive luxations, the PDL space may be absent from all or part of the root and the tooth appears infra-occluded in comparison with the adjacent teeth (Figure 9.14b).

   d. Recommended radiographs: Occlusal, periapical radiographs at different horizontal angles. As demonstrated by Cohenca et al. (Cohenca et al., 2007) the use of a CBCT is extremely important in luxation injuries and particularly in lateral luxations (Figure 9.16). The 3D

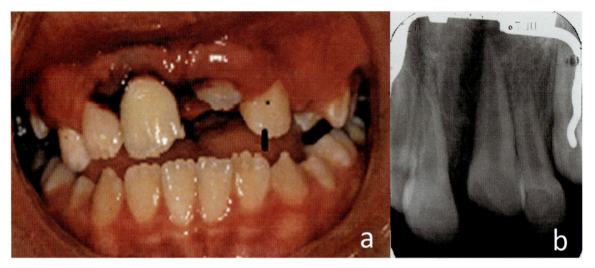

Figure 9.14 Intrusive luxation of the maxillary left central incisor as illustrated (a) clinically and (b) radiographically.

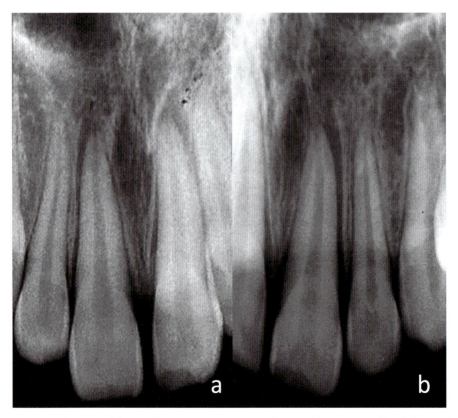

Figure 9.15 (a) Extrusive luxation of the maxillary right central incisor. (b) Lateral luxation maxillary left central incisor. The traumatic displacement of the teeth creates a radiographic appearance of an enlarged periodontal ligament space.

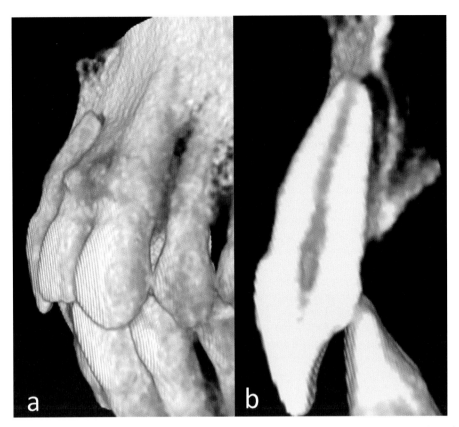

Figure 9.16   Cone beam computed tomography. (a) Transaxial volumetric reconstruction and (b) sagittal plane demonstrating the lateral luxation of the maxillary left central incisor. Courtesy of Dr. Jose Maria Malfaz.

imaging allows for a better diagnosis of alveolar fractures and confirms the correct repositioning of the tooth within the socket.

e. Recommended treatment: for extrusive and lateral luxations, the treatment consists of the immediate repositioning of the tooth and splinting with a flexible splint for 2 weeks. In case of concomitant alveolar fracture, the splinting time might be extended from 3 to 4 weeks. Patients should be prescribed with chlorhexidine rinses and instructed to have soft diet for 2 weeks. In cases of severe luxation and complete root development, endodontic treatment should be initiated no later than 2 weeks after trauma to prevent the onset of external inflammatory root resorption.

Treatment of intrusive luxations differs significantly based on the stage of root development. In immature intruded teeth, spontaneous eruption is expected. In patients ages 12–17 years old with complete root formation, teeth are still capable of spontaneous re-eruption; thus, no immediate repositioning is often the best treatment in regard to marginal periodontal healing. In patients 17 years old and beyond, either surgical or orthodontic extrusion should be performed. In immature teeth, pulp revascularization is possible, but these cases should be closely monitored. In cases of pulp necrosis, apexification and root canal therapy should be considered. Recently, the concept of revascularization of necrotic pulps has been developed for the treatment of immature and undeveloped teeth (Banchs and Trope, 2004; Cotti et al., 2008; Iwaya et al., 2001; Petrino et al., 2010; Thibodeau et al., 2007). If successful, the procedure allows further root development and maturation. Nevertheless, the predictability of this novel approach, particularly for the treatment of immature traumatized teeth, remains unclear, taking in consideration that the long-term prognosis of the tooth depends on the regeneration of the periodontium and not the dental pulp.

In cases of intrusion and complete root development, endodontic treatment should be initiated within 2 weeks, regardless of the degree of intrusion.

f. Patient instructions: Soft diet and good oral hygiene. Chlorhexidine mouth rinse (0.12%) twice a day for 7 days.

g. Urgency: Acute (within a few hours).

h. Follow-up. Splint removal on or before 3 weeks. Clinical and radiographic examination at up to 3 weeks, 6–8 weeks, 6 months, and 1 year.

4. Avulsion.

a. Definition: The complete separation of a tooth from its alveolus by traumatic injury. It implies an extensive damage to the pulp, and the periodontal tissues and the prognosis entirely depends upon the extraoral period and the storage media.

b. Clinical features: Tooth must be completely detached from the socket leaving an empty socket filled with a coagulum.

c. Radiographic features: Periapical radiographs will demonstrate an empty alveolar socket.

d. Recommended radiographs: Periapical radiographs are indicated to confirm the correct position of the avulsed and replanted tooth.

e. Recommended treatment. Time is of the essence. Replantation at the site of injury should always be encouraged as the treatment of choice. In such cases in which the tooth has been already replanted, clean the area with saline or chlorhexidine rinse and verify the position of the tooth radiographically with periapical radiographs. If immediate replantation is not possible, parents should be instructed to place the tooth in a biological storage media such as Hanks balanced salt solution (HBSS) or fresh milk and seek care dental care as soon as possible. Upon patient arrival to the practice or emergency room, local anesthetic should be administered using local infiltration. The root surface should be then irrigated with saline without handling or damaging the root surface. The alveolar socket is then flushed with saline to remove the coagulum and the tooth replanted using light digital pressure. Avoid any curettage of the socket. Verify the position of the tooth radiographically with periapical radiographs. A flexible splint of up to 0.16 mm thick should be applied for 7–14 days. The occlusion should be evaluated and relieved if necessary. The need for root canal therapy depends on two main factors: the stage of root development and the extraoral dry time. In cases of fully matured teeth, endodontic therapy must be initiated within 7–10 days of the time of injury, regardless of the extraoral time and the storage media. In cases of immature teeth that were replanted at the site of injury or were kept in a biological storage media, the tooth should be monitored for a possible pulp revascularization. Soaking these teeth in Minocycline prior to replantation has been shown to increase the chance of pulpal regeneration (Ritter et al., 2004) and allow further maturation of the root (Figure 9.17).

f. Patient instructions: Soft diet and good oral hygiene. Chlorhexidine mouth rinse (0.12%) twice a day for 7 days. Systemic antibiotics for 7 days (Hammarstrom et al., 1986; Sae-Lim et al., 1998). Tetanus booster.

g. Urgency: Acute (first 20 minutes are critical).

h. Follow-up. Splint removal and root canal initiation 7–10 days posttrauma. Clinical and radiographic examination at up to 3 weeks, 6–8 weeks, 6 months, and 1 year.

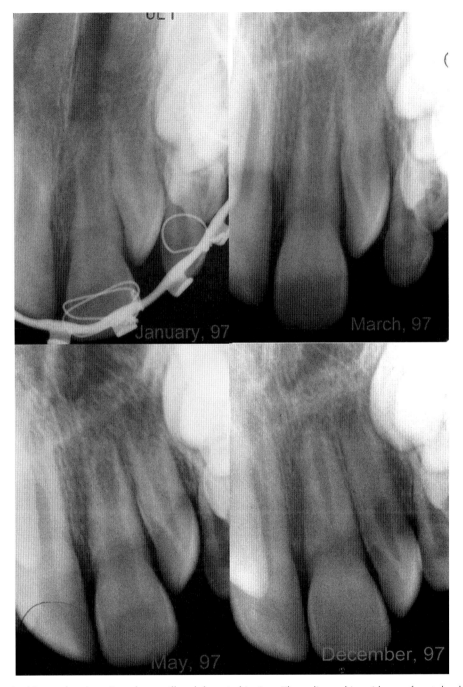

Figure 9.17 Avulsion and replantation of a maxillary left central incisor. The radiographic evidence of root development and maturation are a clear evidence of pulp revascularization.

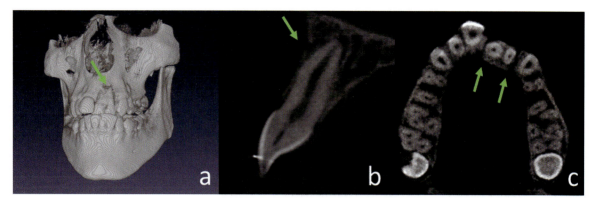

Figure 9.18 Alveolar bone fracture of the maxillary left central and lateral incisors. (a) The transaxial volumetric reconstruction demonstrates the extent of bone injury. (b) The alveolar fracture is observed in the sagittal and (c) axial planes (arrows). Courtesy of Dr. Jose Maria Malfaz.

Injuries to the supporting bone

1. Alveolar fractures.
   a. Definition: Fracture of the alveolar process with or without concomitant involvement of the alveolar socket. Alveolar fractures are often correlated with lateral luxations. Occlusal interference is often present.
   b. Clinical features: Displacement of the alveolar segment. The associated tooth might be displaced from its alveolus, mobile and tender to percussion. The bone segment containing the involved tooth/teeth is mobile.
   c. Radiographic features: The vertical line of the fracture may run along the PDL or in the septum. However, alveolar fractures are very difficult to diagnose on plain periapical, occlusal, or panoramic radiographs.
   d. Recommended radiographs: The use of CBCT is extremely helpful in diagnosing these types of fractures (Figure 9.18) (Cohenca et al., 2007).
   e. Recommended treatment: Reposition the fragment and stabilize the involved teeth with a flexible splint for 3–4 weeks.
   f. Patient instructions: Soft diet and good oral hygiene. Chlorhexidine mouth rinse (0.12%) twice a day for 7 days.
   g. Urgency: Acute (within a few hours).
   h. Follow-up. Splint removal with clinical and radiographic examination at 3–4 weeks. Clinical and radiographic examination at up to 3 weeks, 6–8 weeks, 6 months, and 1 year.
2. Fracture of the mandible or maxillary process.
   a. Definition: A fracture involving the base of the mandible or maxilla and often the alveolar process. The fracture may or may not involve the alveolar socket.
   b. Clinical features: Usually displacement between two alveolar segments within the dental arch. Disturbance in occlusion and deviation upon opening.
   c. Radiographic features: Maxillary fractures are further described by Le Fort classification as follows:
      i. Le Fort I: a horizontal segmented fracture of the alveolar process of the maxilla, in which the teeth are usually contained in the detached portion of the bone.
      ii. Le Fort II: unilateral or bilateral fracture of the maxilla, in which the body of the maxilla is separated from the facial skeleton and the separated portion is pyramidal in shape; the fracture may extend through the body of the maxilla down the midline of the hard palate, through the floor of the orbit, and into the nasal cavity.

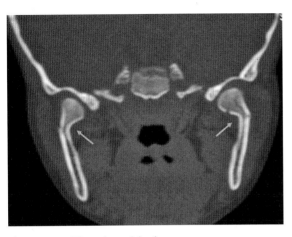

Figure 9.19   Bilateral condylar fractures.

iii.   Le Fort III: a fracture in which the entire maxilla and one or more facial bones are completely separated from the craniofacial skeleton; such fractures are almost always accompanied by multiple fractures of the facial bones.

Mandibular fractures are classified based on two factors: their location, either at the body, the ramus, or the condyle, and angle of the fracture. Chin injuries are often correlated with bilateral condylar fractures (Figure 9.19).

d.   Recommended radiographs: Traditionally, anterior, posterior, and lateral extraoral radiographs are indicated. A panoramic radiograph and CBCT are also extremely helpful in diagnosing these types of fractures (Dolekoglu et al., 2010).

e.   Recommended treatment: Reduction and immobilization are cardinal rules for mandibular and maxillary fractures. This can be accomplished using intermaxillary immobilization for 4 weeks or surgical repositioning and stabilization using mini plates (open reduction). In this case, intermaxillary splinting can usually be avoided.

f.   Patient instructions: Soft diet and good oral hygiene. Chlorhexidine mouth rinse (0.12%) twice a day for 7 days. Antibiotics are recommended.

g.   Urgency: Acute (within few hours).

h.   Follow-up. Clinical and radiographic examination at up to 3 weeks, 6–8 weeks, 6 months, and 1 year.

Injuries to the oral mucosa

1.   Laceration of gingiva or oral mucosa.
2.   Abrasion of gingiva or oral mucosa.

Lacerations and abrasion of soft tissues are commonly part of dental traumatology. Treatment basically depends on extent, depth, and type of tissue (i.e., skin, lip, oral mucosa, gingiva, tongue). Bleeding must be controlled and hemostasis achieved. Although most such injuries are minor in nature, they should be evaluated promptly with a focused history and thorough examination. In addition, facial injuries should be treated early to reduce the likelihood of possible adverse outcomes.

All areas should be thoroughly explored, copiously irrigated, cleaned, and debrided of devitalized tissue before closure. Irrigation lessens the risk of infection. Radiographs are indicated to rule out the possibility of hard tissue being embedded within the soft tissue as demonstrated in Figure 9.2. Nonabsorbable monofilament sutures should be used for skin closure. Nonabsorbable sutures such as braided polyester (polytetrafluoroethylene [PTFE]-coated Tevdek) or absorbable sutures such as polyglactin (Vicryl) are highly recommended for closure of intraoral lacerations.

Patient instructions should include soft diet and good oral hygiene. Chlorhexidine mouth rinse (0.12%) twice a day for 7 days is recommended. Follow-up should be set for suture removal within 5–14 days.

Sequelae of traumatic injuries

1.   Pulp canal obliteration (PCO).
PCO is a common sequela of tooth trauma, particularly in luxated immature teeth. The reported frequency ranges from 35% to 40% (Lee et al., 2003; Nikoui et al., 2003). Robertson et al. (1996) evaluated 82 teeth with history of trauma and subsequent PCO and found that only 8.5% of the tested teeth developed pulpal necrosis based on radiographic evidence of an

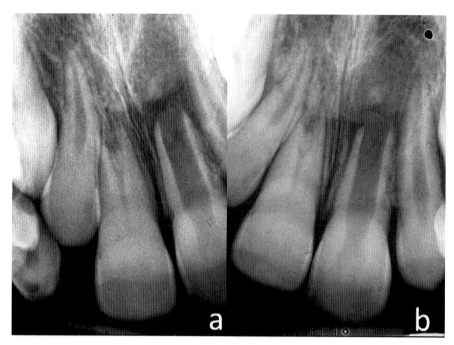

Figure 9.20   Periapical radiographs demonstrating pulp canal obliteration and pulp necrosis on the same patient. (a) Pulp canal obliteration (PCO) of the maxillary right central incisor and (b) radiographic evidence of arrested root development on the maxillary right central incisor.

apical radiolucency. Recently, Oginni et al. evaluated the clinical signs and symptoms associated with teeth with PCO and the status of the periapical tissues using the periapical index (PAI) (Oginni et al., 2009). Sixty-two teeth (33.3%) developed periapical lesions and reacted negatively to sensibility testing. Based on the findings of this study, authors recommended endodontic therapy in teeth presenting with pulp canal obliteration, tenderness to percussion, PAI scores greater than or equal to 3, and a negative response to sensibility testing. In some cases, the same traumatic injury may cause pulp canal obliteration in one tooth and pulp necrosis on the adjacent one (Figures 9.20 and 9.21).

2.   Pulp necrosis and periradicular periodontitis. Pulp Necrosis is a common complication following dental trauma. Pulp exposure due to crown and root fractures may lead to immediate or delayed irreversible changes on the exposed pulp. On the other hand, in cases of injuries to the periodontium, most of the shock is absorbed at the apex of the tooth, causing irreversible damage to the vascular supply of the pulpal tissue. Among the most common types of injuries leading to pulp necrosis are avulsion of fully developed teeth and intrusive luxations (Andreasen et al., 2006a, 2006b, 2006c).

Early diagnosis of pulp necrosis is important to prevent contamination and infection of the space and avoid the onset of inflammatory root resorptions and periradicular periodontitis. Clinically, the most common signs and symptoms include lack of response to sensitivity and vitality tests (pulse oximetry), tenderness to percussion (Andreasen, 1988b), and palpation and crown discoloration. Radiographically, we can observe periradicular radiolucencies consistent with bone resorption due to the periradicular inflammatory response and root resorption. One of the earliest signs of pulp necrosis is lack of development and maturation of the root. It is important to evaluate root maturation in comparison to previous radiographic examinations and observe the development of the injured tooth in comparison to the adjacent, noninjured teeth (Figure 9.22). The acquisition of past radiographs from clini-

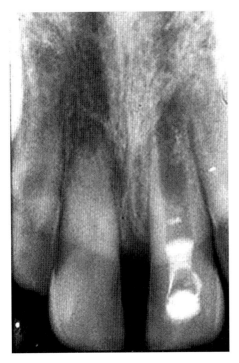

Figure 9.21 Periapical radiograph demonstrating pulp canal obliteration and pulp necrosis on the same patient as a result of the same traumatic injury. While the maxillary right central incisor developed (a) pulp canal obliteration (PCO), the maxillary right central incisor demonstrates (b) radiographic evidence of arrested root development.

cians that had previously seen the patient is often helpful is identifying the progression of radiographic changes and enhances our diagnostic abilities.

3. Root resorption.

Root resorption is defined as a condition associated with either a physiological or a pathological process resulting in a loss of dentin, cementum, or bone. The most common types of resorptions that are highly associated with dental trauma are external replacement root resorption, external inflammatory root resorption, and extracanal invasive root resorption (Figure 9.23).

The radiographic characteristics of root resorptions will be further described on Chapter 7.

Conclusions

Early diagnosis and treatment are essential in dental traumatology and are directly correlated with the outcome and survival of the injured teeth. As part of this diagnostic process, the acquisition of different radiographs, based on the type of injury and the tissues affected, are vital and

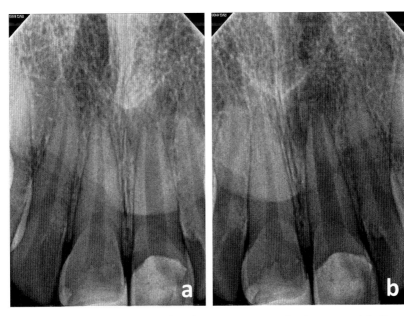

Figure 9.22 Periapical radiographs demonstrating a clear discrepancy on root development and dentin maturation between the maxillary central incisors.

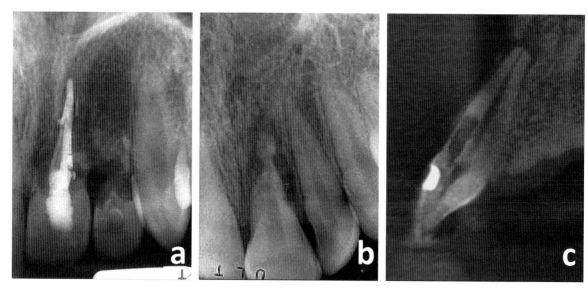

Figure 9.23   Root resorption. (a) External replacement root resorption, (b) external inflammatory root resorption, and (c) extracanal invasive root resorption.

mandatory. Currently, the use of 3D systems such as CBCT has become a valuable imaging system in dental traumatology. By providing a 3D representation of the maxillofacial tissues in a cost- and dose-efficient manner, a better preoperative assessment can be obtained for diagnosis and treatment, thus increasing the outcome of the therapy and avoiding further complications.

References

Andreasen, F.M. (1988a) Histological and bacteriological study of pulps extirpated after luxation injuries. *Endod Dent Traumatol*, 4(4), 170–181.

Andreasen, F.M. (1988b) Histological and bacteriological study of pulps extirpated after luxation injuries. *Endod Dent Traumatol*, 4(4), 170–181.

Andreasen, J.O. and Andreasen, F.M. (1994) Avulsions. In: J.O. Andreasen and F.M. Andreasen, eds., *Textbook and Color Atlas of Traumatic Injuries to the Teeth*, 3rd ed., pp. 383–425. Munksgaard, Copenhagen.

Andreasen, J.O., Bakland, L.K., and Andreasen, F.M. (2006a) Traumatic intrusion of permanent teeth: Part 3. A clinical study of the effect of treatment variables such as treatment delay, method of repositioning, type of splint, length of splinting and antibiotics on 140 teeth. *Dent Traumatol*, 22(2), 99–111.

Andreasen, J.O., Bakland, L.K., and Andreasen, F.M. (2006b) Traumatic intrusion of permanent teeth. Part 2. A clinical study of the effect of preinjury and injury factors, such as sex, age, stage of root development, tooth location, and extent of injury including number of intruded teeth on 140 intruded permanent teeth. *Dent Traumatol*, 22(2), 90–98.

Andreasen, J.O., Bakland, L.K., Matras, R.C., and Andreasen, F.M. (2006c) Traumatic intrusion of permanent teeth: Part 1. An epidemiological study of 216 intruded permanent teeth. *Dent Traumatol*, 22(2), 83–89.

Andreasen, F.M., Andreasen, J.O., and Cvek, M. (2007) Root fractures. In: J.O. Andreasen and F.M. Andreasen, eds., *Textbook and Color Atlas of Traumatic Injuries to the Teeth*. Munksgaard, Copenhagen, pp. 337–371.

Banchs, F. and Trope, M. (2004) Revascularization of immature permanent teeth with apical periodontitis: new treatment protocol? *J Endod*, 30(4), 196–200.

Baumrind, S., Carlson, S., Beers, A., Curry, S., Norris, K., and Boyd, R.L. (2003) Using three-dimensional imaging to assess treatment outcomes in orthodontics: a progress report from the University of the Pacific. *Orthod Craniofac Res*, 6(Suppl 1), 132–142.

Bender, I.B. and Freedland, J.B. (1983a) Clinical considerations in the diagnosis and treatment of intra-alveolar root fractures. *J Am Dent Assoc*, 107(4), 595–600.

Bender, I.B. and Freedland, J.B. (1983b) Adult root fracture. *J Am Dent Assoc*, 107(3), 413–419.

Berkhout, W.E., Beuger, D.A., Sanderink, G.C., and van der Stelt, P.F. (2004) The dynamic range of digital radiographic systems: dose reduction or risk of over-exposure? *Dentomaxillofac Radiol*, 33(1), 1–5.

Bornstein, M.M., Wolner-Hanssen, A.B., Sendi, P., and von Arx, T. (2009) Comparison of intraoral radiography and limited cone beam computed tomography for the assessment of root-fractured permanent teeth. *Dent Traumatol*, 25(6), 571–577.

Brynolf, I. (1970a) Roentgenologic periapical diagnosis: 3. The more roentgenograms—the better the information? *Sven Tandlak Tidskr*, 63(6), 409–413.

Brynolf, I. (1970b) Roentgenologic periapical diagnosis: II. One, two or more roentgenograms? *Sven Tandlak Tidskr*, 63(5), 345–350.

Camps, J., Pommel, L., and Bukiet, F. (2004) Evaluation of periapical lesion healing by correction of gray values. *J Endod*, 30(11), 762–766.

Cohenca, N., Simon, J.H., Roges, R., Morag, Y., and Malfaz, J.M. (2007) Clinical indications for digital imaging in dento-alveolar trauma. Part 1: traumatic injuries. *Dent Traumatol*, 23(2), 95–104.

Cotti, E., Mereu, M., and Lusso, D. (2008) Regenerative treatment of an immature, traumatized tooth with apical periodontitis: report of a case. *J Endod*, 34(5), 611–616.

Cotti, E., Vargiu, P., Dettori, C., and Mallarini, G. (1999) Computerized tomography in the management and follow-up of extensive periapical lesion. *Endod Dent Traumatol*, 15(4), 186–189.

Cotton, T.P., Geisler, T.M., Holden, D.T., Schwartz, S.A., and Schindler, W.G. (2007) Endodontic applications of cone-beam volumetric. *Tomogr J Endod*, 33(9), 1121–1132.

Cvek, M. (1978) A clinical report on partial pulpotomy and capping with calcium hydroxide in permanent incisors with complicated crown fracture. *J Endod*, 4(8), 232–237.

Cvek, M., Andreasen, J.O., and Borum, M.K. (2001) Healing of 208 intra-alveolar root fractures in patients aged 7–17 years. *Dent Traumatol*, 17(2), 53–62.

Danforth, R.A., Peck, J., and Hall, P. (2003a) Cone beam volume tomography: an imaging option for diagnosis of complex mandibular third molar anatomical relationships. *J Calif Dent Assoc*, 31(11), 847–852.

Danforth, R.A., Dus, I., and Mah, J. (2003b) 3-D volume imaging for dentistry: a new dimension. *J Calif Dent Assoc*, 31(11), 817–823.

Degering, C.I. (1970) Radiography of dental fractures. An experimental evaluation. *Oral Surg Oral Med Oral Pathol*, 30(2), 213–219.

Dolekoglu, S., Fisekcioglu, E., Ilguy, D., Ilguy, M., and Bayirli, G. (2010) Diagnosis of jaw and dentoalveolar fractures in a traumatized patient with cone beam computed tomography. *Dent Traumatol*, 26(2), 200–203.

Eggers, G., Mukhamadiev, D., and Hassfeld, S. (2005) Detection of foreign bodies of the head with digital volume tomography. *Dentomaxillofac Radiol*, 34(2), 74–79.

Feliciano, K.M. and De Franca Caldas, A., Jr. (2006) A systematic review of the diagnostic classifications of traumatic dental injuries. *Dent Traumatol*, 22(2), 71–76.

Flores, M.T., Andersson, L., Andreasen, J.O., Bakland, L.K., Malmgren, B., Barnett, F., et al. (2007a) Guidelines for the management of traumatic dental injuries. II. Avulsion of permanent teeth. *Dent Traumatol*, 23(3), 130–136.

Flores, M.T., Andersson, L., Andreasen, J.O., Bakland, L.K., Malmgren, B., Barnett, F., et al. (2007b) Guidelines for the management of traumatic dental injuries: I. Fractures and luxations of permanent teeth. *Dent Traumatol*, 23(2), 66–71.

Flores, M.T., Malmgren, B., Andersson, L., Andreasen, J.O., Bakland, L.K., Barnett, F., et al. (2007c) Guidelines for the management of traumatic dental injuries. III. Primary teeth. *Dent Traumatol*, 23(4), 196–202.

Fuks, A.B., Cosack, A., Klein, H., and Eidelman, E. (1987) Partial pulpotomy as a treatment alternative for exposed pulps in crown-fractured permanent incisors. *Endod Dent Traumatol*, 3(3), 100–102.

Fulling, H.J. and Andreasen, J.O. (1976) Influence of maturation status and tooth type of permanent teeth upon electrometric and thermal pulp testing. *Scand J Dent Res*, 84(5), 286–290.

Fuss, Z., Trowbridge, H., Bender, I.B., Rickoff, B., and Sorin, S. (1986) Assessment of reliability of electrical and thermal pulp testing agents. *J Endod*, 12(7), 301–305.

Glendor, U., Marcenes, W., and Andreasen, J. (2007) Classification, etiology and epidemiology. In: J.O. Andreasen, F.M. Andreasen, and L. Andersson, eds., *Textbook and Color Atlas of Traumatic Injuries to the Teeth*. Munksgaard, Copenhagen, pp. 217–254.

Hammarstrom, L., Pierce, A., Blomlof, L., Feiglin, B., and Lindskog, S. (1986) Tooth avulsion and replantation–a review. *Endod Dent Traumatol*, 2(1), 1–8.

Hatcher, D.C., Dial, C., and Mayorga, C. (2003) Cone beam CT for pre-surgical assessment of implant sites. *J Calif Dent Assoc*, 31(11), 825–833.

Iwaya, S.I., Ikawa, M., and Kubota, M. (2001) Revascularization of an immature permanent tooth with apical periodontitis and sinus tract. *Dent Traumatol*, 17(4), 185–187.

Karabucak, B., Li, D., Lim, J., and Iqbal, M. (2005) Vital pulp therapy with mineral trioxide aggregate. *Dent Traumatol*, 21(4), 240–243.

Lee, R., Barrett, E.J., and Kenny, D.J. (2003) Clinical outcomes for permanent incisor luxations in a pediatric population: II. Extrusions. *Dent Traumatol*, 19(5), 274–279.

Maki, K., Inou, N., Takanishi, A., and Miller, A.J. (2003) Computer-assisted simulations in orthodontic diagnosis and the application of a new cone beam X-ray computed tomography. *Orthod Craniofac Res*, 6(Suppl 1), 95–101; discussion 179–182.

Mandel, U. and Viidik, A. (1989) Effect of splinting on the mechanical and histological properties of the healing periodontal ligament in the vervet monkey (*Cercopithecus aethiops*). *Arch Oral Biol*, 34(3), 209–217.

Nikoui, M., Kenny, D.J., and Barrett, E.J. (2003) Clinical outcomes for permanent incisor luxations in a pediatric population: III. Lateral luxations. *Dent Traumatol*, 19(5), 280–285.

Nolla, C.M. (1960) The development of the permanent teeth. *J Dent Child*, 27, 254–266.

Oginni, A.O., Adekoya-Sofowora, C.A., and Kolawole, K.A. (2009) Evaluation of radiographs, clinical signs and symptoms associated with pulp canal obliteration: an aid to treatment decision. *Dent Traumatol*, 25(6), 620–625.

de Oliveira, D.M., Andrade, E.S., Da Silveira, M.M., and Camargo, I.B. (2008) Correlation of the radiographic and morphological features of the dental follicle of third molars with incomplete root formation. *Int J Med Sci*, 5(1), 36–40.

Petrino, J.A., Boda, K.K., Shambarger, S., Bowles, W.R., and McClanahan, S.B. (2010) Challenges in regenerative endodontics: a case series. *J Endod*, 36(3), 536–541.

Pioto, N.R., Costa, B., and Gomide, M.R. (2005) Dental development of the permanent lateral incisor in patients with incomplete and complete unilateral cleft lip. *Cleft Palate Craniofac J*, 42(5), 517–520.

Ritter, A.L., Ritter, A.V., Murrah, V., Sigurdsson, A., and Trope, M. (2004) Pulp revascularization of replanted immature dog teeth after treatment with minocycline and doxycycline assessed by laser Doppler flowmetry, radiography, and histology. *Dent Traumatol*, 20(2), 75–84.

Robertson, A., Andreasen, F.M., Bergenholtz, G., Andreasen, J.O., and Noren, J.G. (1996) Incidence of pulp necrosis subsequent to pulp canal obliteration from trauma of permanent incisors. *J Endod*, 22(10), 557–560.

Sae-Lim, V., Wang, C.Y., and Trope, M. (1998) Effect of systemic tetracycline and amoxicillin on inflammatory root resorption of replanted dogs' teeth. *Endod Dent Traumatol*, 14(5), 216–220.

Sato, S., Arai, Y., Shinoda, K., and Ito, K. (2004) Clinical application of a new cone-beam computerized tomography system to assess multiple two-dimensional images for the preoperative treatment planning of maxillary implants: case reports. *Quintessence Int*, 35(7), 525–528.

Scarfe, W.C. (2005) Imaging of maxillofacial trauma: evolutions and emerging revolutions. *Oral Surg Oral Med Oral Pathol Oral Radiol Endod*, 100(2 Suppl), S75–S96.

Shrout, M.K., Hall, J.M., and Hildebolt, C.E. (1993) Differentiation of periapical granulomas and radicular cysts by digital radiometric analysis. *Oral Surg Oral Med Oral Pathol*, 76(3), 356–361.

Simon, J.H., Enciso, R., Malfaz, J.M., Roges, R., Bailey-Perry, M., and Patel, A. (2006) Differential diagnosis of large periapical lesions using cone-beam computed tomography measurements and biopsy. *J Endod*, 32(9), 833–837.

Thibodeau, B., Teixeira, F., Yamauchi, M., Caplan, D.J., and Trope, M. (2007) Pulp revascularization of immature dog teeth with apical periodontitis. *J Endod*, 33(6), 680–689.

Trope, M., Pettigrew, J., Petras, J., Barnett, F., and Tronstad, L. (1989) Differentiation of radicular cyst and granulomas using computerized tomography. *Endod Dent Traumatol*, 5(2), 69–72.

Wilson, C.F. (1995) Management of trauma to primary and developing teeth. *Dent Clin North Am*, 39(1), 133–167.

Yilmaz, Y., Guler, C., Sahin, H., and Eyuboglu, O. (2010) Evaluation of tooth-fragment reattachment: a clinical and laboratory study. *Dent Traumatol*, 26(4), 308–314.

Zachrisson, B.U. and Jacobsen, I. (1975) Long-term prognosis of 66 permanent anterior teeth with root fracture. *Scand J Dent Res*, 83(6), 345–354.

Ziegler, C.M., Woertche, R., Brief, J., and Hassfeld, S. (2002) Clinical indications for digital volume tomography in oral and maxillofacial surgery. *Dentomaxillofac Radiol*, 31(2), 126–130.

10 Radiographic Analysis of Acquired Pathological Dental Conditions

Amir Azarpazhooh

This chapter will discuss the lesions that would be acquired after the eruption of the tooth. Some may have no clinical importance. In contrast, some may jeopardize the tooth and cause tooth loss. In this chapter, tooth wear, resorption, pulp calcification, and hypercementosis will be discussed.

Tooth wear

Tooth wear is the result of three processes: (1) abrasion, (2) attrition, and (3) erosion. Tooth wear can be a challenging problem for the clinician due to its subtle early changes, confusing etiology, and the dilemma as to when or how to manage the etiology. (Harpenau et al., 2011). It is well-recognized that individual wear mechanisms rarely act alone but interact with each other. For example, potentiation of abrasion by erosive damage to the dental hard tissues is the major factor in occlusal and cervical wear (Addy and Shellis, 2006).

Attrition

Attrition is a process in which the wear of the occlusal, incisal, or interproximal surfaces of the teeth is produced by interaction and friction between maxillary and mandibular teeth. Attrition leads to the loss of enamel, dentin, or restoration, reduction in tooth length, and significant dimensional changes in facial morphology (Berry and Poole, 1976) (Figure 10.1).

More than 90% of the population have one or more severe attrition facets (Seligman et al., 1988). Generally, a greater attrition has been reported in males than in females (Hugoson et al., 1988; Johansson, 1992; Seligman et al., 1988). Extensive tooth wear among primitive peoples has mainly been attributed to abrasive particles in their diet. In present-day industrialized populations, other factors such as masticatory habits and parafunctions, saliva composition, dietary variables, digestive disturbances, and industrial environmental factors define the extent of attrition and tooth loss (Hugoson et al., 1988). Attrition is a physiological aging process and does not require a particular treatment, except observation. Throughout a lifetime, teeth are not lost in an irregular manner. In fact they are worn away by attrition while the human masticatory system and continuing tooth eruption maintain an efficient function as an evolving compensatory mechanisms (Begg, 1938;

Endodontic Radiology, Second Edition. Edited by Bettina Basrani.
© 2012 John Wiley & Sons, Inc. Published 2012 by John Wiley & Sons, Inc.

Newman, 1999). However, this process may become symptomatic and pathological due to bruxism where a continued dental attrition can lead to a breach of the occlusal enamel, exposing the less wear-resistant dentin. In such a case, the loss of dental hard tissue becomes accelerated and the dental pulp may become involved in extreme conditions (Ingle, 1960). A recent systematic review has found some evidence that correlates attrition and anterior spatial (van 't Spijker et al., 2007). However, no evidence was found suggesting that absent posterior support necessarily leads to increased attrition, or whether there is any relationship between attrition and temporomandibular dysfunction (van 't Spijker et al., 2007). It seems to be a correlation between attrition and self-reported bruxism. In particular, the occurrence of four clinical signs, posterior or anterior dental attrition, abfractions, and occlusal pits, was associated with self-reported bruxers (Tsiggos et al., 2008).

Clinical findings of attrition

Matching occlusal wear between arches, shiny wear facets on restorations, and increased risk for fracture of tooth and restorative structure are among the clinical findings of attrition (Harpenau et al., 2011).

Radiographic findings of attrition

On the radiograph, attrition is viewed as a mild wear of incisal and occlusal surfaces of teeth involved. Depending on the stage of the wear, the crown looks shorter, and volume of the pulp declines due to the deposition of secondary dentine or of amorphous dentine with age (Ketterl, 1983). Widening of periodontal ligament (PDL) can be seen if the tooth is mobile and occasionally there is evidence of hypercementosis (Lam, 2009) (Figure 10.2).

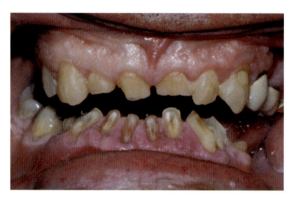

Figure 10.1   Clinical image of maxillary and mandibular anteriors with attrition. Courtesy of Dr. D. Chvartszaid.

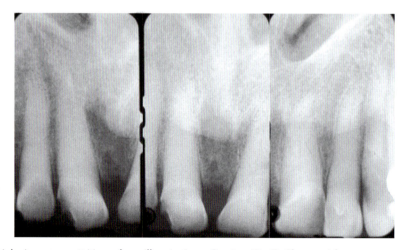

Figure 10.2   Physiologic wear or attrition, of maxillary incisors. Courtesy Dr. D. Chvartszaid.

Clinical management of attrition

Physiologic attrition does not require treatment.

Abrasion

Abrasion is a process in which tooth wear is produced by interaction and friction between teeth and other materials that leads to the loss of enamel, dentin, or restoration. Abrasion of teeth, as a result of brushing with dentifrices, was demonstrated more than a century ago (Miller, 1907). In particular, overly vigorous and improper toothbrushing in a back and forth motion with heavy pressure can cause abrasion with a V-shape wedge in the cervical area of teeth (Grippo et al., 2004, Gillette and Van House, 1980).

This type of abrasion begins apical to the cementoenamel junction and then progresses to dentin. It eventually undermines the enamel with the loss of the original cementoenamel junction (Litonjua et al., 2004). Among other causes for abrasion are improper use of dental floss and toothpicks, partial denture clasps, oral habits such as chewing tobacco, biting on hard objects (such as pens, pencils, or pipe stems), opening hair pins with teeth, and biting fingernails. Abrasion can also be seen among tailors or seamstresses who sever thread with their teeth, shoemakers and upholsterers who hold nails between their teeth, glassblowers, and musicians who play wind instruments (i.e., occupational abrasion) (Grippo et al., 2004). Similar to attrition, based on the level of wear, dentin can be exposed. This communication with the oral cavity can result in pulpal pathosis and an accompanying periapical lesion. However, in most cases, pulpal pathosis and periapical pathosis do not occur because of the ability of the pulp to lay down dentin as the pulp recedes (Meister et al., 1980).

Clinical findings of abrasion

Abrasional lesions can be seen usually as faciocervical concavities that are more broad than deep, in particular among those individuals with an abrasive diet and usually on prominent teeth in the arch such as canines, premolars, and mesiobuccal aspects of first molars. Abrasion may affect several teeth in a row with a "band" of abrasive damage

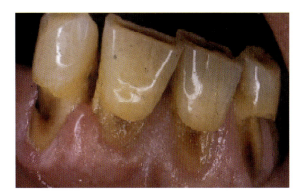

Figure 10.3   Clinical image of mandibular teeth with abrasion. Courtesy of Dr. E. Basrani.

with an increased hypersensitivity (Harpenau et al., 2011). (Figure 10.3)

Radiographic findings of abrasion

A toothbrush abrasion can be seen on radiograph as well-defined semicircular or semilunar shape radiolucent defects in cervical level of the tooth. The borders of defect show increased radiopacity. The pulp chambers appear obliterated (Lam, 2009) (Figures 10.4 and 10.5).

Clinical management of abrasion

Elimination of the cause of abrasion is the priority in the management. Restorative procedure may be indicated in excessive cases.

Erosion

Erosion is a multifactorial process of dissolution of enamel and underlying dentin by acidic substances without bacterial involvement. This chemical process is irreversible, and it leaves teeth susceptible to damage due to wear over the course of a person's lifetime (Wang and Lussi, 2010). The following factors were shown to be triggers for tooth erosion (Dietschi and Argente, 2011; Gandara and Truelove, 1999):

1. behavioral factors such as excessive consumption of acidic food or beverages, or unusual

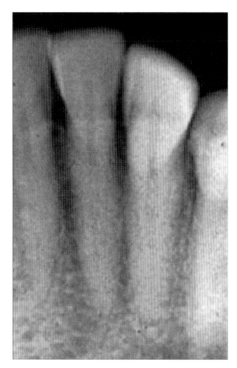

Figure 10.4 Radiographic image of abrasion of the cervical areas of mandibular incisors these incisor teeth. Note the obliteration of the pulp chambers and reduction in size of the root canals. Courtesy of Dr. E. Basrani.

eating and drinking habits such as sipping an acidic drink over a long period of time

2. unbalanced diet, in particular, dietary acids, such as fruit, fruit juices, carbonated drinks, and sports drinks

3. various medical conditions, such as gastric esophageal reflux disorder or with chronic excessive vomiting such as patients with anorexia, bulimia, alcoholism, or gastrointestinal disorders

4. medications such as vitamin C tablets

5. influencing saliva composition and flow rate

Clinical findings of erosion

The clinical appearance of dental erosion includes broad concavities and cupping on smooth surface enamel and increased incisal translucency, which can have undesirable esthetic implications (Gandara and Truelove, 1999). This type of tooth wear can be seen on nonfunctional surfaces and can result in the loss of dental anatomy such as occlusal grooves, cusps, and flat surfaces (Harpenau et al., 2011). Furthermore, loss of enamel can lead to dentin exposure and hypersensitivity, even progressing as far as resulting in pulp exposure in some extreme cases (Gandara and Truelove, 1999).

Radiographic findings of erosion

The findings appear as radiolucent defects on the crown with well-defined or diffused margins (Lam, 2009) (Figure 10.6).

Clinical management of erosion

The clinical signs of dental erosion are initially subtle and the patient remains asymptomatic, unaware, and uninformed (Curtis et al., 2011). However, more advanced situations may require endodontic therapy. Therefore, early detection of the potential causes (such as part of the dietary analysis of high-risk individuals) and the prevention and modification of behavioral factors of dental erosion is an essential component of managing this condition. With restorative treatment of erosion, esthetic consequences can be addressed. However, without eliminating the cause of the erosion, the destructive process will likely to continue.

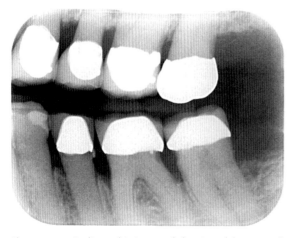

Figure 10.5 Radiographic image of abrasion of the cervical areas of mandibular left molars, evident from excessive and improper use of dental floss. Courtesy of Dr. N. Singh.

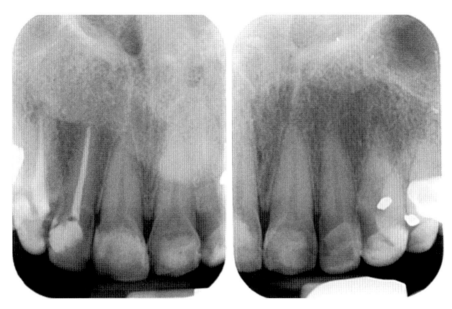

Figure 10.6   Radiographic image of erosion of the cervical areas of maxillary incisors.

Abfraction

Abfraction (from the Latin words "ab," or away, and "fractio," or breaking) is the loss of cervical tooth structure caused by tensile and compressive forces during tooth flexure at a location away from loading (Figure 10.7). These biomechanical loading forces exerted on the teeth can be static, as in swallowing and clenching, or they can be cyclic as in chewing (Grippo, 1991). The clinical appearance of abfraction is a deep, narrow, V-shaped notch in the cervical area (facial aspect) which often affect a single tooth with excursive interferences or eccentric occlusal loads (Harpenau et al., 2011). There is a controversy over abfraction being a distinct clinical entity or a primary factor in cervical lesions (Litonjua et al., 2003). Regardless, abfraction might potentiate wear by abrasion and/or erosion (Addy and Shellis, 2006).

Resorption

Root resorption is the loss of dental hard tissues as a result of clastic activities that is physiological in the primary dentition and a pathologic phenomenon in the permanent dentition (Patel et al., 2010).

Based on the location, root resorption can be classified to internal and external.

Internal root resorption

Internal root resorption is an inflammatory condition that results in the progressive destruction of the internal aspect of the root and dentinal tubules along the middle and apical thirds of the canal walls without adjunctive deposition of hard tissues adjacent to the resorptive sites (Patel et al., 2010). It involves an elaborate interaction between inflammatory cells, resorbing cells, and hard tissue structures (Ne et al., 1999). Histological findings include inflammation of pulpal tissues with the inflammatory infiltrate consisting predominantly of lymphocytes and macrophages, with some neutrophils, dilated blood vessels, and the presence of numerous, large, multinucleated odontoclasts occupying resorption lacunae on the canal walls. The coronal pulp would become necrotic with bacteria being evident either in the necrotic coronal pulp tissue or within the dentinal tubules adjacent to the lesion (Wedenberg and Zetterqvist, 1987). A prerequirement is the disruption of the odontoblast layer and predentin so that the activated clastic cells can

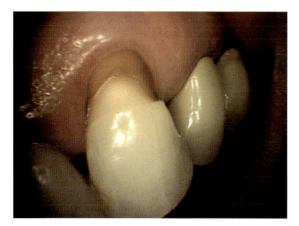

Figure 10.7 Clinical image of abfraction on maxillary left canine. Courtesy of Dr. N. Singh.

adhere to the intraradicular mineralized dentin (Masterton, 1965). A subgroup of internal root resorption is internal replacement resorption, which is defined as the resorption of the intraradicular dentin accompanied by subsequent deposition of a metaplastic bone/cementum-like tissues instead of true dentin (Patel et al., 2010).

Clinical findings of internal root resorption

Internal root resorption can be asymptomatic until the destruction process has advanced significantly, resulting in a perforation. In such a case, necrosis and infection of the entire pulp and symptoms of acute or chronic apical periodontitis can be noticed (Frank and Weine, 1973). In the coronal third of the root canal, internal resorption extending into dentin can exhibit the appearance of pink spot discoloration. However, these pink spots are more commonly seen in cases of external cervical root resorption (see below) (Patel et al., 2009).

Radiographic findings of internal root resorption

The radiographic appearance of internal root resorption is a localized oval-shaped radiolucent enlargement within the pulp chamber that is continuous with the image of the pulp chamber or root canal space (Ne et al., 1999; Patel et al., 2010). Therefore, the pulp chamber or root canal outline cannot be followed through the lesion since the

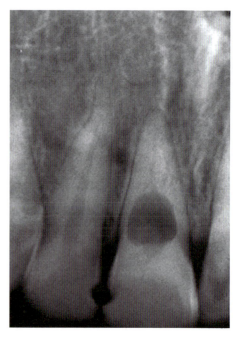

Figure 10.8 Radiographic image of maxillary right central incisor with internal root resorption centered in the root canal system. Note that the radiolucent lesion is continuous with the image of the root canal space and the root canal outline cannot be followed through the lesion. Courtesy of Dr. E. Basrani.

canal walls essentially balloon out (Gartner et al., 1976). In case of an internal root canal replacement resorption, the radiographic feature is an irregular radiographic enlargement of the pulp chamber, with discontinuity of the normal canal space. A fuzzy-appearing material of mild to moderate radiodensity causes the obliteration of canal space (Oehlers, 1951; Patel et al., 2010) (Figure 10.8).

Clinical management of internal root resorption

The resorbing cells in internal resorption are pulpal in origin (Fuss et al., 2003). Therefore, if the tooth is deemed restorable and has a reasonable prognosis, then nonsurgical root canal treatment (with interim calcium hydroxide medication and warm obturation technique) is the treatment of choice. The prognosis varies. It can be from poor (25%) in the presence of perforation to good/excellent (85–95%) in the absence of perforation (Caliskan and Turkun, 1997). However, if the internal resorption has rendered the tooth untreatable or unrestorable, extraction is the only treatment option (Patel et al., 2010).

External root resorption

The mechanisms of external root resorption require injury to precementum such as mechanical damage following dental trauma, surgical procedures, and excessive pressure of an impacted tooth or tumor. However, if the initial resorptive process is followed by bacterial stimulation originating from the periodontal sulcus, the stimulation of resorptive cell would be continued, resulting in external root resorption (Kim and Yang, 2011). External root resorption may be divided into four categories: (1) surface (transient) resorption; (2) progressive inflammatory resorption; (3) cervical resorption; and (4) replacement resorption.

Surface (transient) resorption

The initial injury to precemetum may cause a physiological process called surface resorption. Surface resorption cause small superficial defects in the cementum and small amount of underlying dentin. Without further bacterial stimulation, the resorption process is transient and self-limiting and would stop within 2–3 weeks, when the stimulation of resorptive cell stops. The surface resorption would then undergo repair by deposition of new cementum-like tissue. Surface resorption occurs frequently on traumatized roots and teeth undergoing orthodontic or periodontic without any clinical importance Radiographically, this type of resorption is difficult to observe, and there is generally no (or only slight) changes in the appearance of root. The periodontal membrane and lamina dura remain intact with no radiolucency (Heithersay, 2007).

Progressive inflammatory resorption

Progressive external inflammatory resorption has mainly an orthodontic or endodontic origin. External root resorption associated with orthodontic treatment is related to tissue pressure and should stop once the orthodontic forces are removed (Tronstad, 1988) (Figure 10.9). Therefore, no end-

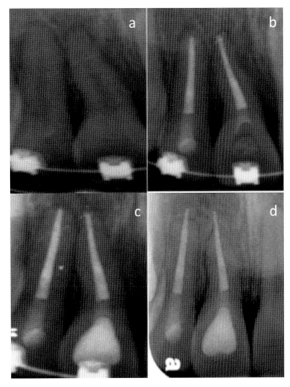

Figure 10.9 External root resorption of maxillary left central and lateral incisors due to orthodontic forces. Courtesy of Dr. M. Rampado.

odontic or operative treatment is necessary once the source of pressure is removed (Fuss et al., 2003).

However, as an endodontic problem, the resorption is related to infection and is seen in teeth with apical periodontitis or in dental trauma. In particular, in luxated teeth, the root resorption is initiated by mechanical trauma, resulting in removal of cementoblasts, precementum, and sometimes cementum. The resorption can be sustained by microbial stimuli from the infected root canal. In such cases, the endodontic treatment is necessary to remove the irritants from the root canal, thus arresting the external inflammatory resorption (Tronstad, 1988).

Clinical findings of external root resorption
Clinically, teeth with external root resorption are usually not symptomatic in the early stages. Therefore, external root resorption is often only detected during routine radiographic examination. As the process progresses, teeth may become symptomatic

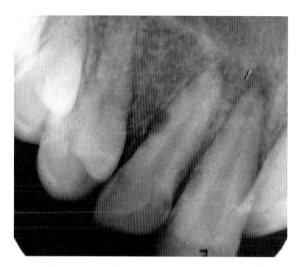

Figure 10.10   External root resorption of maxillary right lateral incisor. Note the undistorted root canal outline. Courtesy of Dr. M Sheikhnezami.

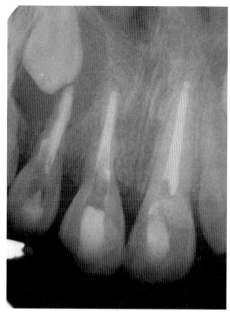

Figure 10.11   External root resorption of maxillary right lateral incisor due to the pressure from impacted canine. Courtesy of Dr. M. Sheikhnezami.

and periradicular abscesses may develop with increasing tooth mobility (Fuss et al., 2003). If external root resorption is undiagnosed and is allowed to progress due to sustained infection, the tooth can be destroyed within months (Tronstad, 1988).

Radiographic findings of external root resorption
The radiographic changes can be seen after a few weeks of clastic activity as periradicular radiolucent areas encompassing areas of the root and the adjacent alveolar bone (Tronstad, 1988). In contrast to internal root resorption, the root canal outline is undistorted and can be traced within the radiolucent lesion because the lesion is superimposed over the root canal. Similarly, with an angled radiograph, the radiolucent lesion would shift, making it distinguishable from internal root resorption (Figure 10.10). When the cause of resorption is due to pressure from impacted tooth, usually maxillary canines affecting lateral incisors (Figure 10.11) and mandibular third molars affecting mandibular second molars (Fuss et al., 2003), or from a tumor (where expansion is slow as is the case with cysts, ameloblastomas, giant cell tumors, and fiber–osseous lesions) (Tronstad, 1988), radiographically, the resorption area is located adjacent to the stimulation factor and is filled with the impacted tooth or the tumor. However, no radiolucent areas can be seen since no infection is involved in the etiological process (Fuss et al., 2003).

Clinical management of external root resorption
Endodontic treatment with long-term calcium hydroxide intracanal medication is the method of choice to remove the irritants from the root canal and to arrest the external inflammatory resorption (Flores et al., 2007). Calcium hydroxide is used to kill bacteria, to favorably influence the local environment at the resorption sites (through the dentinal tubules) by increasing the pH at the site, to inhibit the activity of osteoclastic acid hydrolases in the periodontal tissues, and hence, to prevent a continuation of the external resorptive process. When a continuous PDL space is observed radiographically along the root (in 6–12 months), the root canal is then permanently obturated (Tronstad, 1988).

Cervical root resorption

Cervical resorption is an inflammatory process that follows the injury to the cervical attachment apparatus, in particular below the epithelial attachment (Tronstad, 1988). The source of injury can be dental trauma, chemical irritation caused by bleaching agents, orthodontic treatment, periodontal procedures, or other factors such as bruxism, intracoronal restorations, developmental defects, or systemic diseases (Patel et al., 2009). This unprotected or altered root surface can attract hard tissue-resorbing cells and an inflammatory response maintained by bacterial infection in the gingival sulcus and the surface of the tooth. The pulp tissue is not involved (Tronstad, 1988).

Clinical findings of cervical root resorption
The clinical presentation of cervical root resorption varies considerably depending on the extent of the resorptive process (Heithersay, 2004). Clinically, teeth with cervical root resorption are usually not symptomatic in the early period of the process since the pulp tissue does not play a role in the pathogenesis. Therefore, sensitivity tests are normal, except in very advanced cases where the root canal is perforated and pulp is exposed (Patel et al., 2009). Resorption starts on the root surface in a small denuded area, but when the predentin is reached, the process is resisted (Wedenberg, 1987). Therefore, instead of perforating the canal, the resorptive process spreads around the root in an irregular fashion, proceeding laterally and in an apical and coronal direction, to envelop the root canal (Fuss et al., 2003). In a long-standing resorption that reaches a supragingival area of the crown, granulation tissue of resorption lacunae can be seen through enamel, showing the pink spot discoloration at the crown (Tronstad, 1988)

Radiographic findings of cervical root resorption
Usually, cervical root resorption is detected as a chance radiologic finding because the tooth is usually asymptomatic (Patel et al., 2009). The radiographic finding is a single resorption lacuna in the cervical area of the tooth (Tronstad, 1988). With time, radiolucency may be observed at the alveolar bone adjacent to the resorption lacuna of the dentin (Fuss et al., 2003). Cervical root resorptions are often misdiagnosed as internal root resorption, especially if they are accessible by probing and are projected radiologically over the root canal (Patel et al., 2010). Cervical root resorptions have borders that are ill-defined and asymmetrical, with radiodensity variations within the lesion (mottled appearance in advanced lesions due to deposition of calcified reparative tissue within the lesion [Patel et al., 2009]). In contrast to internal root resorption, the root canal outline is undistorted and can be clearly traced within the

radiolucent lesion because the pulp is not involved and the lesion is superimposed over the root canal. Similarly, with an angled radiograph, the radiolucent lesion would shift, making it distinguishable from internal root resorption (Figure 10.12).

Clinical management of cervical root resorption
Treatment is to expose the resorption lacuna, either surgically or orthodontically, and to remove the granulation tissue. The resorptive defect will then be prepared and restored. If a perforation to the root canal has occurred, then endodontic treatment is necessary (Tronstad, 1988).

Replacement resorption (ankylosis)

Dentoalveolar ankylosis is a loss of cementum, dentin, and PDL with the ingrowth and fusion of bone into the root defect. It is most often seen as a complication to luxation injuries (in particular in avulsed teeth with long extra-alveolar times) and occurs after extensive necrosis of the PDL with formation of bone onto a denuded area of the root surface. If less than 20% of the root surface is involved, reversal of ankylosis may occur. If not, ankylosed teeth are incorporated in the alveolar bone and will become part of the normal remodeling process of the bone; that is, they will gradually resorb and be replaced by bone (Tronstad, 1988).

Clinical findings of replacement resorption
There is a lack of physiological mobility of involved teeth and a metallic percussion sound (Tronstad, 1988). With time, the involved tooth will be infra-occluded (Fuss et al., 2003).

Radiographic findings of replacement resorption
The radiographic findings are the absence of PDL space. The resorption lacuna is filled with remodeled bone that will give the tooth a characteristic moth-eaten appearance due to the ingrowth of bone into dental tissues (Tronstad, 1988). With time, the entire root will be replaced by bone (Fuss et al., 2003) (Figure 10.13).

Clinical management of replacement resorption
Currently, there is no particular treatment. Over time (after years or decades), the crown will break at the gingival crest and fall out (Tronstad, 1988).

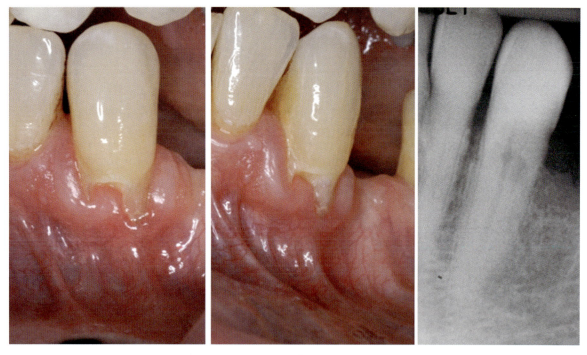

Figure 10.12 Clinical and radiographic images of external cervical resorption of mandibular left canine. Note the undistorted root canal outline. Courtesy of Dr. D. Chvartszaid.

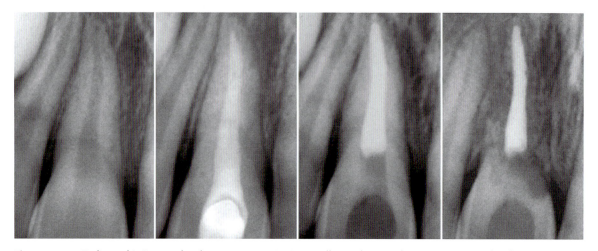

Figure 10.13 Radiographic image of replacement resorption in maxillary right central incisor 3.5 years after the occurrence of trauma. Note the replacement of dental hard tissue with remodeled bone and the remnants of the root filling material. Courtesy of Dr. S. Friedman.

Pulp stone

Pulp stones are discrete physiologic and dystrophic calcifications. Pulp stones can be classified based on their structure as true stones (made of dentine and lined by odontoblasts) and false stones (made of degenerating cells which mineralize) and based on their location as embedded in dentinal wall, adherent to dentinal wall, and free stones within the pulp tissue proper (Goga et al., 2008). They usually occur in the pulp horns and only occasionally in the region of the root canals (Bevelander and Johnson, 1956). The prevalence of pulp stone can be close to 100%, particularly in carious or restored permanent first molars (Goga et al., 2008). In a single tooth, there is a great variation in the number of pulp stones (0 to more than 12) (Bevelander and Johnson, 1956). They also vary in size from 50 μm in diameter to several millimeters when they may occlude the entire pulp chamber (Sayegh and Reed, 1968).

Clinical findings of pulp stones

Pulp stones are not clinically discernible. Moreover, the exact cause of pulp calcifications is not clear (Goga et al., 2008). Periodontal disease (Rubach and Mitchell, 1965), dental caries (Sayegh and Reed, 1968), operative procedure (Sundell et al., 1968), long-term tablet fluoridation (Holtgrave et al., 2001), and cardiovascular diseases (Edds et al., 2005) have been suggested as possible causes, but there is no clear evidence on the cause of this condition.

Radiographic findings of pulp stones

On radiographs, they can be seen as radiopaque structures with a great variation on number, shape, or outline. They can be seen in any type of tooth but significantly higher in molars (Gulsahi et al., 2009; Nayak et al., 2010; Ranjitkar et al., 2002) (Figure 10.14).

Clinical management of pulp stones

There is no clinical significance to pulp stones except the possibility of hindering access to root

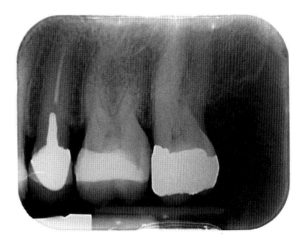

Figure 10.14   Radiographic images of pulp stone in a maxillary left second molar. Note the radiopaque stone within the pulp chamber and the obliterated root canal space.

canals during root canal treatment by blocking access to canal orifices, and altering the internal anatomy. Therefore, the finding of a pulp stone should not be interpreted as a disorder and hence, in the absence of any other sign and symptom, no treatment is necessary (Goga et al., 2008). If the root canal treatment is indicated for other reasons, the pulp stone can be dissected out using burs or ultrasonic tips.

Hypercementosis

Hypercementosis is a non-neoplastic condition, defined as accumulation of excessive cementum in continuation with the normal radicular cementum (Napier Souza et al., 2004). In most cases, its cause is unknown. The origin of hypercementosis has been attributed to the following factors (Pinheiro et al., 2008):

1. Functional stress due to occlusion forces
2. Continuous dental eruption
3. Incorporation of periodontal cementicles during physiological cementum deposition
4. Reactionary deposition in response to periapical inflammatory processes
5. Systemic factors such as atherosclerosis, acromegaly, deforming arthritis, hypertrophic arthritis, thyroid diseases, and Paget's disease.

Clinical findings of hypercementosis

There is no clinical sign or symptoms. The presence of hypercementosis might lead to an abnormal thickness of the root apex that becomes round-shaped and/or with the root appearance being altered macroscopically (Pinheiro et al., 2008).

Radiographic findings of hypercementosis

Hypercementosis is an incidental finding in radiographic examination and can be seen as a large mass of cementum around root. A radiolucent shadow of the periodontal membrane and the radiopaque lamina dura at the outer border of hypercementosis are consistent findings (Napier Souza et al., 2004).

Clinical management of hypercementosis

There is no clinical significance to hypercementosis except the possibility of difficulty extracting such teeth. In such cases, prior sectioning of the teeth may be required. Hypercementosis should not be interpreted as a disorder and hence, in the absence of any other signs and symptoms, no treatment is necessary.

Conclusion

The knowledge of the lesions that can be acquired after the eruption of the tooth is important for dentists. While some of these lesions may not have a significant clinical impact in endodontics, in contrast, some may jeopardize the tooth and cause tooth loss.

References

Addy, M. and Shellis, R.P. (2006) Interaction between attrition,abrasion and erosion in tooth wear. *Monogr Oral Sci*, 20, 17–31.

Begg, P.R. (1938) Progress report of observations on attrition of the teeth in its relations to pyorrhoea and tooth decay. *Austr J Dent*, 42, 315–320.

Berry, D.C. and Poole, D.F. (1976) Attrition: possible mechanisms of compensation. *J Oral Rehabil*, 3, 201–206.

Bevelander, G. and Johnson, P.L. (1956) Histogenesis and histochemistry of pulpal calcification. *J Dent Res*, 35, 714–722.

Caliskan, M.K. and Turkun, M. (1997) Prognosis of permanent teeth with internal resorption: a clinical review. *Endod Dent Traumatol*, 13, 75–81.

Curtis, D.A., Jayanetti, J., Chu, R., and Staninec, M. (2011) Decision-making in the management of the patient with dental erosion. *J Calif Dent Assoc*, 39, 259–265.

Dietschi, D. and Argente, A. (2011) A comprehensive and conservative approach for the restoration of abrasion and erosion: Part I: concepts and clinical rationale for early intervention using adhesive techniques. *Eur J Esthet Dent*, 6, 20–33.

Edds, A.C., Walden, J.E., Scheetz, J.P., Goldsmith, L.J., Drisko, C.L., and Eleazer, P.D. (2005) Pilot study of correlation of pulp stones with cardiovascular disease. *J Endod*, 31, 504–506.

Flores, M.T., Andersson, L., Andreasen, J.O., Bakland, L.K., Malmgren, B., Barnett, F., Bourguignon, C., Diangelis, A., Hicks, L., Sigurdsson, A., Trope, M., Tsukiboshi, M., and Von Arx, T. (2007) Guidelines for the management of traumatic dental injuries: II. Avulsion of permanent teeth. *Dent Traumatol*, 23, 130–136.

Frank, A.L. and Weine, F.S. (1973) Nonsurgical therapy for the perforative defect of internal resorption. *J Am Dent Assoc*, 87, 863–868.

Fuss, Z., Tsesis, I., and Lin, S. (2003) Root resorption—diagnosis, classification and treatment choices based on stimulation factors. *Dent Traumatol*, 19, 175–182.

Gandara, B.K. and Truelove, E.L. (1999) Diagnosis and management of dental erosion. *J Contemp Dent Pract*, 1, 16–23.

Gartner, A.H., Mack, T., Somerlott, R.G., and Walsh, L.C. (1976) Differential diagnosis of internal and external root resorption. *J Endod*, 2, 329–334.

Gillette, W.B. and Van House, R.L. (1980) Ill effects of improper oral hygeine procedure. *J Am Dent Assoc*, 101, 476–480.

Goga, R., Chandler, N.P., and Oginni, A.O. (2008) Pulp stones: a review. *Int Endod J*, 41, 457–468.

Grippo, J.O. (1991) Abfractions: a new classification of hard tissue lesions of teeth. *J Esthet Dent*, 3, 14–19.

Grippo, J.O., Simring, M., and Schreiner, S. (2004) Attrition, abrasion, corrosion and abfraction revisited: a new perspective on tooth surface lesions. *J Am Dent Assoc*, 135, 1109–1118; quiz 1163–5.

Gulsahi, A., Cebeci, A.I., and Ozden, S. (2009) A radiographic assessment of the prevalence of pulp stones in a group of Turkish dental patients. *Int Endod J*, 42, 735–739.

Harpenau, L.A., Noble, W.H., and Kao, R.T. (2011) Diagnosis and management of dental wear. *J Calif Dent Assoc*, 39, 225–231.

Heithersay, G.S. (2004) Invasive cervical resorption. *Endodontic Topics*, 7, 73–92.

Heithersay, G.S. (2007) Management of tooth resorption. *Aust Dent J*, 52, S105–S121.

Holtgrave, E.A., Hopfenmuller, W., and Ammar, S. (2001) Tablet fluoridation influences the calcification of primary tooth pulp. *J Orofac Orthop*, 62, 22–35.

Hugoson, A., Bergendal, T., Ekfeldt, A., and Helkimo, M. (1988) Prevalence and severity of incisal and occlusal tooth wear in an adult Swedish population. *Acta Odontol Scand*, 46, 255–265.

Ingle, J.I. (1960) Alveolar osteoporosis and pulpal death associated with compulsive bruxism. *Oral Surg Oral Med Oral Pathol*, 13, 1371–1381.

Johansson, A. (1992) A cross-cultural study of occlusal tooth wear. *Swed Dent J Suppl*, 86, 1–59.

Ketterl, W. (1983) Age-induced changes in the teeth and their attachment apparatus. *Int Dent J*, 33, 262–271.

Kim, S.Y. and Yang, S.E. (2011) Surgical repair of external inflammatory root resorption with resin-modified glass ionomer cement. *Oral Surg Oral Med Oral Pathol Oral Radiol Endod*, 111, e33–e36.

Lam, E. (2009) Chapter 19: Dental anomalies. In: S.C. White and M.J. Pharoah, eds., *Oral Radiology: Principles and Interpretation*, 6th ed. Mosby/Elsevier, St. Louis, MO.

Litonjua, L.A., Andreana, S., Bush, P.J., Tobias, T.S., and Cohen, R.E. (2003) Noncarious cervical lesions and abfractions: a re-evaluation. *J Am Dent Assoc*, 134, 845–850.

Litonjua, L.A., Andreana, S., Bush, P.J., Tobias, T.S., and Cohen, R.E. (2004) Wedged cervical lesions produced by toothbrushing. *Am J Dent*, 17, 237–240.

Masterton, J.B. (1965) Internal resorption of the dentine; a complication arising from unhealed pulp wounds. *Br Dent J*, 118, 241–249.

Meister, F., JR, Braun, R.J., and Gerstein, H. (1980) Endodontic involvement resulting from dental abrasion or erosion. *J Am Dent Assoc*, 101, 651–653.

Miller, W.D. (1907) Experiments and observations on the wasting of tooth tissue variously designated as erosion, abrasion, chemical abrasion, denudation, etc. *Dent Cosmos*, 49, 109–124.

Napier Souza, L., Monteiro Lima Junior, S., Garcia Santos Pimenta, F.J., Rodrigues Antunes Souza, A.C., and Santiago Gomez, R. (2004) Atypical hypercementosis versus cementoblastoma. *Dentomaxillofac Radiol*, 33, 267–270.

Nayak, M., Kumar, J., and Prasad, L.K. (2010) A radiographic correlation between systemic disorders and pulp stones. *Indian J Dent Res*, 21, 369–373.

Ne, R.F., Witherspoon, D.E., and Gutmann, J.L. (1999) Tooth resorption. *Quintessence Int*, 30, 9–25.

Newman, H.N. (1999) Attrition, eruption, and the periodontium. *J Dent Res*, 78, 730–734.

Oehlers, F.A. (1951) A case of internal resorption following injury. *Br Dent J*, 90, 13–16.

Patel, S., Kanagasingam, S., and Pitt Ford, T. (2009) External cervical resorption: a review. *J Endod*, 35, 616–625.

Patel, S., Ricucci, D., Durak, C., and Tay, F. (2010) Internal root resorption: a review. *J Endod*, 36, 1107–1121.

Pinheiro, B.C., Pinheiro, T.N., Capelozza, A.L., and Consolaro, A. (2008) A scanning electron microscopic study of hypercementosis. *J Appl Oral Sci*, 16, 380–384.

Ranjitkar, S., Taylor, J.A., and Townsend, G.C. (2002) A radiographic assessment of the prevalence of pulp stones in Australians. *Aust Dent J*, 47, 36–40.

Rubach, W.C. and Mitchell, D.F. (1965) Periodontal disease, accessory canals and pulp pathosis. *J Periodontol*, 36, 34–38.

Sayegh, F.S. and Reed, A.J. (1968) Calcification in the dental pulp. *Oral Surg Oral Med Oral Pathol*, 25, 873–882.

Seligman, D.A., Pullinger, A.G., and Solberg, W.K. (1988) The prevalence of dental attrition and its association with factors of age, gender, occlusion, and TMJ symptomatology. *J Dent Res*, 67, 1323–1333.

Sundell, J.R., Stanley, H.R., and White, C.L. (1968) The relationship of coronal pulp stone formation to experimental operative procedures. *Oral Surg Oral Med Oral Pathol*, 25, 579–589.

Tronstad, L. (1988) Root resorption—etiology, terminology and clinical manifestations. *Endod Dent Traumatol*, 4, 241–252.

Tsiggos, N., Tortopidis, D., Hatzikyriakos, A., and Menexes, G. (2008) Association between self-reported bruxism activity and occurrence of dental attrition, abfraction, and occlusal pits on natural teeth. *J Prosthet Dent*, 100, 41–46.

van 't Spijker, A., Kreulen, C.M., and Creugers, N.H. (2007) Attrition, occlusion, (dys)function, and intervention: a systematic review. *Clin Oral Implants Res*, 18(Suppl 3), 117–126.

Wang, X. and Lussi, A. (2010) Assessment and management of dental erosion. *Dent Clin North Am*, 54, 565–578.

Wedenberg, C. (1987) Evidence for a dentin-derived inhibitor of macrophage spreading. *Scand J Dent Res*, 95, 381–388.

Wedenberg, C. and Zetterqvist, L. (1987) Internal resorption in human teeth—a histological, scanning electron microscopic, and enzyme histochemical study. *J Endod*, 13, 255–259.

11 Radiographic Analysis of Periodontal and Endodontic Lesions

Jim Yuan Lai and Bettina Basrani

Introduction

The periodontium is a group of tissues that are involved with the support of the tooth. The tissues are the gingiva, alveolar mucosa, cementum, periodontal ligament, and alveolar and supporting bone (American Academy of Periodontology, 2001). The periodontal ligament space, alveolar bone, and supporting bone are visible radiographically. Radiographs provide important information and are an essential component of a comprehensive periodontal examination.

Normal anatomy of alveolar process and periodontal ligament

Lamina dura

The alveolar process is the bone that houses the tooth and is connected to the basal jaw bone. The alveolar process is composed of the outer cortical plate, the spongiosa which is trabecular or cancellous bone, and an inner cortical plate that faces the tooth which is known as the alveolar bone.

The alveolar bone is identified as the lamina dura radiographically. The lamina dura is a thin well-defined radiopaque line that is continuous around each tooth (Figure 11.1). The appearance of the lamina dura may vary where it may be diffuse or absent. This may be due to the X-ray beam being directed more obliquely or due to superimpositions of various structures. Teeth subjected to heavier occlusal forces may have a wider and denser lamina dura (White and Pharoah, 2009).

Alveolar crest

The alveolar crest is formed where the outer cortical bone meets the alveolar bone. For the first three phases of passive eruption, a histologic study of clinically normal human jaws reported the distance from cementoenamel junction to the alveolar crest ranged (Gargiulo et al., 1961):

- Phase I: 0.04 mm to 3.36 mm (average = 1.08 mm)
- Phase II: 0.35 mm to 5.00 mm (average = 1.55 mm)
- Phase III: 0.88 mm to 3.20 mm (average = 1.71 mm)

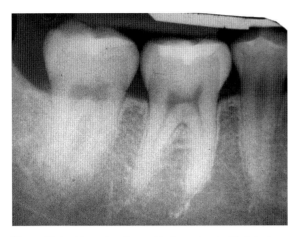

Figure 11.1   Normal radiographic bone level with intact lamina dura.

Some studies have defined the presence of periodontitis if the distance was ≥1 mm while other studies had a threshold of ≥2 mm or ≥3 mm. Recognizing that there is a normal variation, the general consensus is the normal distance from the cementoenamel junction to the alveolar crest is 2.0 mm (Figure 11.1) (Armitage, 1996, Tetradis et al., 2006). The distance may be greater in older patients.

The shape and width of the alveolar crest or interdental septum is dictated by the convexity of the proximal tooth surface and the level of the cementoenamel junction of the adjacent teeth. In the anterior region, the alveolar crest comes to a point due to the close proximity of the teeth. In the posterior region where the interdental space is greater, the alveolar crest is broader and flatter. The angulation of the alveolar crest parallels a line connecting the cementoenamel junction of the adjacent teeth (Ritchey and Orban, 1953).

In a normal and healthy periodontium, the alveolar crest is a thin, continuous radiopaque line that is continuous with the lamina dura (Figure 11.1). Where the alveolar crest meets the lamina dura, the angle is a defined sharp angle (White and Pharoah, 2009).

Periodontal ligament space

The principal tissues involved with attachment of the tooth to the jaw can be divided into two parts.

The soft tissue attachment are gingival fibers inserting into the cementum of the tooth and are not visible radiographically. The second part are periodontal ligament fibers that connect from the cementum to the alveolar bone. The periodontal ligament fibers are primarily collagen fibers, so they are not visible radiographically. The periodontal ligament space, which these fibers occupy, is a narrow radiolucent structure that is delineated by two radiopaque structures, the alveolar bone and tooth root.

The width of the periodontal ligament is 0.15 mm to 0.38 mm. The narrowest portion is around the middle third of the root while the ligament is the widest at the cervical aspect (Coolidge, 1937). Consequently, the periodontal ligament space is wider at the alveolar crest, narrows at the middle third, and then widens again at the apex.

The periodontal ligament reacts to occlusal forces and is able to accommodate physiological forces. There is a thickening of the fiber bundles and consequently, the periodontal ligament space widens. For example, the width of the periodontal ligament in the middle of the alveolus of a premolar in heavy function increases from 0.10 mm to 0.28 mm (Kronfeld, 1931).

Radiographic appearance of periodontitis

Periodontitis is defined as inflammation of the supporting tissues of the teeth (American Academy of Periodontology, 2001). The inflammation results in the destruction of the alveolar bone, periodontal ligament, and the gingival connective tissue attachment. Periodontal pathogens such as *Porphyromonas gingivalis*, *Tannerella forsythia*, and *Aggregatibacter actinomycetemcomitans* initiate this disease but most of the destruction is the result of the host inflammatory response. There are different clinical forms of periodontitis. The most common form is chronic and aggressive periodontitis.

Radiographs are an important adjunct to a clinical examination. They provide useful information about the extent and location of bone loss that have occurred, the width of the periodontal ligament space, local factors such as subgingival calculus, restorations with open margins or overhangs, morphology and length of the root, and crown-to-root ratio (Perschbacher, 2009).

However, there are limitations to the use of radiographs. They only provide a two-dimensional view. Dense bone or the root structure can mask bone loss that has occurred on the facial or lingual surface. Interproximally, the true extent and morphology of interdental craters can be obscured by dense buccal and lingual cortical plates. Typically, there needs to be about 50% bone mineral lost before radiographic changes are detected (Ortman et al., 1982). Clinical attachment loss precedes radiographic evidence of crestal alveolar bone loss by 6–8 months (Goodson et al., 1984). In other words, radiographs underestimate the true extent of destruction that has occurred clinically.

Earliest signs of bone loss include the absence, fuzziness or a break in the crestal lamina dura that may indicate early radiographic changes in periodontitis (Tetradis et al., 2006). However, many stable sites lack an intact lamina dura (Rams et al., 1994). In other words, the absence of the lamina dura is not indicative of disease.

On the other hand, the presence of an intact lamina dura at the alveolar crest indicates a high probability that the site is periodontally stable (Armitage, 1996). If the lamina dura is intact at the apex of the tooth, this strongly suggests a vital pulp (White and Pharoah, 2009).

Other signs of early bone loss are the blunting of the alveolar crest in the anterior region and the rounding or loss of the sharp angle between the lamina dura and alveolar crest in the posterior region (Perschbacher, 2009).

Bone loss is defined when the alveolar crest is more than 2 mm apical to the cementoenamel junction. Bone loss occurs in a horizontal and vertical manner.

Horizontal bone loss is defined when the pattern of the bone loss continues to parallel the line connecting the cementoenamel junction between the adjacent teeth (Figures 11.2 and 11.3). In other words, the alveolar crest remains perpendicular to the root surface. There has been proportionately equal loss of interdental septa, buccal, and lingual bone.

Vertical or angular bone loss is the result of vertical defects where bone loss has occurred in an oblique manner. As a result, the alveolar crest is not parallel to the line between the cementoenamel junctions of the adjacent teeth. Vertical bone loss indicates the presence of vertical or angular osseous

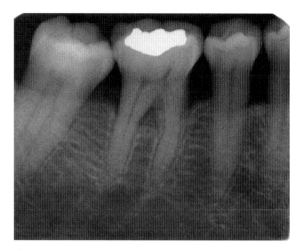

Figure 11.2   Moderate horizontal bone loss with radiolucency in the furcation of the mandibular first molar.

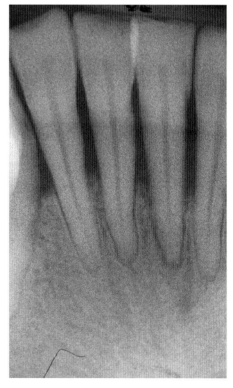

Figure 11.3   Advance horizontal bone loss.

defects where they may be classified as one-, two- and three-walled vertical defects (Figures 11.4 and 11.5).

Severity of the bone loss is based on the extent of bone loss in relationship to the amount of root that remains in the bone. If less than 20% of the root is exposed due to the bone loss, then the severity is described as mild. The severity is moderate when there has been 20–50% bone loss (Figures 11.2 and 11.4). Advance bone loss is when more than 50% bone loss has occurred (Figures 11.3 and 11.5). The severity describes the extent of osseous destruction which is one of the signs of periodontitis. For periodontitis, clinical attachment loss is used to describing severity of that specific disease entity.

When bone loss extends into the furcations of molars, often it is either the buccal or lingual plate that is destroyed. Consequently, the density of the bone between the roots of the molar is less. Sometimes, the furcation invasion in mandibular molars (Figure 11.2) and buccal furcation of the maxillary molars are visible radiographically as a clearly defined radiolucency between the roots.

Mesial and distal furcations of maxillary teeth are more difficult to detect due to the superimposition of the palatal root. These furcations may manifest as small triangular radiographic shadow over the mesial or distal roots known as furcation arrows (Figures 11.6 and 11.7) (Hardekopf et al., 1987).

Radiographs provide information on the amount of periodontal destruction, but it does not provide any information on the disease activity. The radiographic appearance may indicate past destruction with a current stable periodontium with the absence of any periodontitis. On the other hand, the same radiographic appearance may indicate destruction with active progressing disease. Attaining a proper diagnosis will require both radiographs and a comprehensive clinical examination.

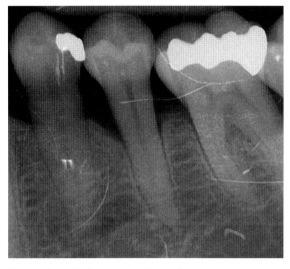

Figure 11.4 Moderate vertical bone loss on the mesial aspects of the mandibular second premolar.

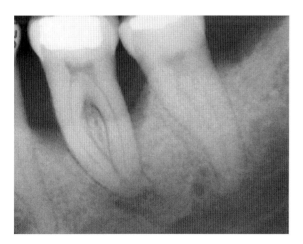

Figure 11.5 Advance vertical bone loss on the distal aspect of the mandibular first molar.

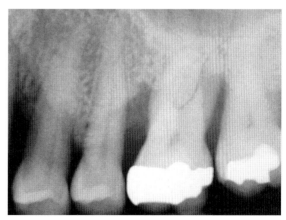

Figure 11.6 Furcation arrow present on the distal aspect of the maxillary first molar.

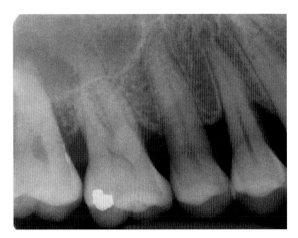

Figure 11.7 Furcation arrows present on the mesial and distal aspects of the maxillary first molar.

Radiographic appearance of endodontic infection and apical periodontitis

Endodontic infection arises when there is a lack of host defense in the root canal system and an invasion of bacteria. This may be due to pulp necrosis as a result of caries, trauma, or periodontal disease (Siqueira and Rocas, 2011).

Toxic metabolites that are expressed from the root apex can trigger a periapical inflammatory lesion. This lesion may be diagnosed as acute or chronic apical periodontitis, periapical abscess, or periapical granuloma.

The radiographic appearance of this lesion may be radiolucent which have been called rarefying osteitis or may be radiopaque which have been called sclerosing osteitis, condensing osteitis, and focal sclerosing osteitis (Lee, 2009).

In general, early signs of lesion may be the widening of the periodontal ligament or a break in the lamina dura. As the lesion evolves, it may become more radiolucent with an ill-defined border around the apex of the tooth or adjacent to a lateral or furcation canal (Berman and Hartwell, 2011). The lamina dura around the involved apex is not seen within the rarefying osteitis.

If the inflammatory lesion is confined to the cancellous bone, the lesion is not visible radiographically. The lesion is only visible radiographically when the lesion has eroded the junction area of the cortex and cancellous bone or perforated the cortex (Bender and Seltzer, 2003).

At other times, there may be sclerotic bone reaction where the lesion has denser and thicker than normal trabecular pattern.

Pulpal infection can drain through the periodontal ligament space and give an appearance of periodontal destruction, termed retrograde periodontitis. Similarly, both pulpal and periodontal infections can coexist in the same tooth, termed combined lesions, where the treatment depends on the degree of involvement of the tissues. Both endodontic and periodontal diseases are caused by a mixed anaerobic infection (Shenoy and Shenoy, 2010).

The most conventional classification used for endodontic-periodontal lesions was given by Simon et al. (1972a, 1972b), separating lesions involving both periodontal and pulpal tissues into the following groups:

1. Primary endodontic lesions
2. Primary endodontic lesions with secondary periodontal involvement
3. Primary periodontal lesions
4. Primary periodontal lesions with secondary endodontic involvement
5. True combined lesions
   a. Primary endodontic lesions
      An acute exacerbation of a chronic apical lesion on a tooth with a necrotic pulp may drain coronally through the periodontal ligament into the gingival sulcus. This condition may clinically mimic the presence of a periodontal abscess. In reality, however, it would be a sinus tract originating from the pulp that opens into the periodontal ligament. Primary endodontic lesions usually heal following root canal therapy. The sinus tract extending into the gingival sulcus or furcation area disappears at an early stage, if the necrotic pulp has been removed and the root canals are well sealed (Figure 11.8) (Rotstein and Simon, 2004).
   b. Primary endodontic lesions with secondary periodontal involvement
      If a primary endodontic lesion remains untreated, it may become secondarily involved with periodontal breakdown. Plaque accumulation at the gingival margin of the sinus tract leads to plaque-induced periodontitis in this area. When

plaque and calculus are detected, the treatment and prognosis of the teeth are different from those of the teeth involved with only endodontic disease. The tooth now requires both endodontic and periodontal

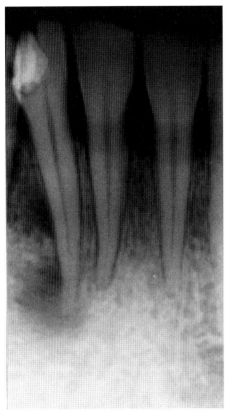

Figure 11.8   Primary endodontic lesion.

treatment. (Rotstein and Simon, 2004) (Figure 11.9).

c. Primary periodontal lesions
These lesions are caused primarily by periodontal pathogens. In this process, chronic periodontitis progresses apically along the root surface. In most cases, pulpal tests indicate a clinically normal pulpal reaction. There is frequently an accumulation of plaque and calculus and the presence of deep pockets may be detected (Figure 11.10).

d. Primary periodontal lesions with secondary endodontic involvement
The apical progression of a periodontal pocket may continue until the apical tissues are involved. In this case, the pulp may become necrotic as a result of infection entering through lateral canals or the apical foramen. In single-rooted teeth, the prognosis is usually poor. In molar teeth, the prognosis may be better. Since not all the roots may suffer the same loss of supporting tissue, root resection can be considered as a treatment alternative (Figure 11.11) (Raja Sunitha et al., 2008).

e. True combined lesions
True combined endodontic periodontal disease occurs less frequently than other endodontic-periodontal problems. It is formed when an endodontic lesion progressing coronally joins an infected periodontal pocket progressing apically. The degree of attachment loss in this type of

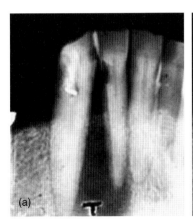
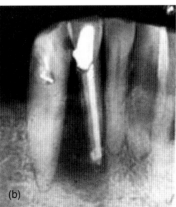
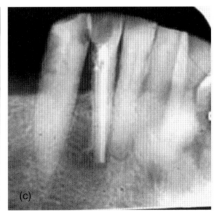

(a)   (b)   (c)

Figure 11.9   (a–c) Primary endodontic lesion with secondary periodontal involvement. (Courtesy of Dr S. Brayton.)

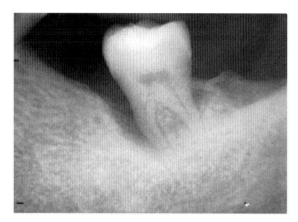

Figure 11.10   Primary periodontal lesion.

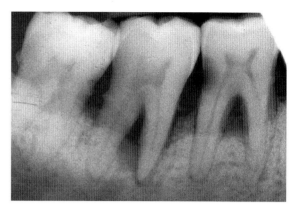

Figure 11.12   True combined lesion.

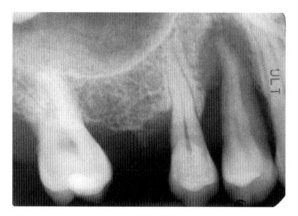

Figure 11.11   Primary periodontal lesion with secondary endodontic involvement.

lesion is invariably large and the prognosis guarded. This is particularly true in single-rooted teeth. In molar teeth, root resection can be an alternative treatment. The radiographic appearance of combined endodontic periodontal disease may be similar to that of a vertically fractured tooth. If a sinus tract is present, it may be necessary to raise a flap to determine the etiology of the lesion (Figure 11.12) (Simon et al., 1972a, 1972b).

Diagnosis of primary endodontic disease and primary periodontal disease usually present no clinical difficulty. In primary periodontal disease, the pulp is vital and is responsive to testing. In primary endodontic disease, the pulp is infected

and is nonvital. However, primary endodontic disease with secondary periodontal involvement, primary periodontal disease with secondary endodontic involvement, or true combined diseases are clinically and radiographically very similar. Accurate diagnosis can be achieved by careful history taking, visual examination, percussion and palpation, and the use of special tests.

Radiographs

Radiographic examination aids in detection of carious lesions, extensive or defective restorations, pulp caps, root fractures, periradicular radiolucencies, thickened periodontal ligament, and alveolar bone loss. Interpretation of early periapical or lateral lesions and early periodontal lesions is of clinical importance in suggesting the cause of the lesion and the proper diagnostic procedures to follow to confirm the cause. Often, the initial phases of periradicular bone resorption from endodontic origin are confined only to cancellous bone. Therefore, it cannot be detected unless the cortical bone is also affected. However, when there is radiographic evidence that bone loss extends from the level of crestal bone to or near the apex of the tooth, the radiograph is of little value in determining the cause.

Fistula tracking

Endodontic or periodontal disease may sometimes develop a fistulous sinus track. Inflammatory exu-

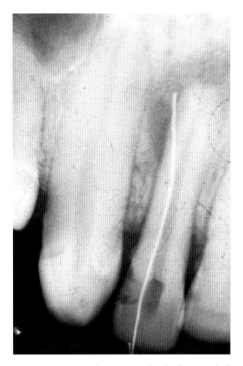

Figure 11.13   Sinus track tracing a fistula from endodontic origin.

dates may often travel through tissues and structures of minor resistance and open anywhere on the oral mucosa or facial skin. Intraorally, the opening is usually visible on the attached buccal gingiva or in the vestibule. Fistula tracking is done by inserting a semirigid radiopaque material into the sinus track until resistance is met. Commonly used materials include gutta-percha cones. A radiograph is then taken, which reveals the course of the sinus tract and the origin of the inflammatory process (Figure 11.13).

Differential diagnosis

Radicular lingual groove

Maxillary incisors are susceptible to developmental anomalies that can lead to periodontal and/or endodontic problems. One such developmental anomaly is the radicular lingual groove (RLG), which is often associated with incorrect diagnosis

and subsequent treatment failure. Radicular lingual grooves have also been termed radicular palatal grooves, cingulo-radicular distolingual grooves, palatal gingival grooves, radicular grooves, and vertical development grooves. The RLG has a funnel-like shape and typically begins on the lingual surface at the level of the cingulum extending to various lengths along the root. The groove is a locus for plaque accumulation, which destroys the sulcular epithelium and deeper parts of the periodontium, finally resulting in the formation of a severely localized periodontal defect.

Radicular lingual grooves can initiate periodontal and pulpal involvement that can be difficult to diagnose and manage. However, if clinicians are aware of the forms in which the condition may occur and can apply the correct treatment modalities, a number of teeth with RLGs may be saved. Computer tomography can be used as a diagnostic tool (Figure 11.14) (More details in Chapter 5) (Gandhi et al., 2011)

Vertical root fracture

Vertical root fracture (VRF) in endodontically treated teeth is one of the most frustrating complications of root canal therapy, which results in tooth or root extraction. The VRF is a longitudinally oriented fracture of the root that originates from its apical end and propagates coronally and is defined as one of the crack types. VRF is usually diagnosed years after all endodontic and prosthetic procedures have been completed. The final diagnosis of VRF is at times complicated for lack of specific signs, symptoms, and/or radiographic features and because several etiologic factors might be involved. Thus, the differential diagnosis from other pathological entities might be difficult. It may mimic a perio and/or endo lesion (Figures 11.15 and 11.16A,B) (Tsesis et al. 2010).

Conclusion

The periodontal-endodontic lesion develops by extension of either periodontal destruction apically combining with an existing periapical lesion or an endodontic lesion marginally, combining with an

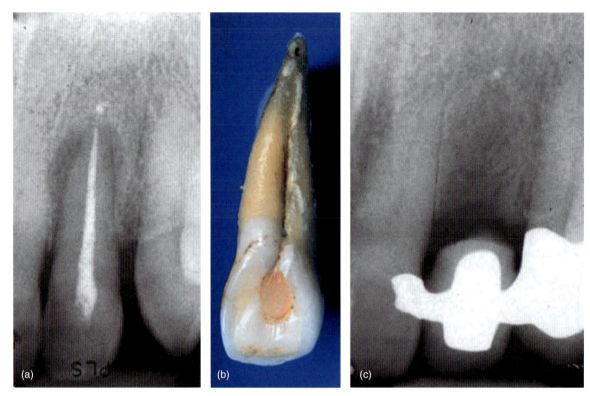

Figure 11.14 (a–c) Lingual groove in maxillary lateral incisor. Root canal was performed but the lesion did not heal; therefore, extraction and replacement was done.

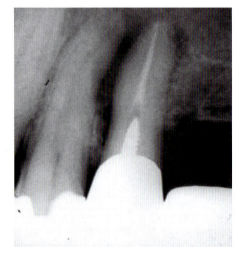

Figure 11.15 Lateral rarefaction in maxillary premolar suggesting a vertical root fracture.

existing periodontal lesion. From the diagnostic point of view, it is important to realize that as long as the pulp remains vital, although inflamed or scarred, it is unlikely to produce irritants that are sufficient to cause pronounced marginal breakdown of the periodontium. Treatment of combined endodontic and periodontal lesions does not differ from the treatment given when the two disorders occur separately. The part of the lesion sustained by the root canal infection can usually be expected to resolve after proper endodontic treatment. The part of the lesion caused by the plaque infection may also heal following periodontal therapy, although little or no regeneration of the attachment apparatus can be expected. This suggests that the larger the part of the lesion caused by the root canal infection, the more favorable the prognosis is for regeneration of the attachment.

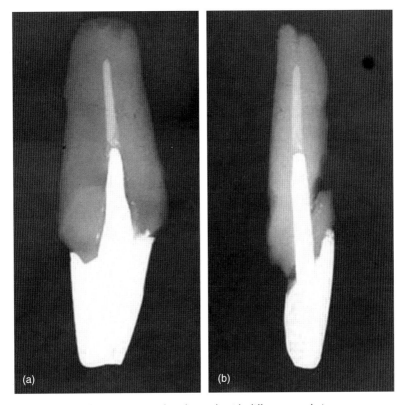

Figure 11.16   A and B. Vertical root fracture seen with radiograph with different angulations.

References

American Academy of Periodontology. (2001) *Glossary of Periodontal Terms*, 4th ed. The American Academy of Periodontology, Chicago, IL.

Armitage, G.C. (1996) Periodontal diseases: diagnosis. *Ann of Periodontol*, 1, 37–215.

Bender, I.B. and Seltzer, S. (2003) Roentgenographic and direct observation of experimental lesions in boneII.1961. *J Endod*, 29(11), 707–712.

Berman, L.H. and Hartwell, G.R. (2011) Diagnosis. In: K.M. Hargreaves and S. Cohen, eds., *Cohen's Pathways of the Pulp*, 10th ed. Elsevier Mosby, St. Louis, pp. 2–39.

Coolidge, E.D. (1937). The thickness of the human periodontal membrane. *J Am Dent Assoc Dent Cosmos*, 24, 1260–1270.

Gandhi, A., Kathuria, A., and Gandhi, T. (2011) Endodontic-periodontal management of two rooted maxillary lateral incisor associated with complex radicular lingual groove by using spiral computed tomography as a diagnostic aid: a case report. *Int Endod J*, 44(6), 574–582.

Gargiulo, A.W., Wentz, F.M., and Orban, B. (1961) Dimensions and relations of the dentogingival junction in humans. *J Clin Periodontol*, 32, 261–267.

Goodson, J.M., Haffajee, A.D., and Socransky, S.S. (1984) The relationship between attachment level loss and alveolar bone loss. *J Clin Periodontol*, 11(5), 348–359.

Hardekopf, J.D., Dunlap, R.M., Ahl, D.R., and Pelleu, G.B. (1987) The "furcation arrow." A reliable radiographic image? *J Clin Periodontol*, 58(4), 258–261.

Kronfeld, R. (1931) Histologic study of the influence of function on the human periodontal membrane. *J Am Dent Assoc*, 18, 1242–1274.

Lee, L. (2009) Inflammatory lesions of the jaws. In: S.C. White and M.J. Pharoah, eds., *Oral Radiology: Principles and Interpretation*, 6th ed. Mosby/Elsevier, St. Louis, pp. 282–294.

Ortman, L.F., McHenry, K., and Hausamann, E. (1982) Relationship between alveolar bone measured by 125I absorptiometry with analysis of standardized radiographs: 2. Bjorn technique. *J Clin Periodontol*, 53, 311–314.

Perschbacher, S. (2009) Periodontal diseases. In: S.C. White and M.J. Pharoah, eds., *Oral Radiology:*

Principles and Interpretation, 6th ed. Mosby/Elsevier, St. Louis, pp. 282–294.

Raja Sunitha, V., Emmadi, P., Namasivayam, A., Thyegarajan, R., and Rajaraman, V. (2008) The periodontal–endodontic continuum: a review. *J Conserv Dent*, 11(2), 54–62.

Rams, T.E., Listgarten, M.A., and Slots, J. (1994) Utility of radiographic crestal lamina dura for predicting periodontitis disease activity. *J Clin Periodontol*, 21(9), 571–576.

Ritchey, B. and Orban, B. (1953) The crests of the interdental speta. *J Clin Periodontol*, 24, 75–87.

Rotstein, I. and Simon, J.H. (2004) Diagnosis, prognosis and decision making in the treatment of combined periodontal-endodontic lesions. *Periodontol 2000*, 34, 265–303.

Shenoy, N. and Shenoy, A. (2010) Endo-perio lesions: diagnosis and clinical considerations. *Indian J Dent Res*, 21(4), 579–585.

Simon, J.H., Glick, D.H., and Frank, A.L. (1972a) The relationship of endodontic-periodontic lesions. *J Clin Periodontol*, 43, 202.

Simon, J.H., Glick, D.H., and Frank, A.L. (1972b) The relationship of endodontic-periodontic lesions. *J Periodontol*, 43, 202–208.

Siqueira, J.F. and Rocas, I.N. (2011) Microbiology and treatment of endodontic infections. In: K.M. Hargreaves and S. Cohen, eds., *Cohen's Pathways of the Pulp*, 10th ed. Elsevier Mosby, St. Louis, pp. 559–600.

Tetradis, S., Carranza, F.A., Fazio, R.C., and Takei, H.H. (2006) Radiographic aids in the diagnosis of periodontal disease. In: M.G. Newman, H.H. Takei, and P.R. Klokkevold, eds., *Carranza's Clinical Periodontology*, 10th ed. Saunders, St. Louis, pp. 561–578.

Tsesis, I., Rosen, E., Tamse, A., Taschieri, S., and Kfir, A. (2010) Diagnosis of vertical root fractures in endodontically treated teeth based on clinical and radiographic indices: a systematic review. *J Endod*, 36(9), 1455–1458.

White, S.C. and Pharoah, M.J. (2009) *Oral Radiology: Principles and Interpretation*, 6th ed. Mosby/Elsevier, St. Louis.

12 Radiographic Imaging in Implant Dentistry

Amir Azarpazhooh and Jim Yuan Lai

Discussion of this chapter is specifically focused on radiographic imaging of implant therapy for single tooth replacement or for a small partially edentulous span. The key to the successful outcome of implant dentistry is osseointegration. Osseointegration is where vital bone is in direct and intimate contact with the titanium surface of the dental implant (Adell et al., 1981).

Various success criteria have been developed that involve clinical and radiographic findings (Albrektsson et al., 1986; Buser et al., 1990; Mombelli and Lang, 1994). They include:

- No pain, discomfort, altered sensation or infection attributable to the implants
- Individual unattached implants are immobile when tested clinically
- No probing depth greater than 5 mm
- No probing depth of 5 mm with bleeding on probing
- Absence of a continuous radiolucency around the implant
- Mean vertical bone loss is less than 0.2 mm annually following the first year of function.

Osseointegration is a histological and microscopically phenomenon, so clinically, use of radiographs is important in determining the location of the bone in relationship to the implant.

Normal radiographic findings around dental implants

Use of periapical and bitewing radiographs is often adequate to assess the quality and quantity of bone around the implants that have been restored and are in function.

Adequate bone-to-implant contact is indicated by the absence of continuous radiolucency around the implant. With respect to marginal peri-implant bone level, during the first year of function and depending on the type of implant system, bone remodeling may lead to marginal bone loss of 1.5 mm (Adell et al., 1981). This often coincides with the level of the first thread. After the first year, there should be negligible progressive bone loss of less than 0.2 mm annually (Albrektsson et al., 1986) (Figures 12.1a,b and 12.2a,b).

Radiographic assessment of implants should be performed annually during the first 3 years by the inexperienced clinician. Afterwards,

Endodontic Radiology, Second Edition. Edited by Bettina Basrani.
© 2012 John Wiley & Sons, Inc. Published 2012 by John Wiley & Sons, Inc.

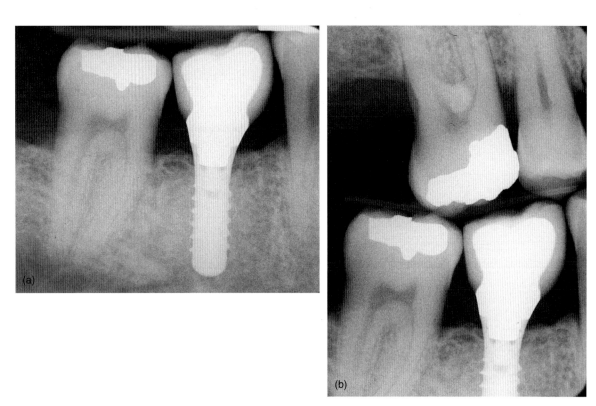

Figure 12.1 (a) Implant with normal bone level. (b) Implant with normal bone level.

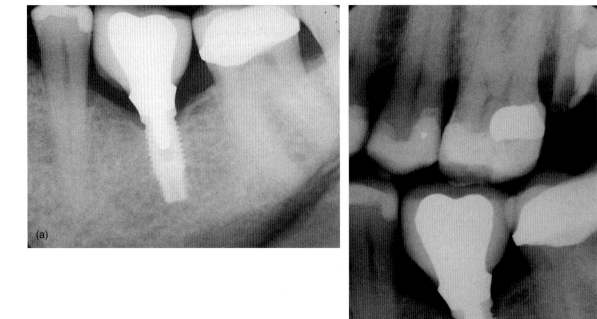

Figure 12.2 (a) Implant with normal bone level; (b) Implant with normal bone level.

assessments may be individualized as one gains more clinical experience (Gröndahl and Lekholm, 1997a).

Abnormal radiographic findings around dental implants

Abnormal radiographic findings do not necessary mean that the dental implant has failed. However, it does warrant further investigation. A decision as to whether further treatment is needed will depend on the clinical findings and how implant therapy fits in the overall treatment plan.

Often the early signs of implant failure are subtle and may not be visible radiographically. However, if there is peri-implant radiolucency, there is a high positive predictive value of 83% to radiographically identify failing implants. Only 5% of implants were found to be failing without any radiographic

evidence (Gröndahl and Lekholm, 1997b) (Figures 12.3a,b–12.6).

Preoperative radiographic planning for implant surgery

When planning for surgical placement of dental implants, it is crucial to obtain information on bone volume and quality, topography, and adjacent anatomical structures (nerves, vessels, roots, nasal floor, and sinus cavities). While some information can be gathered by clinical examination, appropriate radiographic imaging is a common clinical task and is one of the most important parameters a practitioner can assess. Therefore, it is considered a prerequisite for preoperative planning in implant treatment (Park, 2010).

The American Academy of Oral and Maxillofacial Radiology (AAOMR) considers complete

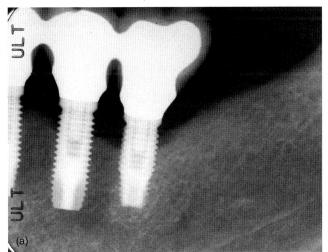
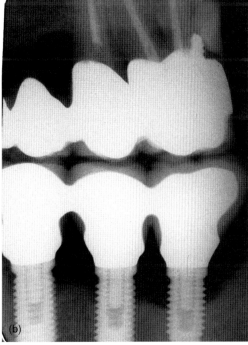

Figure 12.3   (a) Implants with bone loss. (b) Implants with bone loss.

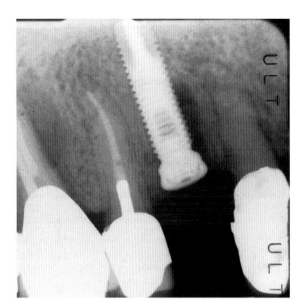

Figure 12.4 Implant with radiolucency on its mesial aspect.

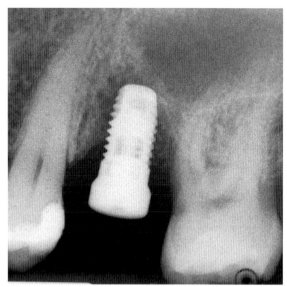

Figure 12.6 Implant with radiolucency on its mesial and distal aspect.

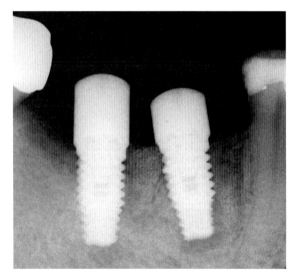

Figure 12.5 Mesial implant has radiolucency on its mesial and apical aspect.

imaging to reveal information about the following (White et al., 2001):

1. presence of disease,
2. the location of anatomic features that should be avoided when placing the implant (e.g., the maxillary sinus, nasopalatine canal, inferior alveolar canal, mental canal and foramen, and anterior extensions of inferior alveolar canal),
3. the osseous morphology (including knife-edge ridges, the submandibular fossa, developmental variations, postextraction irregularities, enlarged marrow spaces, cortical integrity and thickness, and trabecular bone density),
4. the anatomical quantification (including the dimensions available for implant placement and, equally important, the orientation axis of alveolar height)

Standard radiographic imaging techniques in implant dentistry include intraoral, panoramic, and profile (lateral) radiographs. Until the late 1980s, these conventional radiographic techniques have been the accepted standard. Since then, there has been significant development in cross-sectional imaging techniques and in certain special indications, such techniques (i.e., spiral tomography and multiplanar reformatted computed tomography (CT), and cone beam computed tomography [CBCT]) may be necessary. This section will provide a brief overview of the imaging modalities utilized in implant planning, placement, and evaluation for single tooth replacement or small partially edentulous span.

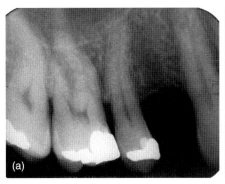 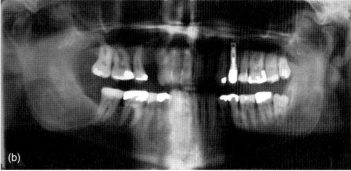

Figure 12.7   (a) Periapical radiograph to assess the maxillary first premolar site for an implant—note the mesial curvature of the second premolar that may interfere with implant placement. (b) Panoramic radiograph to assess the maxillary first premolar site for an implant—Overall view of maxilla and mandible—note the location of right maxillary sinus, sinus has no pathology, impacted mandibular wisdom tooth, presence of a dental implant that appears to have an open margin.

Intraoral radiography

Periapical radiography

Periapical radiographs are used before, during, and after implant placement and restoration. The periapical radiography is available in all dental practices. The paralleling technique with F-speed film and rectangular collimation with palate or occlusal plane placed horizontally (respectively for maxilla and mandible) is a recommended technique of the acquisition of the radiographic image (Harris et al., 2002) (Figure 12.7a).

A periapical radiograph needs to be positioned as parallel as possible to the long axis of the implant to minimize image distortion and magnification. In this way, a high-quality detailed image with more accurate measurements in both vertical and horizontal directions can be obtained at a very low cost and with a low radiation exposure (associated effective doses of <0.006 mSv per radiograph to the patient) (Harris et al., 2002). Such image can compare well to more advanced cross-sectional imaging techniques (outlined below) for longitudinal and linear distance measurement (Wakoh et al., 2006). A slight vertical angulation of 9 degrees from the long axis of the implant may be necessary for proper bony and inner thread visualization. However, it should be noted that a vertical angle exceeding 13 degrees will cause some overlap of the thread images (Hollender and Rockler, 1980).

In some situations (such as shallow vestibule), intraoral anatomical configurations may interfere with the proper placement of a periapical film apically to image the entire implant. In such cases, two radiographs, including a bite-wing-type projection to assess bone response around the coronal portion and a bisecting angle technique to image the entire length of the implant, is recommended. It should be noted that a bisecting angle projection may obviously exceed the 13 degrees maximum as outlined above (Truhlar et al., 1993). Except in such a particular situation, the use of the bisecting angle technique is discouraged. It should be remembered that with the periapical radiographs, only a limited field of bone/dentition can be imaged and a cross-sectional view of the alveolar process cannot be examined (Wyatt and Pharoah, 1998).

Extraoral imagining techniques

Panoramic radiography

Panoramic radiography has contributed significantly to maxillofacial diagnoses in the last 30 years (Angelopoulos et al., 2008). The panoramic radiography has been used frequently as the first choice of imaging modalities for preimplant evaluation and placement. It is rapid and relatively inexpensive modality used to gain an excellent general overview of the dentition and jaws with minimum radiation exposure to patients (associated effective doses of <0.003 mSv) (Harris et al., 2002). Panoramic radiographs can provide relatively clear images of the jaws due to the correct alignment of the head and teeth (except for edentulous patients) (Wyatt and Pharoah, 1998). However, the accuracy of the image varies greatly with patient positioning. Therefore, in order to avoid positioning artifacts, proper positioning (meato-orbital plane horizontal, head symmetrical, lower jaw protruding, lower and upper incisors inside the image layer and neck extended) is critical (Harris et al., 2002).

Panoramic radiographs can provide basic information on the shape of the jaws and dimension of the bone, and the location and dimension of the important adjacent anatomical structures such as maxillary sinus, nasal cavity floor, inferior alveolar canal, and mental foramen (Figure 12.7b). In addition, panoramic radiographs are useful in screening for any pathological conditions or residual roots.

However, they have inherent limitations that can influence the accuracy of measurement/diagnosis in implant dentistry:

1. A magnification up to 25% has been reported for panoramic images that is more pronounced in horizontal direction (up to 16%) than in the vertical direction (up to 10%) (Reddy et al., 1994). Therefore, horizontal measurements on panoramic films are more unreliable than vertical measurements (Truhlar et al., 1993).
2. Parallax errors may cause images of facial structures to be cast inferior to those of lingually positioned structures in the same horizontal plane, thus possibly leading to a less than optimum placement of an implant (White et al., 2001).
3. They are unreliable in determining bone density and bone quality due to the superimposition of airway shadows, soft tissue shadows and ghost images.
4. They cannot show the presence of anatomical variants such as large marrow spaces or anterior loops of the mandibular canal (White et al., 2001).
5. Just like any other two-dimensional imaging technique, no information can be gathered

with the panoramic radiography on bone width. Therefore panoramic radiographs are not suitable for implant placement in relation to the submandibular gland fossa, the sublingual gland fossa, the incisive fossa, the inferior alveolar canal, the maxillary sinus, and the floor of the nose (Wyatt and Pharoah, 1998).
6. They are also not suitable for assessing bone adjacent to implants during follow-up due to the poor resolution qualities that prevent detection of fine changes in horizontal bone height or peri-implant changes (Friedland, 1987; Hedesiu et al., 2008).
7. They cannot show the axis of orientation of the alveolar bone (White et al., 2001).

Considering these limitations, panoramic imaging alone is not sufficient in order to provide all the necessary information for optimum implant selection and therefore, it should be augmented with tomography (either conventional or computed as described below) (White et al., 2001).

Tomographic radiography and CT

Before the development of cross sectional imaging, two-dimensional imaging modalities as outlined before were the only options available to clinicians in the planning and placement of implants. While they are still useful in many cases, the superimpositions, projection geometry, and the lack of third dimension of bone depth are limitations that can resulted in an inaccurate or unreliable diagnosis (Angelopoulos et al., 2008). The simultaneous and controlled movement of the film and X-ray beam results in the blurring of structures outside the desired image layer. Tomography can produce cross-sectional slices of jaws (as small as 1 mm) and provide a means of assessing jawbone width for implant placement (Wyatt and Pharoah, 1998). The tomography performed is conventional (either linear, circular, trispiral, elliptical, and hypocycloidal) or complex motion tomography where the tube and cassette motion is controlled by a computer (computer-assisted or CT). Conventional tomographic views are most useful (free of streaking artifacts) when complex tube/film motions (such as spiral or hypocycloidal patterns) are used instead of linear movement. CT systems offer the following advantages when compared to conventional tomograms (White et al., 2001):

1. CT provides a high-contrast image with a well-defined image layer free of blurring with uniform magnification,
2. With CT, it is easier to identify bone grafts or hydroxyapatite materials used to augment maxillary bone in the sinus region
3. With CT, it is possible to have multiplanar views and three-dimensional reconstruction,
4. With CT, there is a shorter acquisition time (and hence lower radiation dose when multiple sites are being evaluated on an individual arch)

However, conventional tomography usually costs less and requires less radiation than CT and should be used for most cases in which the technology and expertise are available rather than in cases in which bone grafts or complex trauma are involved, for which CT might be more appropriate (White et al., 2001).

The potential diagnostic benefits of CT prior to surgery are to identify the following:

1. bone volume
2. jaw topography
3. bone structures
4. location of important anatomical landmarks
5. the optimal locations of implant sites in relation to the anatomical conditions for best aesthetics, function, and loading conditions
6. particular postoperative monitoring where some kind of complications have occurred (such as nerve damage, postoperative infections in relation to nasal and/or sinus cavities close to implants).

CT systems are also of value in the preoperative planning stage for various augmentation protocols (Harris et al., 2002).

Cone beam CT

Medical CT has a relatively higher cost and higher radiation dose compared to other imaging modalities (associated effective doses of <0.5 mSv per jaw) (Harris et al., 2002). They work by having the X-ray head rotate several times around the patient's head (range of 4–64 revolutions or slices) to acquire the image. Since a small gap will exist between each parallel slice, after mathematical reconstruction of the multiple slices, a built-in imaging error will exist (Winter et al., 2005).

A new advancement in cross-sectional imaging is the development of CBCT, specifically for craniofacial area. This system relies on a cone-shaped X-ray beam source and a digital detector that move synchronously and in opposite directions (Angelopoulos et al., 2008). With only one single rotation to capture the entire object, a high number of projections are rapidly captured, reducing the scanning time to 10–40 seconds resulting in less patient movement (Jabero and Sarment, 2006).

Later, a reconstruction algorithm renders cross sections to generate a 3D volumetric data set. This data set can be used to provide primary reconstruction images in three orthogonal planes (axial, sagittal, and coronal) (Scarfe et al., 2006). The resonstructed images can then be displayed in any clinically meaningful way such as panoramic and cross-sectional images of the maxilla and mandible, or temporomandibular joint sagittal and coronal images (Angelopoulos et al., 2008).

In comparison to conventional medical CT, the CBCT has been shown to have similar diagnostic performance for evaluating preoperative bone density (Aranyarachkul et al., 2005) and bone width measurement (Loubele et al., 2007). It has more accuracy for distance measurement (maximum error of 0.65 mm for CBCT vs. 1.11 mm for conventional CT) (Kobayashi et al., 2004), higher resolution in any direction for visualization of details of the small bony structures (Loubele et al., 2007), and 3–18 times less effective radiation exposure (Chau and Fung, 2009; Mah et al., 2003).

Therefore, CBCT may be a better alternative to conventional CT for preoperative radiographic assessment of potential dental implant sites. Also, because CBCT images are reformatted slices of the maxilla and mandible, they are free of magnification, superimposition of neighboring structures, and other problems inherent to panoramic radiology. This may result in very clear images that better depict important anatomical structures, such as the mandibular canal (Figures 12.8 and 12.9) (Angelopoulos et al., 2008).

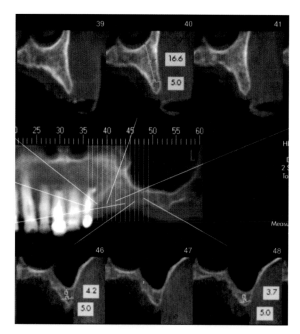

Figure 12.8 Cone beam CT scan of maxilla—note the location of the sinus floor in relationship to the alveolar ridge, the cross-section view of the alveolar ridge.

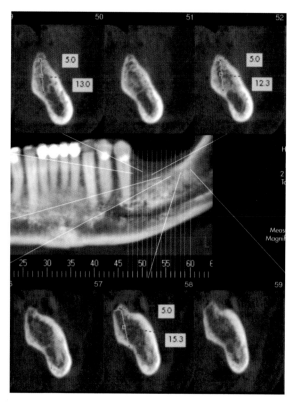

Figure 12.9 Cone beam CT scan of mandible—note the location of the mandibular canal, submandibular fossa, the cross-section view of the alveolar ridge.

Application of imaging techniques

Imaging for implant treatment planning

Decision on the appropriate imaging is balanced between obtaining the essential diagnostic information and the as low as reasonably achievable (ALARA) principle on radiation exposure.

When planning for a single tooth or small partially edentulous span, the initial radiograph needed is the panoramic radiograph. Panoramic radiographs serve to screen for any pathology and provides an initial view of the implant site in relationship to the vital structures with minimal radiation exposure to the patient (Frederiksen et al., 1994). However, because of magnification and distortion, periapical radiographs are required to obtain greater image detail and accurate measurements (Wyatt and Pharoah, 1998).

CT or CBCT are not necessarily needed for every case, and clinicians should decide on the basis of the clinical examination and treatment requirements, and on information obtained from conventional radiographs whether or not cross-sectional imaging will be of particular benefit to the particular patient. For example, these more advanced imaging need to be considered for the following situations (Harris et al., 2002):

1. when there is a risk of damage to important anatomical structures,
2. when there is a need for more information in borderline clinical situations of limited available bone height and/or bone width for successful implant treatment, or
3. when there is a need to improve implant positioning and axial direction that will optimize biomechanical, functional, and aesthetic treatment results.

When using advance imaging such as CBCT, the use of a radiographic stent or guides is particularly useful. The radiographic guide has radiopaque markers which may be in the form of gutta percha, metal cyliners, and radiopaque barium sulfate that is incorporated into the acrylic resin. The image of the radiographic guide is superimposed on the radiographic image which indicates the relationship between the bone to the final prosthesis. The information can then be translated into a surgical guide (Figure 12.10a–d).

Imaging during stage I implant surgery

In cases where implant placement is not close to any vital structures, taking additional radiographs during the stage I surgery is not needed. However, there are certain clinical situations where it is appropriate to take a periapical radiograph with the direction indicator inserted into the osteotomy site. These include:

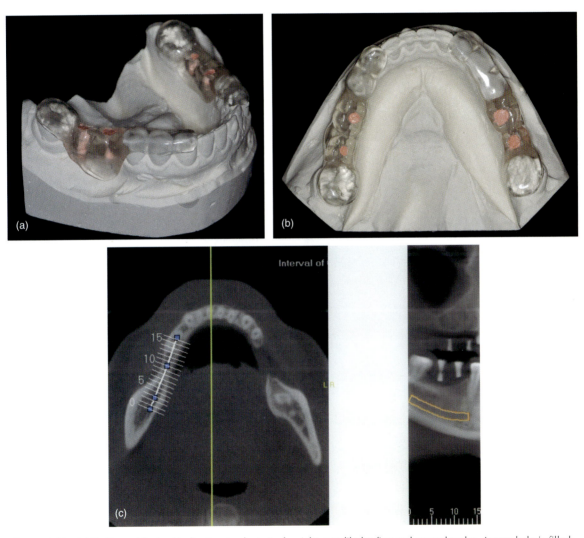

Figure 12.10 (a) Radiographic stent indicating implant site for right mandibular first and second molar. Access hole is filled with gutta percha. (b) Occlusal view of the access holes of the radiographic stent. Access hole is filled with gutta percha. (c) Cone beam CT scan of mandible—note patient is wearing the radiographic stent. The gutta percha indentify the mesial-distal angulation of the access holes. (d) Cone beam CT scan of mandible—Slice 7 and 11 indicated the relationship of the access hole with respect to the buccal-lingual dimension of the alveolar ridge and the location of the mandibular canal. Note the location of the mental foramen in slice 11.

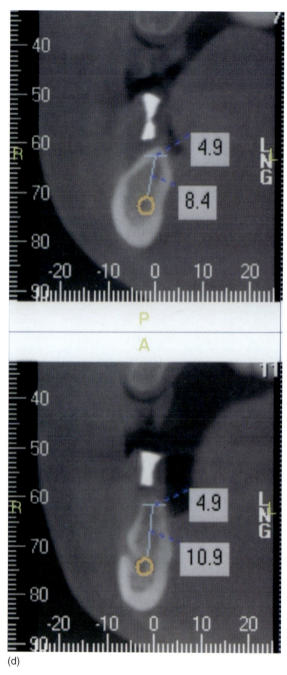

(d)

Figure 12.10   (Continued)

1. Narrow mesial-distal distance between the two adjacent teeth or when the root of the tooth converges toward the planned implant site, proper angulation of the osteotomy site is critical.
2. Close proximity to vital structures such as the floor of the sinus, mandibular canal, and mental foramen.
3. If placing multiple implants, periapical radiographs can be taken to ensure parallelism between the implants (Figure 12.11a,b).

When the radiographs are taken during the initial drill sequence, there is opportunity to make adjustments without compromising the osteotomy site.

Imaging at abutment and prosthetic component connections

The long-term clinical success of implant prostheses relies on an absolute and passive fit of an abutment to an implant to allow for the even distribution of occlusal forces at the whole implant surface, resulting in nonaxial loading of implants and fixation screws (Papavassiliou et al., 2010). While various clinical methods such as probing with dental explorers, visual control, use of periotest device, and so on, have been suggested for the control of the fit, the radiographic examination of marginal gaps at the implant–abutment interface is a common clinical task in prosthodontic treatment (Figures 12.12 and 12.13). Radiographic analysis affiliated with a certain degree of clinical experience possesses features for an adequate clinical management of restoration defects (Konermann et al., 2010).

They are also useful to detect implant and abutment screw fractures and other mechanical problems. A properly exposed and developed periapical film positioned as parallel as possible to the long axis of the implant is the radiograph of choice. The X-ray diagnosis of gap at the interface can be significantly influenced by the inclination of the X-ray tube in relation to the long axis of the implant. With an increase in vertical angulation, the ability to detect the gap diminishes. In fact, a gap is not detectable at angulations higher than 20 degrees

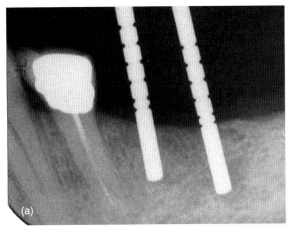
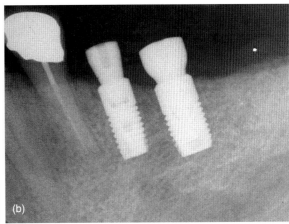

Figure 12.11 (a) Direction indicators placed in the osteotomy site to demonstrate the parallelism between the two implant sites. The mesial direction indicator also demonstrates the osteotomy is not converging to the root of the first premolar. (b) Final implant placement of two implants—Note the parallelism and the implants are away from any vital structures.

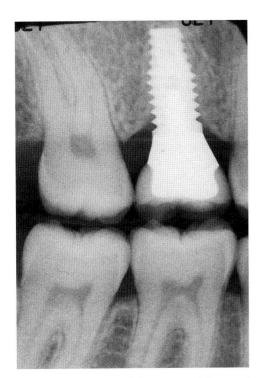

Figure 12.12 The crown and abutment are fully seated on the implant shoulder.

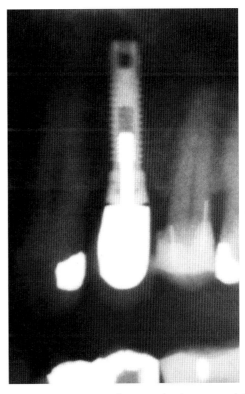

Figure 12.13 Open margin between the abutment and the implant shoulder which indicates a poorly fitting prosthesis.

(i.e., bisecting angle technique). Therefore, to achieve accurate results, the use of a paralleling device is advocated in order to achieve greater detection ability (Papavassiliou et al., 2010).

Conclusion

Use of radiographic imaging is critical for implant therapy. Radiographic imaging is used during treatment planning, during the stage I surgery, abutment connection, and monitoring of osseointegrated implants. Selection of the appropriate radiographic imaging should be guided by the ALARA principle on radiation exposure.

References

Adell, R., Lekholm, U., Rockler, B., and Branemark, P.-I. (1981) A 15-year stude of osseointegrated implants in the treatment of the edentulous jaw. *Int J Oral Surg*, 10, 387–416.

Albrektsson, T., Zarb, G., Worthington, P., and Eriksson, A.R. (1986) The long-term efficacy of currently used dental implants: a review and proposed criteria of success. *Int J Oral Maxillofac Implants*, 1(1), 11–25.

Angelopoulos, C., Thomas, S.L., et al. (2008) Comparison between digital panoramic radiography and cone-beam computed tomography for the identification of the mandibular canal as part of presurgical dental implant assessment. *J Oral Maxillofac Surg*, 66(10), 2130–2135.

Aranyarachkul, P., Caruso, J., et al. (2005) Bone density assessments of dental implant sites: 2. Quantitative cone-beam computerized tomography. *Int J Oral Maxillofac Implants*, 20(3), 416–424.

Buser, D., Weber, H.P., and Brägger, U. (1990) The treatment of partially edentulous patients with ITI hollow-screw implants: presurgical evaluation and surgical procedures. *Int J Oral Maxillofac Implants*, 5(2), 165–175.

Chau, A.C. and Fung, K. (2009) Comparison of radiation dose for implant imaging using conventional spiral tomography, computed tomography, and cone-beam computed tomography. *Oral Surg Oral Med Oral Pathol Oral Radiol Endod*, 107(4), 559–565.

Frederiksen, N.L., Bensen, B.W., and Sokolowski, T.W. (1994) Effective dose and risk assessment from film tomography used for dental implant diagnostics. *Dentomaxillofac Radiol*, 23, 123–127.

Friedland, B. (1987) The clinical evaluation of dental implants—a review of the literature, with emphasis on the radiographic aspects. *J Oral Implantol*, 13(1), 101–111.

Gröndahl, K. and Lekholm, U. (1997a) The predictive value of radiographic diagnosis of implant instability. *Int J Oral Maxillofac Implants*, 12(1), 59–64.

Gröndahl, K. and Lekholm, U. (1997b) The predictive value of radiographic diagnosis of implant instability. *Int J Oral Maxillofac Implants*, 12(1), 59–64.

Harris, D., Buser, D., et al. (2002) E.A.O. guidelines on the use of diagnostic imaging in implant dentistry. A consensus workshop organized by the European Association for Osseointegration in Trinity College Dublin. *Clin Oral Implants Res*, 13(5), 566–570.

Hedesiu, M., Balog, C., et al. (2008) The accuracy of alveolar crest dimensions measurement for dental implants. In vitro study. *Rev Med Chir Soc Med Nat Iasi*, 112(1), 224–228.

Hollender, L. and Rockler, B. (1980) Radiographic evaluation of osseointegrated implants of the jaws. Experimental study of the influence of radiographic techniques on the measurement of the relation between the implant and bone. *Dentomaxillofac Radiol*, 9(2), 91–95.

Jabero, M. and Sarment, D.P. (2006) Advanced surgical guidance technology: a review. *Implant Dent*, 15(2), 135–142.

Kobayashi, K., Shimoda, S., et al. (2004) Accuracy in measurement of distance using limited cone-beam computerized tomography. *Int J Oral Maxillofac Implants*, 19(2), 228–231.

Konermann, A.C., Zoellner, A., et al. (2010) In vitro study of the correlation between the simulated clinical and radiographic examination of microgaps at the implant-abutment interface. *Quintessence Int*, 41(8), 681–687.

Loubele, M., Guerrero, M.E., et al. (2007) A comparison of jaw dimensional and quality assessments of bone characteristics with cone-beam CT, spiral tomography, and multi-slice spiral CT. *Int J Oral Maxillofac Implants*, 22(3), 446–454.

Mah, J.K., Danforth, R.A., et al. (2003) Radiation absorbed in maxillofacial imaging with a new dental computed tomography device. *Oral Surg Oral Med Oral Pathol Oral Radiol Endod*, 96(4), 508–513.

Mombelli, A. and Lang, N.P. (1994) Clinical parameters for the evaluation of dental implants. *Periodontology 2000*, 4, 81–86.

Papavassiliou, H., Kourtis, S., et al. (2010) Radiographical evaluation of the gap at the implant-abutment interface. *J Esthet Restor Dent*, 22(4), 235–250.

Park, J.B. (2010) The evaluation of digital panoramic radiographs taken for implant dentistry in the daily practice. *Med Oral Patol Oral Cir Bucal*, 15(4), e663–e666.

Reddy, M.S., Mayfield-Donahoo, T., et al. (1994) A comparison of the diagnostic advantages of panoramic radiography and computed tomography scanning for placement of root form dental implants. *Clin Oral Implants Res*, 5(4), 229–238.

Scarfe, W.C., Farman, A.G., et al. (2006) Clinical applications of cone-beam computed tomography in dental practice. *J Can Dent Assoc*, 72(1), 75–80.

Truhlar, R.S., Morris, H.F., et al. (1993) A review of panoramic radiography and its potential use in implant dentistry. *Implant Dent*, 2(2), 122–130.

Wakoh, M., Harada, T., et al. (2006) Reliability of linear distance measurement for dental implant length with standardized periapical radiographs. *Bull Tokyo Dent Coll*, 47(3), 105–115.

White, S.C., Heslop, E.W., et al. (2001) Parameters of radiologic care: an official report of the American Academy of Oral and Maxillofacial Radiology. *Oral Surg Oral Med Oral Pathol Oral Radiol Endod*, 91(5), 498–511.

Winter, A.A., Pollack, A.S., et al. (2005) Cone beam volumetric tomography vs. medical CT scanners. *N Y State Dent J*, 71(4), 28–33.

Wyatt, C.C. and Pharoah, M.J. (1998) Imaging techniques and image interpretation for dental implant treatment. *Int J Prosthodont*, 11(5), 442–452.

Part 3

Sequence of Endodontic Treatment

Chapter 13   Radiographic Considerations during the Endodontic Treatment

Chapter 14   Electronic Apex Locators and Conventional Radiograph in Working
Length Measurement

Chapter 15   Vertical Root Fractures: Radiological Diagnosis

Chapter 16   Healing of Chronic Apical Periodontitis

13 Radiographic Considerations during the Endodontic Treatment

Bettina Basrani

Introduction

Radiology is an indispensable tool in the clinical practice of endodontics because most structures harboring disease are not visible to the naked eye. As a result, radiographs are needed during several aspects of the treatment, and their proper interpretation and analysis is crucial to the establishment of a favorable outcome (Torabinejad and Walton, 2009) (Figure 13.1A,B).

Standard two-dimensional radiographs used for the management of endodontic problems yield limited information because the images produced often are accompanied by geometric distortion and anatomical noise. Goldman et al. (1972), in his classic paper, mentioned that radiographs are not so much read as interpreted and that this process can be ambiguous and inconsistent. Dentists are always asking: is there an area of radiolucency? How large is the area? Where is the apex of the tooth? (Figure 13.2).

In endodontics, radiographs are essential in diagnosis, treatment planning, treatment procedures, prognosis, follow-up, legal documentation, and education. In this chapter, the art of interpreting everyday radiographs will be explained in detail. (Note that through this chapter, the term "radiographs" will suggest conventional receptors as well as digital sensors.)

Diagnosis

Radiographs are important, if not the most important, tools available to the clinician; and they help identify the problem–the tooth–and help develop the treatment plan. At least one current preoperative radiograph taken using the paralleling technique is mandatory in identifying the presence and nature of pathosis.

Some common rules are important to follow when radiographs are used to assess diagnosis: If the tooth in question is fully mature and vital and your diagnostic testing reveals an irreversible pulpitis, no significant changes may be apparent on the radiograph. Teeth with necrotic pulps do not routinely have rarefactions associated with their roots, and apical rarefactions of pulpal origin will routinely demonstrate the loss of the apical lamina dura in association with the rarefaction (Figure 13.3) (Gutmann et al., 1992).

Endodontic Radiology, Second Edition. Edited by Bettina Basrani.
© 2012 John Wiley & Sons, Inc. Published 2012 by John Wiley & Sons, Inc.

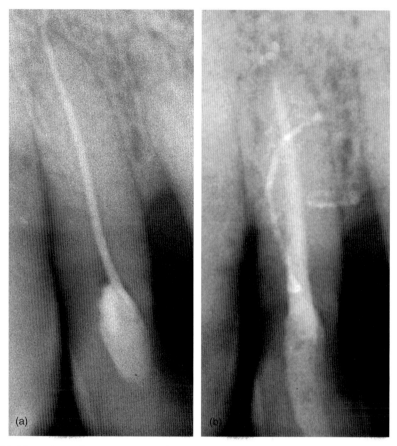

(a)   (b)

Figure 13.1   (a and b) The radiographs contain more information than can readily be seen by the naked eye. Noticeable in this retreatment case is the complex anatomy of the lateral incisor (Courtesy of Dr G. Yared).

From the clinical point of view, it is important to remember that necrosis can sometimes be seen by the naked eye. In other words, when a crown that we "see" is discolored, it may be an indication of pulpal necrosis; or when we "see" a sinus track on the gingiva, it may indicate the presence of infection originating from a necrotic pulp. By the same standard, an apical rarefaction that we "see" radiographically may indicate necrosis. While patients demonstrating the clinical signs of irreversible pulpitis may not show demonstrable radiographic changes, the radiograph does have the potential to show etiological contributing factors, such as caries or a deep restoration. Establishing a diagnosis in cases such as this can at times be more challenging.

During the diagnostic procedures, it is crucial to assess tooth restorability. Radiographs are also helpful in assessing and in explaining to the patient the risks and benefits of the proposed treatment.

The preoperative (or diagnositc) radiograph should also be used to assess the root canal anatomy, and the difficulty of the case should be evaluated. A supplemental bite-wing (Figure 13.4) radiograph is useful to detect caries, to determine the depth of a calcified pulp chamber, or to reveal a pulp chamber obscured by a large radiopaque restoration. A second periapical radiograph taken at a different horizontal projection is also helpful in determining the number and shape of the roots when multirooted teeth are involved.

When a sinus track or fistula is present (Figure 13.5A,B), it can sometimes be traced back to an area of pathosis. This is accomplished by threading a new gutta-percha cone (size 30 or 40) through the track and exposing a periapical radiograph. Gener-

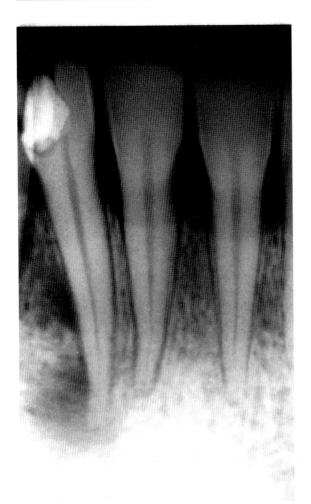

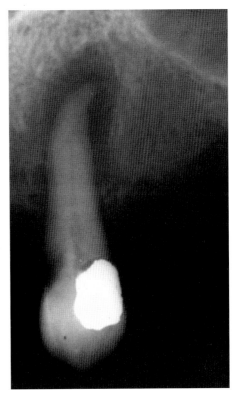

Figure 13.3   Radiograph showing the lost of the lamina dura at the apex, indicating pulp pathosis.

Figure 13.2   This radiograph shows an apical and lateral rarefaction. Accurate interpretation of these areas is essential for correct diagnosis.

ally, it is not necessary to anesthetize during this step. If the sinus track cannot be penetrated with a gutta-percha point, it may be necessary to reopen it with an explorer tip or periodontal probe and then introduce a new cone.

The clinician must realize that periradicular pathosis and/or bone destruction may be present, but not radiographically visible. Radiographic bone loss is not evident until there is significant erosion of the cortical plate (Bender and Seltzer, 2003) (Figure 13.6A,B).

There are some limitations of conventional radiography for endodontic diagnosis (Patel et al.,

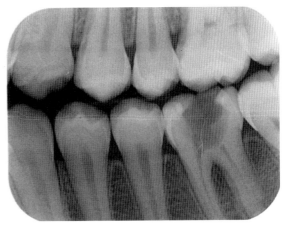

Figure 13.4   Bite-wing radiograph can be taken as a complimentary diagnosis aid.

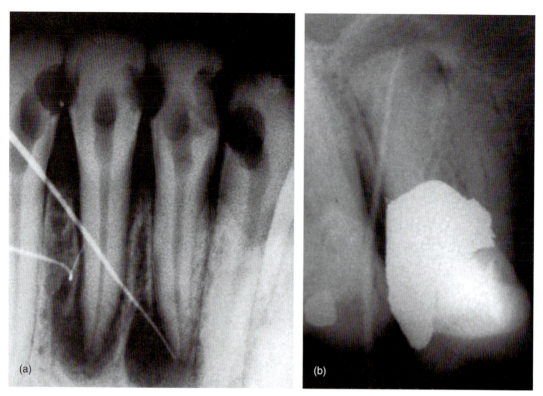

Figure 13.5 (a and b) Sinus track traced with a gutta percha cone.

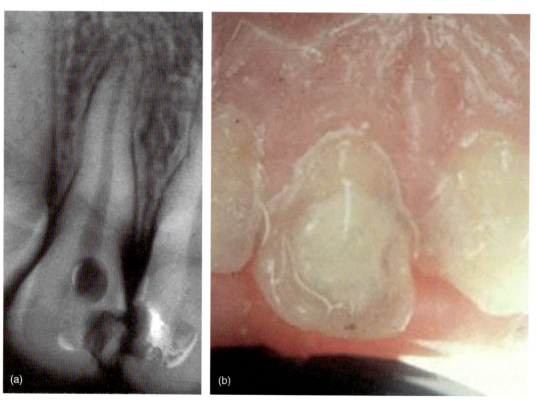

Figure 13.6 (a and b) Radiograph showing maxillary lateral incisor with an acute abscess with minimal bone destruction.

2009). The most important one is the loss of three-dimensional anatomy: Conventional images compress three-dimensional anatomy into a two-dimensional image or shadowgraph, greatly limiting diagnostic performance (Webber and Messura, 1999). Important features of the tooth and its surrounding tissues are visualized in the mesiodistal (proximal) direction only. Similar features presenting in the buccolingual plane (i.e., the third dimension) may not be fully appreciated.

On occasions, deliberate and controlled alteration of the radiation geometry can be beneficial and provide additional information not always visible on images taken with standard angulations. For example,

Changing horizontal angulation separates anatomical features and periapical radiolucencies: This effect can be used to dissociate the incisive foramen and mental foramen from adjacent tooth apices (Figure 13.7A,B) (Fava and Dummer, 1997).

Changing vertical angulation is useful on distinguishing lingual roots, normal landmarks, and apical pathology, and allows for more accurate visualization of their apices. This effect can be used to determine whether anatomical landmarks lay buccally or lingually (Fava and Dummer, 1997). However, it must be appreciated that increases in vertical angulation will lead to a shortening in the length of tooth images,

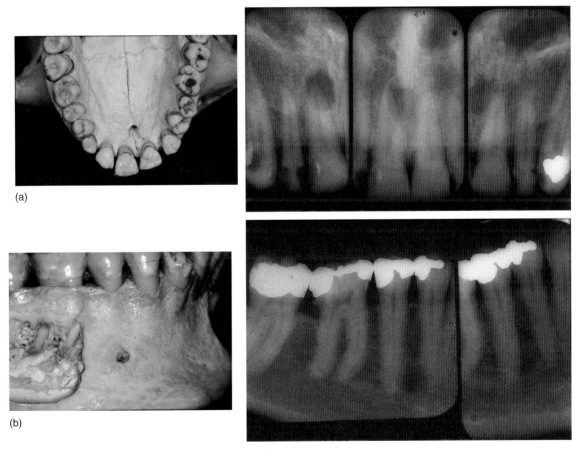

(a)

(b)

Figure 13.7   (a) Anatomical superimposition. Superimposition of the nasopalatine foramen. Tooth roots change position more than foramen with changes in direction of central ray (Courtesy of Dr. C. Torneck). (b) Anatomical superimposition with mental foramen. Being buccal to the tooth roots, the mental foramen will move more in the direction of the change in the direction of the central ray than the teeth (Courtesy of Dr. C. Torneck).

with buccal roots appearing shorter than lingual roots in multirooted teeth because they are further from the receptor (Fava and Dummer, 1997).

Preoperative radiograph and anatomy

During the preoperative steps, it is important to analyze and categorize the tooth with the different degree of difficulty (average, moderate, or high risk) (form adapted from the risks and difficulty form used by the University of Toronto) (Table 13.1). A special consideration and analysis should be given to the radiographic consideration of the canal(s). The following points need to be examined:

- *Angle of curvature*: There are many techniques to evaluate the canal curvature. The first and most common method was reported by Schneider in 1971. The degree of canal curvature was defined as the acute angle between the long axis of the canal and a line from the point of initial curvature to the apical foramen. In 1982, Weine proposed another method that defined the angle of curvature differently. The acute angle between lines passing through the apical and coronal portions was measured. Pruett et al. (1997) pointed out that the shape of any root canal curvature could be more accurately described by using two parameters, angle of curvature and radius of curvature (Gu et al., 2010).

- *Radius of curvature*: The radius is defined as the length of a line segment between the center and circumference of a circle or sphere and represents the abruptness of curvature. The shorter the radius, the more abrupt the curvature (Figure 13.8A,B).

- *Distance*: From the start of the curvature to the apex: The smaller the distance, the more abrupt the curvature.

- *Number of canals*:
  - When a radiograph reveals a root canal space that is not at the center of the root, an

Table 13.1   Analysis of endodontic case difficulty and risk (Adapted from the risks and difficulty form used by the University of Toronto).

Criteria and sub criteria	Average risk	Moderate risk	High risk
1. Radiograph/receptor placement	☐ No limitations/ restrictions	☐ Restrictive floor/palate	☐ Gagging
2. Tooth appearance in preoperative radiograph	☐ Clearly discernible	☐ Superimposed but visible	☐ Superimposed obscured
3. Anatomy	☐ Normal	☐ Taurodontism, microdens	☐ Fusion, dens in dente
4. Isolation	☐ Normal considerations	☐ Large coronal deficiency	☐ No coronal tooth structure
5. Access	☐ Normal considerations	☐ Pulp stones/calcified chamber	☐ Artificial crown present
6. Root curvature	☐ Single, mild	☐ Single, moderate curve	☐ Double/severe curve (>30)
7. Root canal morphology	☐ Apparently normal	☐ Subdivision/treatable	Complex/C-shape/ >25 mm
8. Canals expected	☐ 1 or 2 anterior/premolar	☐ 1 to 3 molar	☐ >3 molars
9. Root formation	☐ Apex closed	☐ Apex fairly open	☐ Apex widely open
10. Radiographic presentation of canal(s)	☐ Normal presentation	☐ Narrow	☐ Not discernible area(s)
11. External resorption	☐ None evident	☐ Present without perforation	☐ Present with perforation
12. Other resorption	☐ None	☐ Apical	☐ Internal
13. History of trauma	☐ None/concussion	☐ Luxation	☐ Avulsion
14. Root fracture	☐ None	☐ Apical 1/2	☐ Coronal 1/2

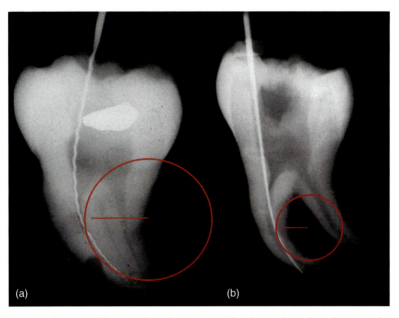

Figure 13.8 (a and b) Image showing different radius of curvatures. The shorter the radius, the more abrupt the curvature is.

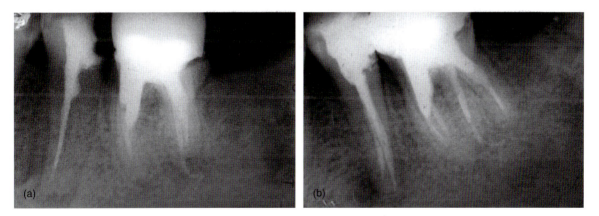

Figure 13.9 (a and b) Radiograph reveals a root canal space that is not at the center of the root. Therefore, an extra canal should be suspected (Courtesy of Dr. Hilu).

extra canal should be suspected. If there is only one canal, it will appear in the center of the root regardless of the angulations (Figure 13.9).

○ In a single rooted tooth, a sharp or rapid change in the visible density of the root canal space usually indicates that one large canal that has split into two canals (Figure 13.10) (Gutmann et al., 1992).

○ If a rapid change in density occurs in the apical third of the root, it is possible that the canal exists on the buccal or lingual surface of the root (Figure 13.11A–D) (Gutmann et al., 1992).

Radiographs and Different Teeth Groups (Hargreaves and Cohen, 2011)

Maxillary central incisor

The root canal system outline of this tooth reflects the external surface outline. It is the only tooth where the mesial-distal dimension and the buccal-lingual dimension are similar.

Maxillary lateral incisor

This tooth is wider mesiodistally than buccolingually. The probability of a sharp apical curvature is high. Buccal or lingual root curvature is not visible on the standard (direct) view. Changing the horizontal angulation will allow this common occurrence to be identified, although such images are often poorly defined. Buccal curves move in the opposite direction to the angulation of the beam; a mesial angulation will produce a movement of the root apex toward the distal aspect. Lingual curves will move toward the direction of angulation. When identification of root curvature is critical, such as when surgery is planned, or when the precise location of canal irregularities or fractured instruments is required, the use of the triangular scanning technique (Bramante et al., 1980) can be beneficial (explained in detail in Chapter 2), as visualization of the opposite maxillary lateral incisor can also give some information on the anatomy, given that teeth are usually symmetric (Torabinejad and Walton, 2009).

Maxillary canine

The root canal system is similar to that of the maxillary incisor. It is wider labiolingually than mesiodistally. The average length is 26.5 mm. This is the longest tooth in the mouth. It can be problematic

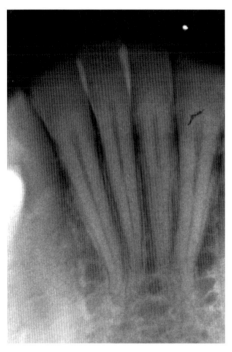

Figure 13.10   Changes in the radiolucency of the canals indicates that the canals may split in two.

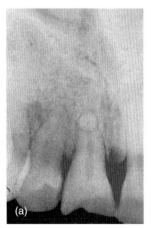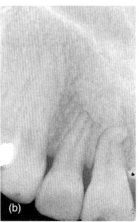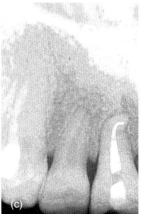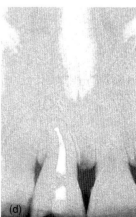

(a)   (b)   (c)   (d)

Figure 13.11   (a–d) Rapid change in density occurs in the apical third of the root; it is possible that the canal exists on the buccal.

to visualize the apex in the radiograph. By increasing the vertical angulation of the X-ray tube, it may help foreshorten the root and give a more accurate idea of the periodontal ligament space, lamina dura, and the end of the root.

First maxillary premolars

The majority of the first premolars have two canals located in the buccal and lingual surfaces. Changing 20 degrees on the horizontal projection has great value to separate the two canals.

Maxillary molars

Maxillary first molar is one of the most complex in root canal anatomy, making it very difficult and challenging to treat. A major reason is associated with radiography. The frequent superimposition of portions of the other roots on each other, superimposition of bony structure (such as sinus floor or zygomatic process) on root structures, and shape and depth of the palate can obstruct the visualization of the roots. This problem can be solved by proper changes in the angulation of the root. On many occasions, and particularly when using the bisecting angle technique, superimposition of the zygomatic process of the maxilla over the root apices of molar teeth occurs, resulting in the characteristic arch-like radiopacity which hinders radiographic interpretation. To lessen this imaging difficulty, modification by decreasing the vertical angulation can be considered. In addition, when using the bisecting angle technique, the vertical orientation of the receptor is dictated by the local anatomy. So in situations where the receptor forms an angle with the long axis of the teeth, most commonly occurring in the palatal arch of the maxilla, placement of a cotton roll will help the positioning of the receptor. Alternatively, a film holder that positions the receptor in a parallel orientation to the teeth and guides the X-ray beam (e.g., Rinn holder) can be used to minimize this anatomical obstruction. (Special radiographic techniques are explained in detail in Chapter 2.)

Lower central and lateral incisors

The mandibular incisors, because of their small size and internal anatomy, may be the most difficult to access and prepare. The possibility of second canals is high (around 40%). The canal found first after access will always be the buccal canal, therefore the access needs to be extended toward the lingual to find the second canal. Changing the horizontal angulation separates the canals and allows their identification (Figure 13.12A,B).

Mandibular canines

The root canal system is very similar to that of the maxillary canine, except that the dimensions are smaller. The root canal outlines are narrower in the mesial-distal dimensions but usually very broad buccolingually. Occasionally, they may have two roots, located in buccal and lingual surfaces.

Mandibular premolars

This teeth group shares the same issue as the mandibular incisors, namely the possibility of two canals in the buccal-lingual dimension. Changing the horizontal angulation to 20 degrees to mesial or to distal is often needed. The more apical the bifurcation, the more challenging the subsequent treatment (Figure 13.13).

Mandibular molars

Because mandibular molars are the earliest permanent teeth to erupt, they usually are very highly restored, and they are subject to heavy occlusal stress. The radiographic image of the pulp chamber is frequently calcified. The tooth has usually two roots with one, two, or three canals per root. Horizontal angulation can be altered to separate the two canals in the mesial or distal roots. The mesial root in mandibular molars is commonly considered to have two canals, with an isthmus in between. Within this system, the presence of an accessory mesial canal has been identified with a prevalence ranging from 0% to 17%. Although the high-prevalence accessory mesiobuccal canals in maxillary molars have been well characterized, the lower-prevalence accessory mesial canals in mandibular molars are not well recognized by clinicians. The accessory mesial canals invariably originate within the subpulpal groove or isthmus connecting the two main canals, making their detection very challenging (Karapinar-Kazandag et al., 2010) (Figure 13.14).

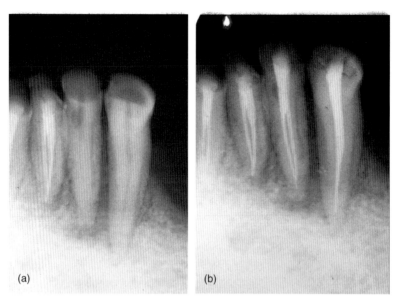

Figure 13.12   (a and b) Lower incisor with two canals (courtesy of Dr. Ricardo Portigliatti).

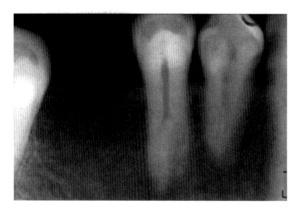

Figure 13.13   Lower premolar with two canals.

C-shape canals

The prevalence of C-shaped canals in mandibular molars is estimated to be between 2.7% and 9.0% in Whites, but is as high as 31.5% among Asian populations. Endodontic treatment of the pathosis involving a mandibular molar may be difficult because of variations in the root canal system. Canal shaping and obturation can be hampered because of the presence of a lateral canal, transverse anastomosis, or an apical delta in the C-shaped canal. Access to root canals with instruments and clearing of debris in the C-shaped canal are more complicated than in second mandibular molars without such anatomy. To prevent such complications, knowledge of the shape and length of the pulp canal is essential. Furthermore, this information can help ensure successful debridement, instrumentation, obturation, and restoration. Although detection of a C-shaped canal is important in the early stages of treatment, these canals are not easily diagnosed using dental radiography because findings that indicate fusion between mesial and distal roots are often equivocal. More accurate diagnoses can be achieved by making use of three-dimensional imaging techniques such as high-resolution computed tomography (Jung et al., 2010) (Figure 13.15).

Preoperative radiograph and access: "access for success"

The objectives of the access preparation are

- To provide a smooth free-flowing channel from the orifice to the apex.
- To confirm etiology of pulpal pathosis.
- To assess restorability.

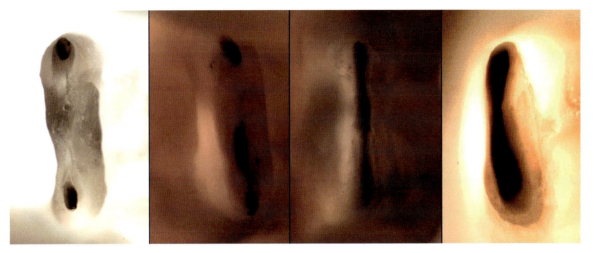

Figure 13.14 Photographs of the subpulpal groove observed in mandibular molars with (a) two canals, (b and c) three canals, and (d) an open isthmus (Courtesy of Dr. Karapinar Kazandag).

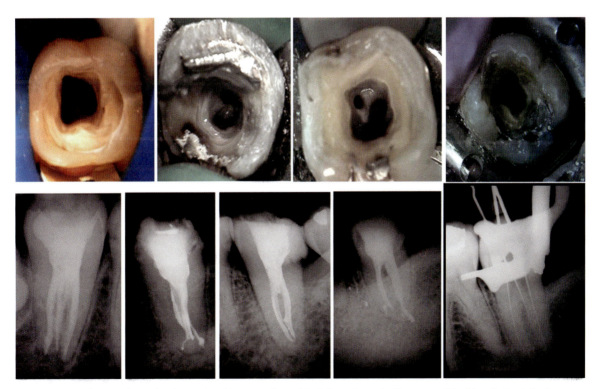

Figure 13.15 Photographs and radiographs of lower molars with C-shaped canals (Courtesy of Dr. Ricardo Portigliatti).

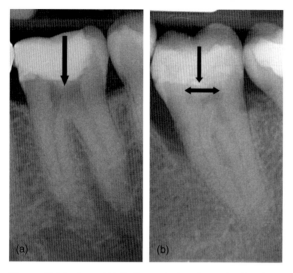

Figure 13.16   (a and b) Radiograph showing pulp chambers with different degrees of calcification and how the access preparation should be considered.

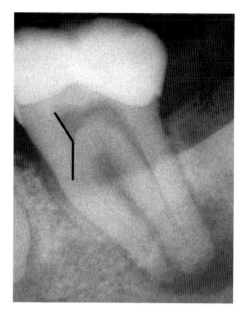

Figure 13.17   Radiograph showing the angle of emergence of the mesial canals.

The preoperative radiograph and an initial supplemental bitewing can be good aids to the design of the access preparation. The following points need to be considered:

1. Pulp chamber: Wide or calcified: When working in a wide pulp chamber, a round bur can be introduced in the chamber until an empty space is felt. However, when working in a calcified chamber, the round bur needs to be used very carefully and the dentinal layers removed slowly (Figure 13.16).
2. Angle of emergence of canals: In order to achieve a straight line access to the apex, the angle of emergence needs to be analyzed, and the amount of dentin that is to be removed must be determined (Figure 13.17).

When having difficulty with the access and the canal(s) cannot be found, a radiograph is taken and the access is verified. In these cases, the knowledge of internal anatomy, along with correct skills and resources, such as microscope and ultrasonic tips, can help to localize and negotiate the canal. It is necessary to penetrate with a bur where the canal is supposed to be. At this time, a radiograph can be taken without rubber dam (so the clamp will not obscure the vision). Then by applying the SLOB rule (same lingual, opposite buccal) (explained in detail in Chapter 2), interpretation of the direction can be made. If the canal is still not localized, a bur or a file attached with wax or cotton pellet can be placed in the access cavity and a new angled radiograph can be taken. This film will assist in correcting the orientation of the access. If an endodontic instrument is placed in the canal, total isolation with rubber dam is mandatory (Figures 13.18A–D and 13.19A–C).

Accidents during access

A perforation of the chamber wall or floor is an accident that needs immediate attention. The clinical indicator of the presence of a perforation is sudden, and there is persistent bleeding in the canal (Figure 13.20).

A small file can be placed in the canal, and a radiograph can be taken to verify the perforation. If the perforation occurred in either the buccal or the lingual surface, it may be hidden in the regular film; therefore, an off angle radiograph is recommended (Figure 13.21A–D). A small file could be inserted into the suspected perforated area and

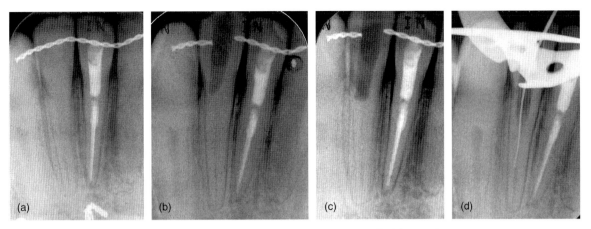

Figure 13.18   (a–d) Sequence of radiographs taken during access preparation to find the canal.

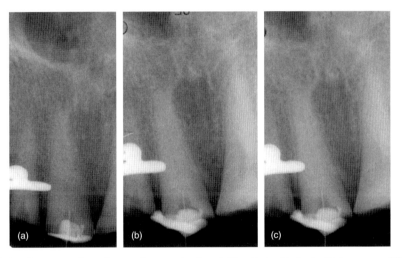

Figure 13.19   (a–c) Another case, where the canal cannot be found. The file is attached with temporary filling material to the access and a series of radiographs are taken (Courtesy of Dr. G. Yared).

connected to the apex locator. If the apex locator indicates immediately that it has detected the apex which is usually not there, it probably means that a perforation was created. Commonly, if the apex locator indicator moves slowly while introducing the file, it is more likely that the file is inside the canal rather than in a perforation. (More details on apex locators can be found in Chapter 14.)

In molars, perforations usually occur in the floor of the pulp chamber. By analyzing the preoperative radiograph and measuring the distance between the enamel (cusp tips) and the pulp floor, this accident can be prevented (Figure 13.22). The perforation at the furcation level can be visualized in the radiograph as a radiolucent shadow in the bone with reduction of the radiographic density of the surrounding dentine. Once the perforation is identified, the hemorrhage should be controlled and the perforation should be sealed as soon as possible or referral be made to a specialist for perforation repair and continuation of the treatment (Figure 13.23).

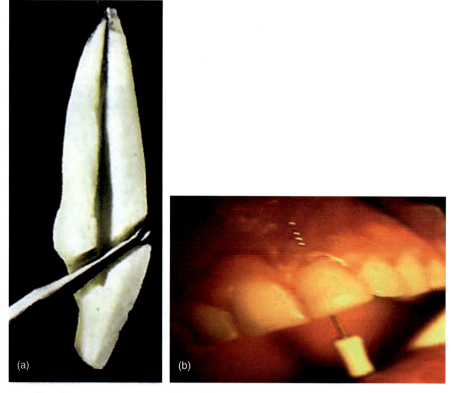

Figure 13.20 (a and b) Schematic representation of a perforation during access prep. Clinical picture of a buccal perforation.

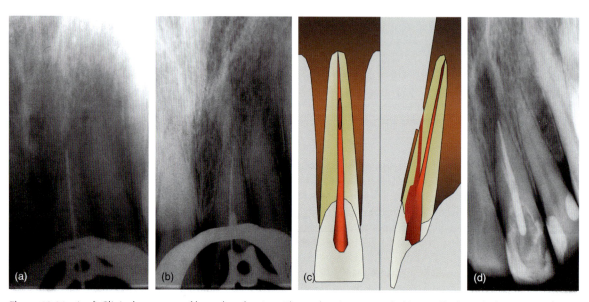

Figure 13.21 (a–d) Clinical sequence of buccal perforation. The perforation was sealed internally through the root canal. Schematic representation of the perforation (Courtesy of Dr. Portigliatti).

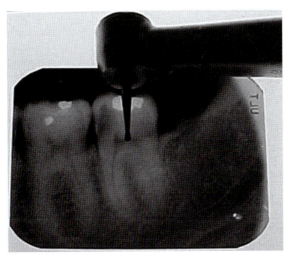

Figure 13.22   Superimposition of the high-speed bur and the preoperative radiograph to verify the distance to the pulp floor.

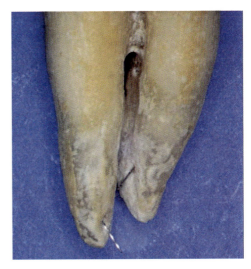

Figure 13.24   Limitation of the two-dimensional images to assess working length. The picture is showing that the canal terminus does not coincide with the anatomic apex.

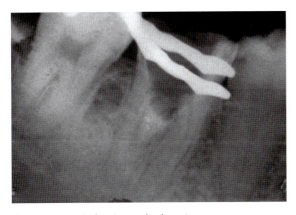

Figure 13.23   Perforation at the furcation area.

Radiograph for verification of the working length

Working radiographs are made while the rubber dam is in place. The desired working length for the biomechanical preparation and resultant obturation of the root canal system is one of the most important phases of endodontic therapy. Traditionally, radiographs are used to confirm working length of the root and to evaluate the subsequent obturation of the root canal system (Stein and Corcoran, 1992).

Although electronic apex locators (EALs) are very accurate in determining the working length (see details in Chapter 14), it is recommended that a working length radiograph be taken to verify this measure and the tooth anatomy (Figure 13.24).

This radiograph, taken with a small file placed in the canal, will be the first indicator of the real anatomy of the root. The presence of sharp or double curvatures needs to be taken into consideration when the instrumentation technique is chosen (Figure 13.25).

After measuring the preoperative radiograph to estimate the length of the canal, and confirming this length with an EAL, a file is selected and a radiograph is taken with the file in the canal. A file smaller than #15 is not recommended because it will not be visible in the radiograph. This radiograph will show the relationship between the file and the apex of the tooth.

If the file is seen trespassing the apex by more than 2 mm, a new radiograph with an adjusted measurement should be taken at this point (Figure 13.26).

An angulated radiograph can be taken if more than one canal per root is suspected (Clark, 1916). When treating teeth with buccal and lingual canals, application of the buccal object rule is essential to properly locate the correct working length (this

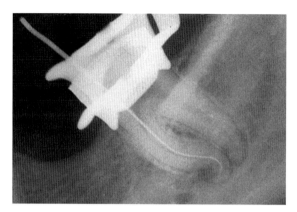

Figure 13.25 Small file placed in the canal shows the double curvature in a lower molar (Courtesy of Dr. Yared).

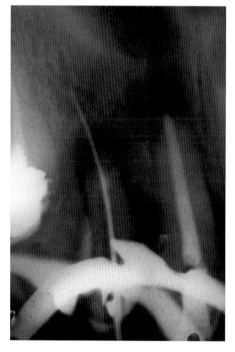

Figure 13.26 Radiograph showing endodontic file trespassing the apex more than 2 mm.

technique is explained in detail in Chapter 2) (Figure 13.27A–H).

The beam angulation will affect the appearance of the image of the rubber dam clamp on the radiograph. The lingual arm of the rubber dam always appears closer to the apex, and it will move in the same direction as the central ray (Figure 13.28A–D).

In cases where the roots of mandibular molars are short, superimposition of the clamp can interfere with the image of the roots. In these cases, an angulated radiograph is recommended. A more negative vertical angulation will elongate the radiographic appearance of the roots helping to provide an unobstructed view (Figure 13.29A–F).

Inserting the film with the rubber dam in place and the files in the canals is not an easy task. Specially designed holders are available for this purpose. In some cases, hemostat pliers can be used to properly place the receptor (see Chapter 2).

The decision of when to take the working length radiograph may vary depending on factors such as the diagnosis (vital vs. necrotic pulp), the degree of the root development, and the technique used for instrumentation (crown down or step back).

It is recommended that measurements of the working length be taken after the coronal enlargement is finalized, so that the files can have a better straight line access to the apex and so that this measurement will not change in the future. In addition, if cusps are going to be reduced or flatted, this step needs to be done before the working length determination radiograph is taken.

Once the radiograph is taken, it is important to analyze the following two aspects:

1. Is the real length (RL) the same as the estimate length (EL)? (RL = EL) or
2. Is RL greater than or less than the EL? (RL> or < than EL) (Figure 13.30).

Canal preparation

Once working length is established, cleaning and shaping of the apical portion can be started. Different systems and techniques are available to clean and shape the root canal system. Usually, no radiographs are needed at this stage. However, if a mishap occurs during this phase, a radiograph is mandatory to diagnose the problem and evaluate the possible outcome of the tooth.

The errors that most often occur during canal preparation include loss of working length (blockage), deviation from normal canal anatomy (ledge, zip, and elbow), and inadequate canal preparation, perforation, and/or separation of root canal instrument.

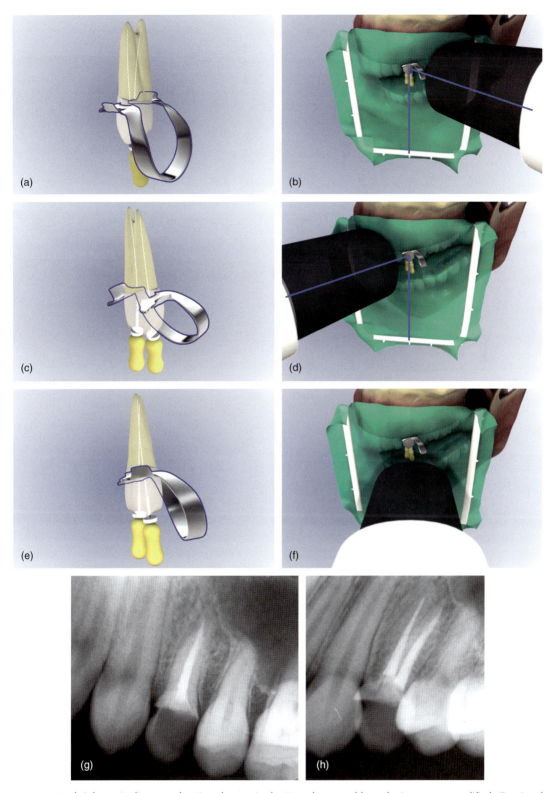

Figure 13.27 (a–f) Schematic diagrams showing changes in the X-ray beam and how the images are modified. (Reprinted with permission from the University of Toronto.) (g–h) Radiograph showing superimposition of the two canals with the orthoradial views and the separation of the two canals during a mesial angulation).

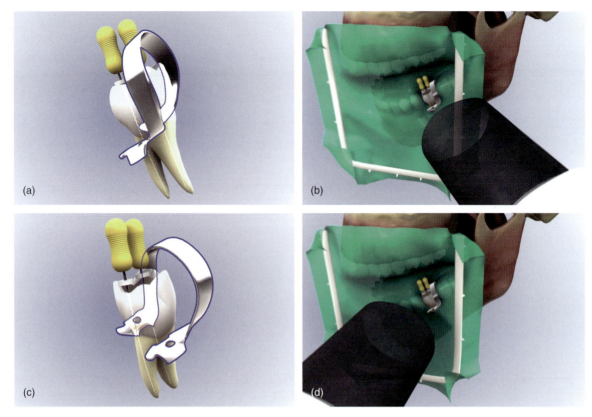

Figure 13.28   (a–d) Lingual arm of the rubber dam (always appearing closer to the apex) will move in the same direction than the head of the radiograph machine (Reprinted with permission from the University of Toronto.)

Special radiographic techniques can be used for these situations and are explained Chapter 2.

Radiograph for verification of master apical file (MAF)

Once the canal preparation has been completed, a radiograph is taken with the MAF in place. The MAF is the largest file that achieves the working length. This radiograph is vital to confirm that the length of the MAF is to working length and the shapes of the canals are adequately tapered (Figure 13.31).

Intracanal medication

If the root canal will be performed in more than one appointment, the use of intracanal medication is recommended. The most commonly used intracanal dressing is calcium hydroxide ($Ca(OH)_2$). Calcium hydroxide has similar radiopacity to the dentin. Therefore, if a radiograph is taking with $Ca(OH)_2$ in place, interpretation of these images needs to be done carefully, because the canal can appear calcified but actually is filled with the temporary medication (Figure 13.32).

Cone fit radiograph

This radiograph is taken by placing the master cone in the prepared canal just before obturation. An accurate cone fit picture assures that the tooth will be properly obturated if the clinician has achieved an ideal tapered preparation. This radiograph should reveal a cone which is not kinked or deformed in any way (Figure 13.33).

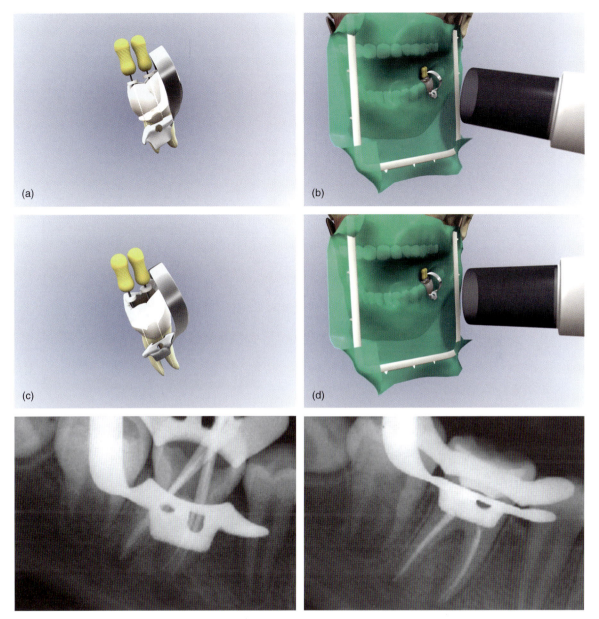

Figure 13.29 (a–d) Schematic diagrams showing short roots in lower molars; the presence of clamp can interfere with the image of the roots. In these cases, an angulated radiograph is recommended (Reprinted with permission from the University of Toronto). (e and f) Radiographs showing a clinical situation where the angulation needs to be changed in order to have a clear view of the end of the roots.

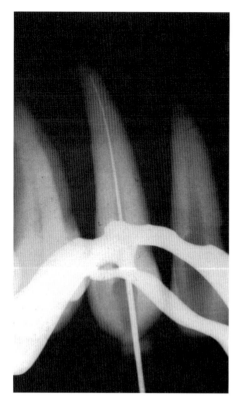

Figure 13.30 Trail file radiograph.

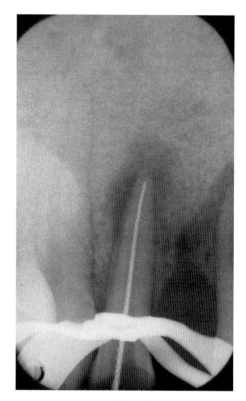

Figure 13.31 Master apical file radiograph.

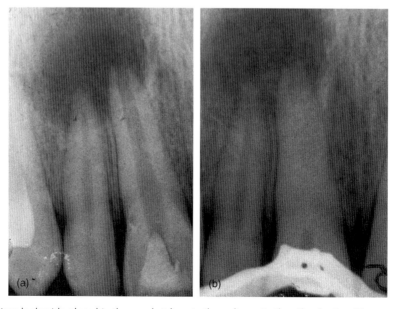

Figure 13.32 Calcium hydroxide placed in the canal. It has similar radiopacity than the dentine (Courtesy of Dr. Pascon).

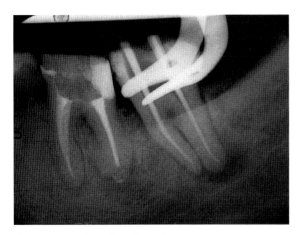

Figure 13.33 Cone fit radiograph.

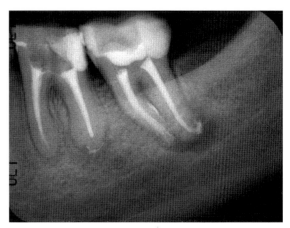

Figure 13.34 Postoperative radiograph.

Postoperative radiograph

Postoperative radiographs should be taken with the same technique as the preoperative radiograph. In this radiograph, the evaluation of the obturation is made. Length, density, configuration, and the general quality of the obturation in each canal are determined. This final radiograph will be the one that the clinician will use during follow-up appointments and with which comparisons will be made (Figure 13.34).

Recall

The same principles used for diagnostic and postoperative radiographs apply to recall radiographs. The traditional method of assessing the success of endodontic therapy involves clinical examination and the use of recall radiographs (see also Chapter 16). At some time following the completion of endodontic therapy, a radiograph of the treated tooth is taken and compared with the radiographs taken at the time of treatment. Radiographs are used to assess the periapical bone in order to determine whether the tooth has healed, is still in the process of healing, or has signs of persistent infection. The dentist's decision regarding this success or failure is important because it may determine the subsequent disposition of the case. Additional angled radiographs are often required to assess diagnosis

(Zakariasen et al., 1984) (Figures 13.35 and 13.36A,B). (See more details in Chapter 16.)

Documentation

Clinicians must be aware of how to file reports correctly and of the importance of documentation for dental records and as legal documents. It is necesary to document the exposure of dental radiographs, the number of receptors exposed, as well as the quality of the radiographs, as this may all be an important issue in a malpractice suit. An informed consent should be completed because it is the dentist's responsibility to discuss the need for radiographs and treatment procedures with the patient.

For valid informed consent, the patient must be provided with the following information in lay terms (www.csi.edu/facultyAndStaff_/webTools/sites/Bowcut58/courses/570/ch40.ppt):

1. The risks and benefits of the radiographs
2. The person who will be exposing the radiographs
3. The number and type of radiographs
4. The consequences of not having the radiographs
5. Any alternative diagnostic aids that may provide the same information as the radiographs

The dental record must include the number and type of radiographs exposed, the rational for exposing the radiographs, and the diagnostic interpretation.

Special consideration in endodontic radiography

Angulation of X-ray beam

The head of a dental X-ray machine can be moved in two planes. When the head is moved about a horizontal axis, the beam can be directed upward or downward and thus alter the vertical angulation. This movement can be used to localize an object in relation to a horizontal line as with the buccal or lingual position of the inferior dental canal and the apices of mandibular teeth.

When the head is moved about a vertical axis, the beam can be directed mesially or distally and thus alter the horizontal angulation. This movement can be employed to localize objects in relation to a vertical line, as with the superimposed roots of a maxillary premolar tooth where a mesial or distal shift in angulation will reveal both roots (Fava and Dummer, 1997).

The maximum information will be obtained with the exposure of at least two radiographs of a tooth, one taken at the normal angle and the other with an altered angulation. In endodontics, such changes in angulation can be useful to determine the number of canals, establish the position of root curvatures, locate and distinguish the position of root apices in relation to anatomical landmarks, distinguish between anatomical landmarks and radiolucent apical pathology, determine the position of iatrogenic errors (perforations, fractured instruments, etc.), distinguish between internal and external root resorption, locate foreign bodies following trauma, and establish the position and type of root fractures or resorptive processes.

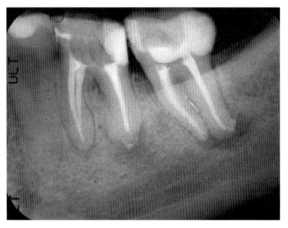

Figure 13.35   Recall radiograph.

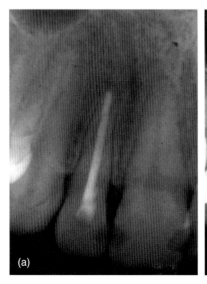
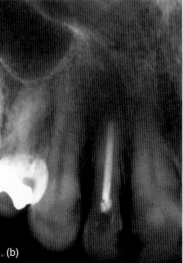

(a)   (b)

Figure 13.36   25-year recall radiograph (Courtesy of Dr. María Teresa Cañete).

Although having the potential to improve diagnosis, radiographs taken with eccentric beam angulations and altered receptor placement are inherently less clear, as the images lose the normal sharpness expected from standard receptors. However, this is balanced by the increased diagnostic yield that is achieved (Fava and Dummer, 1997).

Alteration in vertical angulation

Foreshortening or elongation

These are distortions in the vertical angulation. Under normal circumstances, the optimal relationship of the beam, tooth, and receptor occurs when the tooth and receptor are parallel and at right angles to the X-ray beam. This provides an image which is free from distortion (alteration in shape and size) apart from the effect that occurs as a result of the unavoidable increase in circumference of the X-ray beam which can be minimized, but not entirely eliminated, by using a long cone technique. The routine use of receptor holders and beam-aiming devices will facilitate the creation of accurate radiographs which are free from distortion, and it is essential that such receptors are taken as a routine for diagnosis and during endodontic procedures. Unfortunately, although free from distortion, images created by the standard angulations can result in superimposition of adjacent anatomical landmarks or pathological features leading to difficulties during interpretation (Figure 13.37A,B).

Alteration in horizontal angulation

To identify how a radiograph was taken in regard to its horizontal angulation (mesial or distal), the following details need to be observed:

1. Clamp wings: The wing that appears close to the apex is usually the palatal wing in maxillary or lingual wing in the mandible (Figure 13.38).
2. Tips of the cusps: The tips of the palatal (max) cusps or mandibular/lingual cusps are closer to the root apex (Figure 13.39).
3. Superimposition of roots in maxillary molars: The palatal root will be superimposed to the mesial buccal root if the radiograph was taken from mesial and vice versa (Figure 13.40).
4. Superimposition in contacts: In an orthoradial radiograph, the contact between the teeth will be very clear. When the angle is changed to the mesial, the mesial contacts will be clear, and the distal contacts will be superimposed (Figure 13.41).
5. Clarity of images: In a straight radiograph, the bone can be seen clearly. If angulate to mesial, the bone and lamina dura will be clear in the mesial area of the tooth and unclear at the distal aspect (Figure 13.42).

Infection control in dental radiography

Dental radiography presents unique infection control problems because of the potential for

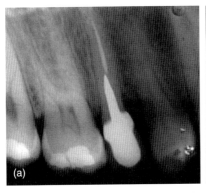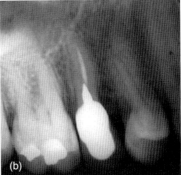

Figure 13.37   Radiograph elongated.

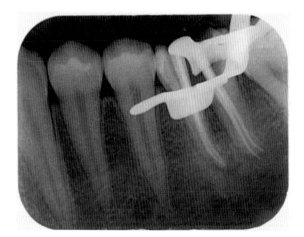

Figure 13.38   Radiograph showing wing of the clamp closer to the apical third of the root is the lingual one.

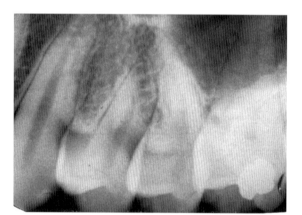

Figure 13.39   Radiograph showing the tip of the cusp closely to the apex is the palatal or lingual cusp.

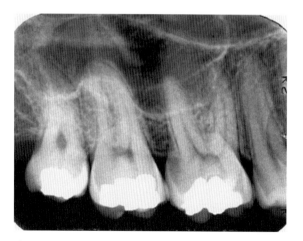

Figure 13.40   Radiograph showing superimposition of palatal root onto the mesiobuccal root.

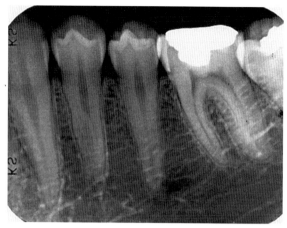

Figure 13.41   Distal contacts superimposed.

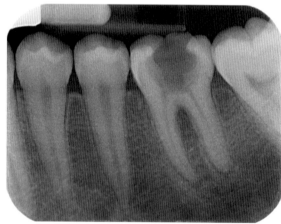

Figure 13.42   Bone and lamina dura will be clear in the mesial area.

operator contamination and cross contamination of other patients and of other members of the dental team. Constant movement by the operator from the oral cavity to the exposure controls outside the operatory to the darkroom and finally to receptor mounting increases the risk of exposing others to infectious diseases

The first step in preparation of the operatory is to determine the surfaces to be covered or disinfected with a high-level surface disinfectant. In general, surfaces that cannot be easily cleaned and disinfected should be protected by a barrier (most commonly plastic or foil barriers). Surface barriers are preferred to be on electrical switches because of the possibility of the cleaner and disinfectant causing an electrical short. The tube head, position-indicating device (PID), control panel, and exposure button must all be covered or carefully disinfected (www.csi.edu/facultyAndStaff_/webTools/sites/Bowcut58/courses/570/ch40.ppt).

References

Bender, I.B. and Seltzer, S. (2003) Roentgenographic and direct observation of experimental lesions in bone: I. 1961. *J Endod*, 29(11), 702–706.

Bramante, C.M., Berbert, A., and Bernardineli, N. (1980) Recursos Técnicos Radiográficos Aplicados À Endodontia. *Rev Bras Odontol*, 37, 8–24.

Clark, C.A. (1916) A method for ascertaining the relative position of unerupted teeth by means of film radiograph. *Proc R Soc Med*, Odontology Section, 3, 85–89.

Fava, L.R.G. and Dummer, P.M.H. (1997) Periapical radiographic techniques during endodontic diagnosis and treatment. *Int Endod J*, 30, 250–261.

Goldman, M., Pearson, A.H., and Darzenta, N. (1972) Endodontic Success—who's Reading The Radiograph? *Oral Surg Oral Med Oral Pathol*, 33(3), 432–437.

Gu, Y., Lu, Q., Wang, P., and Ni, L. (2010) Measurement of root canal curvatures in three-rooted mandibular first molars. *J Endod*, 36(8), 1341–1346.

Gutmann, J.L., Dumsha, T., Lovdahl, P.E., and Hovland, E.J. (1992) *Problem Solving in Endodontics: Prevention, Identification, and Management*, 2nd ed. Mosby, St. Loius, MO.

Hargreaves, K.H. and Cohen, S. (2010) *Cohen's Pathways of the Pulp Expert Consult*, 10th Ed. Mosby, St Louis.

Jung, H.J., Lee, S.S., Huh, K.H., Yi, W.J., Heo, M.S., and Choi, S.C. (2010) Predicting the configuration of a C-shaped canal system from panoramic radiographs. *Oral Surg Oral Med Oral Pathol Oral Radiol Endod*, 109(1), E37–E41.

Karapinar-Kazandag, M., Basrani, B.R., and Friedman, S. (2010) The operating microscope enhances detection and negotiation of accessory mesial canals in mandibular molars. *J Endod*, 36(8), 1289–1294.

Patel, S., Dawood, A., Ford, T.P., and Whaites, E. (2007) The potential applications of cone beam computed tomography in the management of endodontic problems. *Int Endod J*, 40(10), 818–830. Epub 2007 August 14. Review.

Patel, S., Dawood, A., Whaites, E., and Pitt Ford, T. (2009) New dimensions in endodontic imaging: Part 1. Conventional and alternative radiographic systems. *Int Endod J*, 42(6), 447–462.

Pruett, J.P., Clement, D.J., and Carnes, D.L. Jr. (1997) Cyclic fatigue testing of nickel-titanium endodontic instruments. *J Endod*, 23, 77–85.

Schneider, S.W. (1971) A comparison of canal preparations in straight and curved root canals. *Oral Surg Oral Med Oral Pathol*, 32, 271–275.

Stein, T.J. and Corcoran, J.F. (1992) Radiographic "working length" revisited. *Oral Surg Oral Med Oral Pathol*, 74(6), 796–800.

Torabinejad, M. and Walton, R.E. (2009) *Endodontics: Principles and Practice*. 4th ed. Elsevier Health Sciences, St. Louis, MO. Illustrated.

Velvart, P., Hecker, H., and Tillinger, G. (2001) Detection of the apical lesion and the mandibular canal in conventional radiography and computed tomography. *Oral Surg Oral Med Oral Pathol Oral Radiol Endod*, 92(6), 682–688.

Webber, R.L. and Messura, J.K. (1999) An in vivo comparison of diagnostic information obtained from tuned-aperture computed tomography and conventional dental radiographic imaging modalities. *Oral Surg Oral Med Oral Pathol Oral Radiol Endod*, 88(2), 239–247.

Weine, F. (1982) *Endodontic Therapy*, 3rd ed. CV Mosby, St. Louis, MO.

Zakariasen, K.L., Scott, D.A., and Jensen, J.R. (1984) Endodontic recall radiographs: how reliable is our interpretation of endodontic success or failure and what factors affect our reliability? *Oral Surg Oral Med Oral Pathol*, 57(3), 343–347.

14 Electronic Apex Locators and Conventional Radiograph in Working Length Measurement

Gevik Malkhassian, Andres Plazas, and Yosef Nahmias

Introduction

The success of endodontic treatment is highly dependent on the adequate three-dimensional cleaning, shaping, disinfection, and obturation of the root canal system. It is universally accepted that the correct determination of the working length (WL) is one of the crucial steps in the process of a successful treatment.

It is believed that root canal preparation and filling should be kept inside the root canal system to prevent damage to the periradicular tissues. On the other hand, selecting a point shorter than apical constriction may leave infected tissue apically, which may cause the persistence of the disease (Schilder, 1967; Seltzer et al., 1969).

The glossary of endodontic terminology of the American Association of Endodontists (American Association of Endodontists 2003) defines the WL as "the distance from a coronal reference point to the point at which canal preparation and obturation should terminate."

In order to define an apical end point during a course of root canal therapy, it is imperative to know the anatomy of the apical portion of the root.

Several anatomical landmarks exist at the apical segment of each root (Figure 14.1; Table 14.1).

Traditionally, radiographic images were extensively used to help locate the apical end of the roots. The radiographic apex, which was believed to commonly coincide with apical foramen and was easy to detect radiographically, was considered as the end of the root canal. However, several investigators (Green, 1956, 1960; Kuttler, 1955; Pineda and Kuttler, 1972) have shown that less than 50% of the time, the apical foramen coincides with the anatomical apex (Figure 14.1). Such variations are not easily detectable in two-dimensional radiography, even with minimum distortion. Therefore, considering the radiographic apex as the terminus seems not ideal. Although two different anatomical entities, traditionally, the apical constriction is known as the cementodentinal junction (CDJ) (Grove, 1928, 1930; Kuttler, 1958). However; the location of the apical constriction that coincides with CDJ is known to be variable (Dummer et al., 1984). The apical constriction is easily detectable in histological sections. It is a challenge to detect it clinically or radiologically. Moreover, the apical constriction varies in its

Endodontic Radiology, Second Edition. Edited by Bettina Basrani.
© 2012 John Wiley & Sons, Inc. Published 2012 by John Wiley & Sons, Inc.

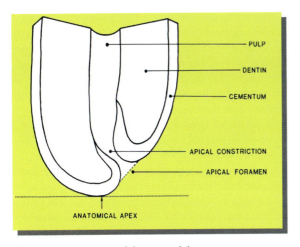

Figure 14.1   Anatomy of the apex of the root.

Table 14.1   Some definitions from *Glossary of Endodontic Terms* (2003).

Anatomy of the apical section	Definition
Anatomic apex	The tip or end of the root as determined morphologically
Apical foramen or major foramen	The main apical opening of the root canal.
Apical constriction or minor foramen (minor apical diameter, minor diameter)	The apical portion of the root canal having the narrowest diameter; position may vary but is usually 0.5–1.0 mm short of the center of the apical foramen.
Cementodentinal junction (CDJ)	The region at which the dentin and cementum are united commonly. Its position can range from 0.5–3.0 mm from the anatomic apex.
Radiographic apex	The tip or end of the root as determined radiographically; its location can vary from the anatomical apex due to root morphology and distortion of the radiographic image.

topography. It has been classified into simple, diverging, multiple, and parallel constrictions (Dummer et al., 1984). According to these findings it may be concluded that the constriction and its position differ not only in form but also in their presence within root canal space as an anatomical reference.

The majority of the endodontists and clinicians would agree that the apical constriction or minor foramen is where the apical end of the root canal preparation and filling should terminate. The rationale is that minor foramen is the narrowest section of the canal close to the apex with the minimum blood supply where the pulp tissue and the periodontal ligament (PDL) meet and that during root canal treatment, it provides the smallest wound site which is the most favorable for healing (Ricucci and Langeland, 1998).

WL measurement methods

Several methods have been used to determine the WL: (1) knowledge of anatomy and average root canal lengths, (2) apical sensitivity reported by patient when the instrument passes through the apical foramen, (3) tactile sensation of the apical constriction with endodontic file, (4) bleeding point as detected by the use of paper points showing bleeding in the most apical portion of the canal, and (5) radiographic technique by using an endodontic instrument within the root canal.

Most of these methods have some limitations and are not sufficiently reliable to be considered as the main measuring technique. Teeth lengths are variable. Apical sensitivity may be absent due to the use of local anesthetic. The tactile sensation of the apical constriction depends on countless factors (Palmer et al., 1971); for example, it might be only helpful in detection of the apical constriction in less than 60% of the cases (Seidberg et al., 1975). An incorrect radiographic technique can cause major distortion of the image (Vande Voorde and Bjorndahl, 1969).

Radiographic technique

Grove explained that using radiographic technique in the determination of WL is achieved by insertion of an endodontic instrument, usually a file, into the canal to a predetermined length, using a table showing the average length of each of the teeth and taking a radiograph and then adjusting the length as required (Grove, 1928, 1930). This method also has been described in detail by Ingle (1957), and it has been reported to be considered as the most successful method of WL determination compared to the other techniques available to that date (Bramante and Berbert, 1974).

Limitations with radiographic technique

Although the radiographic technique is considered the traditional technique and is still used for determining the WL, it has several limitations.

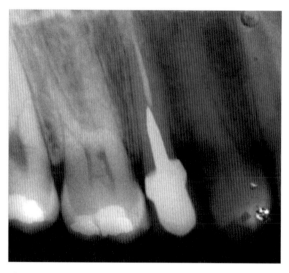

Figure 14.2   Distorted radiograph, elongated image.

The rationale for using this technique is based on the suggestion that the apical constriction may be located at 1 mm short of the radiographic apex. However; it is not all inclusive, and in some cases, the apical foramen can even be located as far as 3 mm short of the radiographic apex (Kuttler, 1955; Pineda and Kuttler, 1972).

It provides only a two-dimensional image of a three-dimensional object. It is also technique sensitive and relies entirely on the experience of the operator. Variables such as radiographic technique, angulations, inadequate radiographic exposure, will result in distorted or completely useless radiographic images (Figure 14.2). It is sometimes necessary to take several radiographs that will expose the patient to the unnecessary radiation levels; for example, identification of buccal and lingual canals may be challenging because of superimposition of those over each other in a radiographic straight angle image (Figure 14.3a,b). The interpretation of the radiographic image can also be very subjective and an important factor in accuracy of the technique. The radiographic technique provides a two-dimensional image which is subject to error, and some anatomical landmarks could be superimposed on each other, for example, the superimposition of the zygomatic arch over the roots of maxillary molars or mandibular torus over the roots of mandibular premolars (Figure 14.4a,b), which impede the proper location of the radiographic apex on those teeth. The zygomatic arch

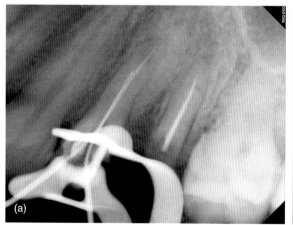
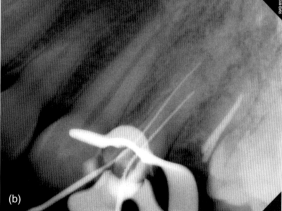

Figure 14.3   (a) Superimposed files over each other in buccal and palatal canals. (b) The same image taken from another angle to see the files separately.

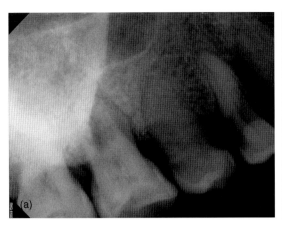
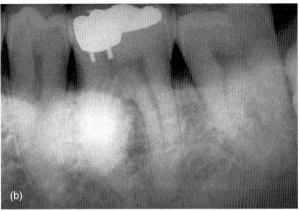

Figure 14.4   (a) Superimposition of the zygomatic arch over the roots of maxillary molars. (b) Superimposition of the Torus Mandibularis over the roots of mandibular premolars.

has been reported to be superimposed in approximately 20% and 42% on the apices of the first and second maxillary molars, respectively (Tamse et al., 1980). The presence of apical resorption can also create a problem for adequate WL measurement using this technique. Based on the fact that root resorption can alter the apical constriction, Weine (2004) suggested subtracting an extra 0.5 mm from the WL in teeth exhibiting radiographic evidence of apical resorption. This may ensure that both the instrumentation and filling materials will be kept confined within the root canal space.

History of apex locators

The idea of using electronic locators was born when Custer in 1918 used the electric current to measure the length of the root canals. In 1942, Suzuki conducted experiments of iontophoresis with silver nitrate and ammonium in dogs using direct current and discovered that the electrical resistance between the PDL and oral mucosa had a constant value of 6.5 k ohms (Suzuki, 1942). Sunada in 1962 introduced this principle to the clinic area. He postulated that, according to the results obtained by Suzuki, it would be possible to design a device to measure the length of the root canal electronically. He used an ohmmeter with one electrode connected to the oral mucosa and another electrode connected to an endodontic file. As the file moved into the canal, he found that

when the tip of the file was just touching the PDL at apical foramen level, the device registered 40 μA regardless of patient age or the shape and length of the tooth (Figure 14.5a–c). With his findings, he explained that it was necessary to pass the file through the apical foramen to obtain accurate measurements. This would eliminate variables that could produce erroneous measurements (Sunada, 1962).

Based on these basic principles, the first apex locators were introduced. In reality, these devices operate using the human body as one of the components to complete the electric circuit. One of the electrodes of the apex locator is connected to an endodontic file while the other is connected through a clip to the labial mucosa of the patient (Figures 14.6 and 14.7). Once the file is inserted into the root canal, the circuit is partially complete, and as the file reaches to the apex, then the electric circuit is completed, and the exact position of the apical foramen is located (Pilot and Pitts, 1997) (Figure 14.8a–c).

The first generation of apex locators used direct current. Unfortunately, they were very inaccurate and unpredictable. Therefore, in 1969, the Japanese medical company Onuki designed a device that used alternating current. This apex locator was called Root Canal Meter and worked at a frequency of 150 Hz. Today, it is speculated that these devices primarily measure impedance of the electrode; therefore, electrolytic substances as sodium hypochlorite cause erroneous measurements when

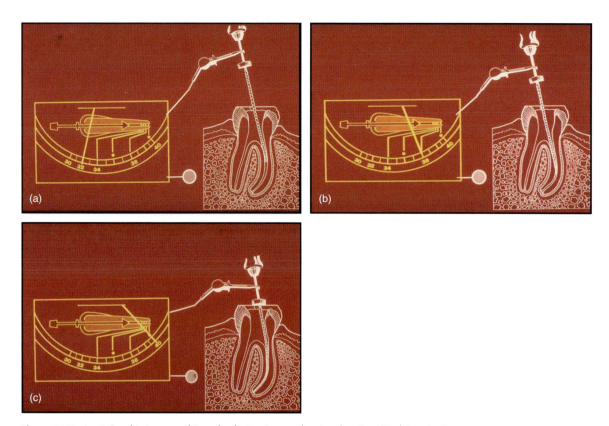

Figure 14.5   (a–c) Graphic images of Sunada electronic apex locator showing WL determination.

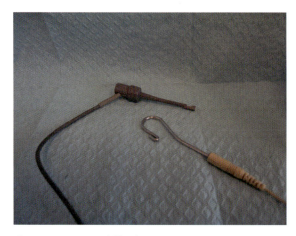

Figure 14.6   Lip and file clips.

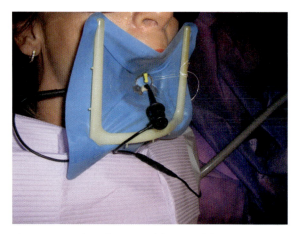

Figure 14.7   Clinical picture of the use of the apex locator.

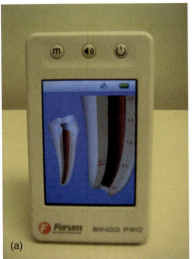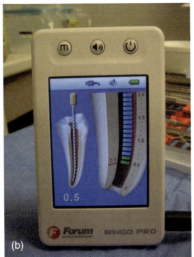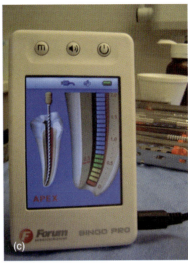

Figure 14.8   Clinical use of Bingo electronic apex locator. (a) Before. (b) At working length. (c) Beyond the working length.

using these devices (Kobayashi, 1997). As the technology was advancing, new appliances appeared on the market. Some used the detection of changes in electrical frequency for measuring the root canals; others used the voltage gradient method. However, the presence of electrolytes within the root canals prevents proper operation of all these devices. A significant breakthrough was achieved with the introduction of a new generation of the apex locators. This third generation of electronic apex locators (EALs) such as Endex calculates the difference between two electrical impedances in the canal, using an alternating current composed of two different frequencies. This apex locator can accurately measure the length of the root canals even in the presence of electrolytes (Fouad et al., 1993). It is reported that the Endex can find the apical foramen in more than 90% of the cases (Frank and Torabinejad, 1993).

In 1991, the EALs that worked based on "the ratio method" were introduced. These apex locators were not affected by the presence of electrolytes in the canals. In this method, EALs work in such a way that if there is an electrolyte in the canal, two impedances are measured simultaneously by two electric currents with different frequencies. Thus, if one of the impedances changes because of the presence of electrolyte in the canal,

the second impedance also changes in the same proportion. Therefore, the ratio between the two frequencies is not affected even in the presence of electrolytes (Kobayashi, 1997). The Root ZX (Morita Japan) is designed based on this principle (Figure 14.9). This device has the advantage of not having to be calibrated for each patient and makes it one of the most efficient and versatile to use. Clinical studies demonstrate its accuracy by 96% of cases (Shabahang et al., 1996).

All apex locators are equipped with a display screen or some indicators and a type of alarm that visually and audibly indicate both the proximity and the location of the apical foramen (Figure 14.10a,b).

Different studies have resulted in an accuracy of between 8% and 94% (Fouad et al., 1993; Frank and Torabinejad, 1993). Shabahang et al. (1996) found that the Root ZX could locate the apical foramen with a tolerance of ±0.5 mm in vital teeth, in 96.2% of the time. Ibarrola et al. (1999) concluded that if the canals are widened before using the apex locator, the results are more consistent. Pagavino et al. (1998) found that the Root ZX could find the apical foramen in 100% of cases, with a tolerance of ±1 mm. Saad and al-Nazhan (2000) suggest using apex locators in conjunction with digital radiovisiography to help reduce the amount of radiation.

They only recommend taking a digital radiograph with the master cone in the canal, after having determined the WL electronically.

Clinical technique

Different operators may use the apex locators slightly differently. Hence, a common technique

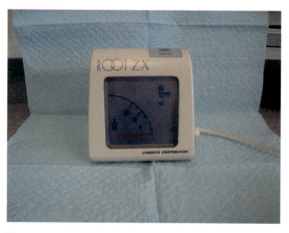

Figure 14.9   Root ZX electronic apex locator.

has only been described here. But the concept of using the apex locator stays the same.

Routinely, regular endodontic therapy procedures usually start with anesthetizing the region and rubber dam isolation. Then an access cavity is prepared, the pulp tissue is removed from the chamber, and the canal orifices are located then the chamber and the canals are irrigated with hypochlorite solution. Then a small K-file No 8 or 10 is introduced into the canal until it reaches the estimated working length (EWL) based on the predetermination using the preoperative radiograph. The files can also be introduced to EWL following coronal preflaring of the canals. It is always helpful to remove calcifications and dentinal shavings which may have a negative impact on the accuracy of EALs. It is suggested that preflaring of the root canals prior to WL measurement using EAL may increase the accuracy of these devices (de Camargo et al., 2009; Ibarrola et al., 1999).

After checking the battery of the apex locator and calibrating it if required (as noted earlier, most new models do not need to be calibrated), make sure that the lip clip is in stable contact with the lip. An endodontic 25-mm length file is inserted into the canal. Then a second electrode is connected

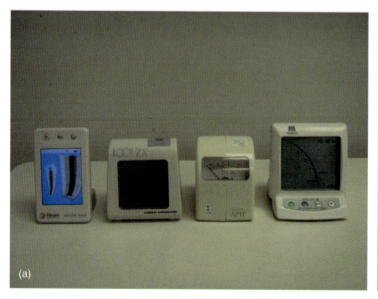

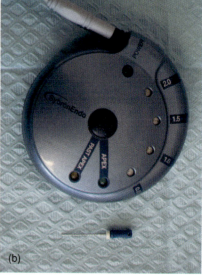

(a)   (b)

Figure 14.10   (a) Four different types of electronic apex locators from left to right: Bingo, Root ZX, Osada APIT, Root ZX II. (b) Sybron Endo Mini Apex Locator next to a 21 mm H-file.

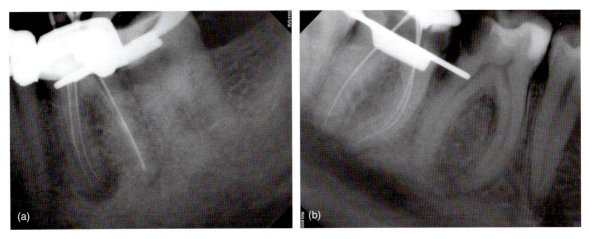

Figure 14.11   (a and b) Confirmation of WL determination by radiographs.

to the file. At this point the apex locator is beginning to indicate that the file is short, beyond, or at WL. It needs to be adjusted accordingly until it indicates that the file is at WL. It is recommended to introduce the file initially slightly beyond the foramen in order to make sure that the file has reached the PDL and then pull the file back to adjust the WL at the apical constriction. It is noteworthy that if there are sudden changes in the reading, it is possible that there is flooding or a lot of liquid in the chamber or the file is touching a metal restoration. Drying the chamber using a gentle blow of air or using a piece of cotton pellet may overcome to this problem.

Special attention must be made to remove any metal restoration that can come into contact with the files that are used to make measurements. The contact of these files with metallic elements transmits electricity directly to the adjacent periodontal area. Therefore, the apex locator will provide a wrong measure. It is usually beneficial to take a radiograph to confirm what the apex locator has detected (Figure 14.11a,b). However, in the hands of an experienced clinician, it is not always needed (Saad and al-Nazhan, 2000).

Advantages of apex locators

There are several advantages reported using EALs. First, they are beneficial in reducing the number of radiographs required to determine WL (Nahmias et al., 1983; Saad and al-Nazhan, 2000). Some dentists determine the WL only by using the apex locators; others use only one radiograph to confirm the initial measurement. Thus, by decreasing the total number of required radiographs, the patient's exposure to radiation is also reduced. It can be especially invaluable in cases where the patient is at high risk when exposed to radiation.

Another advantage is by providing a greater precision in locating the apical foramen compared to the radiographic method. It is not uncommon that the apical foramen and the radiographic apex do not coincide (Green, 1956, 1960). Therefore, the radiographic interpretation of the instrument in the canal with respect to the foramen is questionable. It has been reported that only in 40% of the specimens was it possible to locate the foramen with radiographic methods (Plant and Newman, 1976). Instead the foramen was located accurately in 93.8% of cases when electronic measurements were used. It was concluded that the apex locators are highly accurate when used correctly.

The apex locators can be used at any stage and if required for several times during the instrumentation to verify whether the WL remains stable or not and can be adjusted accordingly.

The endodontic procedure may be shorter in time when EALs are used instead of conventional radiographs. A 54% reduction of the time compared with traditional radiographic technique has been reported (Cash, 1975).

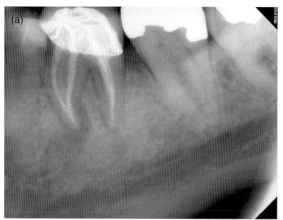 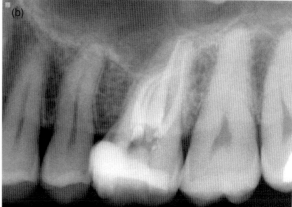

Figure 14.12   (a and b) Cases of multirooted obturated root canals.

In multirooted teeth, the radiographic method can be complicated for WL measurement. EALs could be very helpful in lessening the uncertainties in these cases (Figure 14.12a,b).

Apex locators are invaluable in detection of perforations (Fuss et al., 1996; Kaufman et al., 1997).

In patients with an acute gag reflex, taking radiographs can be extremely challenging. Electronic WL measurement can provide an invaluable assistance in these situations.

Limitation of apex locators

Occasionally, apex locators provide false measurements. A list of such situations is presented:

1. Apex locators do not work properly in the presence of metallic restorations, profuse bleeding, saliva in contact with file, and in case of open apices.
2. Some patients have sensed electrical impulses when apex locators are used, although not common (Nahmias et al., 1983).
3. Patients who have a pacemaker must consult their physician to determine whether or not it is safe to use the apex locator (Woolley et al., 1974).
4. They are relatively expensive. The modern apex locators are more expensive than their predecessors. However; due to their valuable assistance, they are considered essential to the dentist.

5. The technique requires the operator to be familiar with the equipment and learn how to interpret it. Like any new instrument, the apex locators require a period of learning to use them effectively.

Comparing EAL to radiographs

Apex locators and conventional radiographs

Accurate WL determination is a crucial part of successful root canal treatment (Ricucci, 1998). The apical constriction is regarded as an ideal apical end point for instrumentation and obturation in root canal therapy (Dummer et al., 1984); unfortunately, the location and shape of the apical constriction are variable and are not radiographically detectable (ElAyouti et al., 2001; Ricucci and Langeland, 1998). In addition to radiographic measurements, electronic WL determination has become increasingly important. The electronic method reduces many of the problems associated with radiographic measurements. Its most important advantage over radiography is that it can measure the length of the root canal to the apical foramen, not to the radiographic apex (Kobayashi, 1995).

Based on a study on extracted teeth using Root ZX apex locator, it was reported that Radiographic WL determination alone resulted in overestimation in 51% of the root canals while the percentage of overestimation was reduced to 21% by using EAL

(ElAyouti et al., 2002). The authors concluded that complementing radiographic WL determination with EAL may help to avoid overestimation beyond apical foramen.

Kim et al. (2008) found that the accuracy of Root ZX when used alone was 84%, but in combination of Root ZX and radiograph, the accuracy was 96%.

Vieyra et al. (2010) found that radiographs located minor foramen correctly 20% of the time in anterior and premolar teeth, and 11% of the time in molar teeth.

Patino-Marin et al. (2011) found that the apex locators were more accurate than conventional radiography in determining the WL in primary teeth.

Krajczar et al., (2008) based on an in vitro study on MB canals of upper first molars, concluded that EAL was more accurate than radiological method alone.

In two different studies, when accuracy of the different apex locators were compared with digital radiography, the apex locators showed to be more accurate than digital radiography in determining the WLs (Cianconi et al., 2010; Real et al., 2011).

As a result, it seems logical to conclude that EALs are more accurate than radiographic techniques alone in determination of WL during root canal treatments.

Apex locators and digital radiography

"Digital radiography uses sensors to produce electronic radiographic images that can be viewed on a monitor and that allow for a reduction in radiation exposure; sensors can be integrated with intraoral digital cameras and patient management database software" (American Association of Endodontists, 2003). Digital radiographs are captured and saved in a digital format so they do not need usual chemicals for image processing (Figure 14.13a–c). The digital formatting allows the clinician to have the ability to use different image

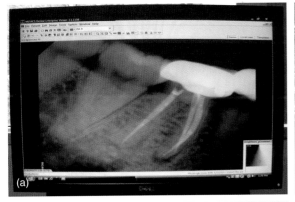
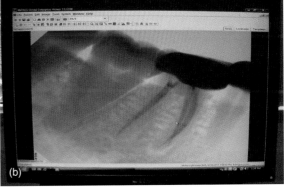
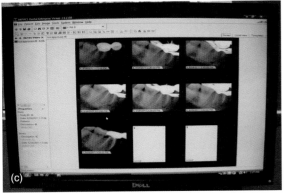

Figure 14.13   (a–b) Digital display of a radiograph on the monitor.

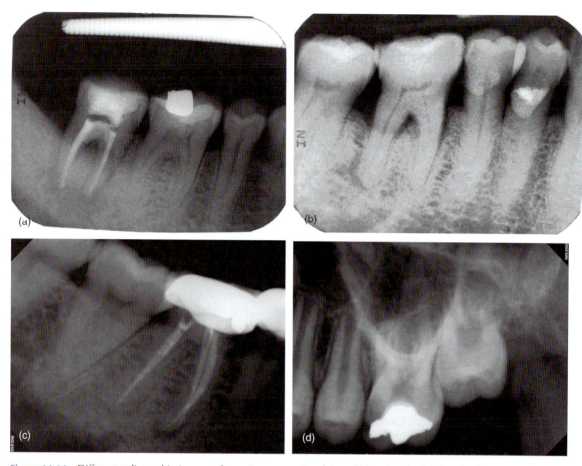

Figure 14.14   Different radiographic images taken using conventional (a and b) and with digital technologies (c and d).

densities with the capability of better image analysis. Moreover, the brightness and the contrast of the image could be adjusted if needed (Burger et al., 1999; Loushine et al., 2001). However, it seems that using digital radiography is not superior to conventional radiography techniques regarding WL measurements (Figure 14.14a–d). In one study, a 64.9% accuracy in determining the WL by digital radiography has been reported compared to apex locators (Real et al., 2011). In another study, it was concluded that the EALs were more reliable than digital radiographs in locating the apical foramen (Cianconi et al., 2010).

It has been suggested that even small doses of radiation might have some deleterious effects (Goaz and White, 1987; Poyton, 1968). Digital radiographs have the advantage of reducing the

exposure dosage to the patient. As a result, in order to reduce the radiation dose, the use of digital radiographs instead of conventional radiographs in combination with EAL's is advised for WL determination (Saad and al-Nazhan, 2000).

Apex locator's employment in the detection of perforations

Perforations are one of the significant factors affecting the prognosis of root canal treatment (de Chevigny et al., 2008). They can happen due to pathological factors like resorption or caries or be caused during regular root canal treatment or during post space preparation (Fuss and Trope, 1996). They may occur at the floor or wall of the pulp chamber or at any level of the root canal (Figure 14.15). Perforations are sometimes difficult to diagnose particularly if accompanied by abnormal bleeding from the site. Traditionally, radiographs have been used, but their use is limited (Fuss et al., 1996) especially if the perforation site is on the buccal or lingual aspect of the root. After the introduction of EALs, it was noted that they can be very helpful in locating and diagnosing perforations (Nahmias et al., 1983) (Figure 14.16a,b).

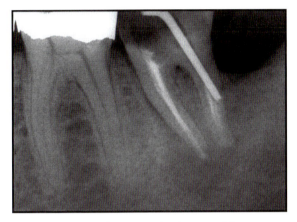

Figure 14.15   A perforation on distal aspect of the mandibular second molar.

In order to detect a perforation, a simple technique has been described. A small file could be inserted into the suspected area and connected to the apex locator. If the apex locator indicates immediately that it has detected the apex which is usually not there, it probably means that a perforation was created. Commonly, if the apex locator indicator moves slowly while introducing the file, it is more likely that the file is inside the canal rather than in a perforation (Figure 14.17a,b). In a study using different models of EALs, it was found that radiographs were less reliable than apex locators in the identification of perforation locations (Fuss et al., 1996). In another in vitro study using three different type of EALs, it was reported that EALs were acceptable tools for the detection of root perforations clinically (Kaufman et al., 1997).

The effect of different parameters on performance of EALs

Moisture, different irrigants, or solutions in the canal

WL measurements using the first two generation models of EALs were considered to be inaccurate in the presence of conductive fluids, moisture and

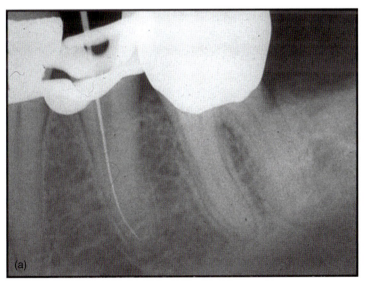

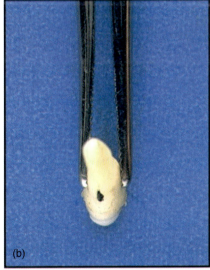

(a)   (b)

Figure 14.16   (A) The file seems to be in the canal. (B) After extraction, a perforation on the buccal aspect of the root was confirmed.

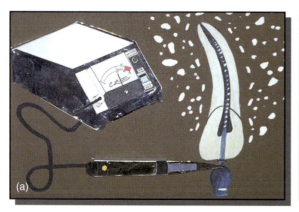 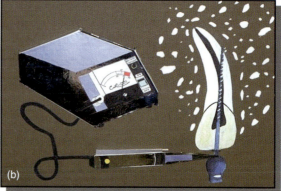

Figure 14.17 (A) Schematic view of an apex locator indicating file is in the canal. (B) The abrupt change in the measurement shows the presence of the perforation.

electrolytes such as blood and sodium hypochlorite in the canal (Fouad and Krell, 1989; Fouad et al., 1993; Huang, 1987). However, with the introduction of later generations of apex locators, this problem was overcome, and most EALs perform well in the presence of different solutions and electrolytes (Carvalho et al., 2010; Jenkins et al., 2001; Kang and Kim, 2008; Meares and Steiman, 2002). As a result of these reports and studies, it can be concluded that the new generations of EALs could be confidently used for WL measurement in the presence of tissue fluids or different electrolytes.

Type and size of the file

The accuracy of the measurement appears not to be affected by the size of the canal or that of the measuring instrument (Briseno-Marroquin et al., 2008; Nguyen et al., 1996).

In another in vitro study, the effect of different type of files made of stainless-steel or nickel-titanium were assessed in conjunction with Root ZX, and no difference was noted in accuracy of WL determination between those types of files (Thomas et al., 2003).

Preflaring of the root canals

It is suggested that preflaring of the root canals prior to WL measurement using EAL may increase

the accuracy of these devices. Most of the apex locators performed better in determining WL measurement after initial preflaring of the root canals (de Camargo et al., 2009; Ibarrola et al., 1999).

Primary teeth

Investigations to test the ability of EALs in determining WL on primary teeth were started around 2008 (Bodur et al., 2008; Leonardo et al., 2009; Tosun et al., 2008). All the studies (regardless of using in vitro or in vivo conditions) concluded that EALs were accurate enough to be used in primary teeth during root canal treatment even in the presence of external root resorption (Angwaravong and Panitvisai, 2009; Beltrame et al., 2010; Bodur et al., 2008; Leonardo et al., 2009; Mello-Moura et al., 2010; Odabas et al., 2011; Patino-Marin et al., 2011; Tosun et al., 2008).

Fractures

Many clinicians would agree that detecting and locating the position of the root fractures pose a dilemma in a routine daily practice. The ability of EALs to detect horizontal, vertical, and oblique root fractures were investigated mainly on extracted single-rooted teeth, and the results showed that the EALs were able to accurately determine the position of horizontal root fractures but were unreliable to detect the position of vertical root fractures (Azabal et al., 2004; Ebrahim et al., 2006a; Goldberg et al., 2008).

Pulp status (vitality)

The presence of vital or necrotic tissue in the root canals does not affect the reliability of the EALs when tested in vivo (Akisue et al., 2007; Dunlap et al., 1998).

Apical foramen size

In the presence of a large apical foramen either enlarged inadvertently during a course of root canal treatment, or due to the presence of external root resorption at the apex, or because of partially developed apical root segment, EALs can be valuable tools to establish a reasonable WL (Goldberg et al., 2002; Kang and Kim, 2008; Nguyen et al., 1996). However, some limitations have been reported on the performance of EALs in these situations. For example, some initial studies showed that some apex locators may be more reliable than the other ones (Fouad et al., 1993). Using small files in widened foramens may affect the reliability of the measurements (Ebrahim et al., 2006b). The diameter of apical constriction may affect the accuracy of the EALs, and it was reported that the WL measurements of root canals with apical foramens larger than a size 100 K-file were not reliable (Herrera et al., 2007).

Retreatment of previously treated teeth

The results of two studies also indicated that EALs are useful in determining the WL of root canals during retreatment of previously treated root canals (Aggarwal et al., 2010; Goldberg et al., 2005).

Conclusion

Radiographic techniques were used conventionally as the main tools by practitioners during endodontic WL measurements for many years. The introduction and evolvement of electronic WL measurement devices have provided another reliable means to help practitioners in their routine daily root canal treatment procedures. Although both techniques have their own limitations, the great advantages of EALs have made them an important part of a daily endodontic practice. It has been suggested that more predictable results can be achieved by combination of EALs and radiographic techniques in WL measurement.

References

Aggarwal, V., Singla, M., and Kabi, D. (2010) An in vitro evaluation of performance of two electronic root canal length measurement devices during retreatment of different obturating materials. *Journal of Endodontics*, 36, 1526–1530.

Akisue, E., Gavini, G., and De Figueiredo, J.A.P. (2007) Influence of pulp vitality on length determination by using the Elements Diagnostic Unit and Apex Locator. *Oral Surgery, Oral Medicine, Oral Pathology, Oral Radiology, and Endodontics*, 104, e129–e132.

American Association of Endodontists (AAE). (2003) *Glossary of Endodontic Terms*, 7th ed. American Association of Endodontists, Chicago, IL.

Angwaravong, O. and Panitvisai, P. (2009) Accuracy of an electronic apex locator in primary teeth with root resorption. *International Endodontic Journal*, 42, 115–121.

Azabal, M., Garcia-Otero, D., and de la Macorra, J.C. (2004) Accuracy of the Justy II Apex locator in determining working length in simulated horizontal and vertical fractures. *International Endodontic Journal*, 37, 174–177.

Beltrame, A.P.C.A., Triches, T.C., Sartori, N., and Bolan, M. (2010) Electronic determination of root canal working length in primary molar teeth: an in vivo and ex vivo study. *International Endodontic Journal*, 44, 402–406.

Bodur, H., Odabas, M., Tulunoglu, O., and Tinaz, A.C. (2008) Accuracy of two different apex locators in primary teeth with and without root resorption. *Clinical Oral Investigations*, 12, 137–141.

Bramante, C.M. and Berbert, A. (1974) A critical evaluation of some methods of determining tooth length. *Oral Surgery, Oral Medicine, and Oral Pathology*, 37, 463–473.

Briseno-Marroquin, B., Frajlich, S., Goldberg, F., and Willershausen, B. (2008) Influence of instrument size on the accuracy of different apex locators: an in vitro study. *Journal of Endodontics*, 34, 698–702.

Burger, C.L., Mork, T.O., Hutter, J.W., and Nicoll, B. (1999) Direct digital radiography versus conventional radiography for estimation of canal length in curved canals. *Journal of Endodontics*, 25, 260–263.

Carvalho, A.L.P., Moura-Netto, C., Moura, A.A.M.D., Marques, M.M., and Davidowicz, H. (2010) Accuracy of three electronic apex locators in the presence of different irrigating solutions. *Brazilian Oral Research*, 24, 394–398.

Cash, P.W. (1975) Letter: endo research challenged. *Journal of the American Dental Association (1939)*, 91, 1135–1136.

Cianconi, L., Angotti, V., Felici, R., Conte, G., and Mancini, M. (2010) Accuracy of three electronic apex locators compared with digital radiography: an ex vivo study. *Journal of Endodontics*, 36, 2003–2007.

de Camargo, E.J., Zapata, R.O., Medeiros, P.L., Bramante, C.M., Bernardineli, N., Garcia, R.B., de Moraes, I.G., and Duarte, M.A.H. (2009) Influence of preflaring on the accuracy of length determination with four electronic apex locators. *Journal of Endodontics*, 35, 1300–1302.

de Chevigny, C., Dao, T.T., Basrani, B.R., Marquis, V., Farzaneh, M., Abitbol, S., and Friedman, S. (2008) Treatment outcome in endodontics: the Toronto study—phases 3 and 4: orthograde retreatment. *Journal of Endodontics*, 34, 131–137.

Dummer, P.M., Mcginn, J.H., and Rees, D.G. (1984) The position and topography of the apical canal constriction and apical foramen. *International Endodontic Journal*, 17, 192–198.

Dunlap, C.A., Remeikis, N.A., Begole, E.A., and Rauschenberger, C.R. (1998) An in vivo evaluation of an electronic apex locator that uses the ratio method in vital and necrotic canals. *Journal of Endodontics*, 24, 48–50.

Ebrahim, A.K., Wadachi, R., and Suda, H. (2006a) Accuracy of three different electronic apex locators in detecting simulated horizontal and vertical root fractures. *Australian Endodontic Journal: The Journal of the Australian Society of Endodontology Inc*, 32, 64–69.

Ebrahim, A.K., Yoshioka, T., Kobayashi, C., and Suda, H. (2006b) The effects of file size, sodium hypochlorite and blood on the accuracy of Root ZX apex locator in enlarged root canals: an in vitro study. *Australian Dental Journal*, 51, 153–157.

ElAyouti, A., Weiger, R., and Lost, C. (2001) Frequency of overinstrumentation with an acceptable radiographic working length. *Journal of Endodontics*, 27, 49–52.

ElAyouti, A., Weiger, R., and Lost, C. (2002) The ability of root ZX apex locator to reduce the frequency of overestimated radiographic working length. *Journal of Endodontics*, 28, 116–119.

Fouad, A.F. and Krell, K.V. (1989) An in vitro comparison of five root canal length measuring instruments. *Journal of Endodontics*, 15, 573–577.

Fouad, A.F., Rivera, E.M., and Krell, K.V. (1993) Accuracy of the Endex with variations in canal irrigants and foramen size. *Journal of Endodontics*, 19, 63–67.

Frank, A.L. and Torabinejad, M. (1993) An in vivo evaluation of Endex electronic apex locator. *Journal of Endodontics*, 19, 177–179.

Fuss, Z. and Trope, M. (1996) Root perforations: classification and treatment choices based on prognostic factors. *Endodontics & Dental Traumatology*, 12, 255–264.

Fuss, Z., Assooline, L.S., and Kaufman, A.Y. (1996) Determination of location of root perforations by electronic apex locators. *Oral Surgery, Oral Medicine, Oral Pathology, Oral Radiology, and Endodontics*, 82, 324–329.

Goaz, P.W. and White, S.C. (1987) *Radiation Biology. Oral Radiology: Principles and Interpretation*, 2nd ed. Mosby, St. Louis, MO.

Goldberg, F., De Silvio, A.C., Manfre, S., and Nastri, N. (2002) In vitro measurement accuracy of an electronic apex locator in teeth with simulated apical root resorption. *Journal of Endodontics*, 28, 461–463.

Goldberg, F., Marroquin, B.B., Frajlich, S., and Dreyer, C. (2005) In vitro evaluation of the ability of three apex locators to determine the working length during retreatment. *Journal of Endodontics*, 31, 676–678.

Goldberg, F., Frajlich, S., Kuttler, S., Manzur, E., and Briseno-Marroquin, B. (2008) The evaluation of four electronic apex locators in teeth with simulated horizontal oblique root fractures. *Journal of Endodontics*, 34, 1497–1499.

Green, D. (1956) A stereomicroscopic study of the root apices of 400 maxillary and mandibular anterior teeth. *Oral Surgery, Oral Medicine, and Oral Pathology*, 9, 1224–1232.

Green, D. (1960) Stereomicroscopic study of 700 root apices of maxillary and mandibular posterior teeth. *Oral Surgery, Oral Medicine, and Oral Pathology*, 13, 728–733.

Grove, C.J. (1928) A new simple standardized technique producing perfect fitting impermeable root canal fillings extending to the dento-cemento junction. *Dental Items of Interest*, 50, 855–857.

Grove, C.J. (1930) Further evidence that root canals can be filled to the dentinocemental junction. *The Journal of the American Dental Association*, 17, 293–296.

Herrera, M., Abalos, C., Planas, A.J., and Llamas, R. (2007) Influence of apical constriction diameter on Root ZX apex locator precision. *Journal of Endodontics*, 33, 995–998.

Huang, L. (1987) An experimental study of the principle of electronic root canal measurement. *Journal of Endodontics*, 13, 60–64.

Ibarrola, J.L., Chapman, B.L., Howard, J.H., Knowles, K.I., and Ludlow, M.O. (1999) Effect of preflaring on Root ZX apex locators. *Journal of Endodontics*, 25, 625–626.

Ingle, J.I. (1957) Endodontic instruments and instrumentation. *Dental Clinics of North America*, 1, 805–822.

Jenkins, J.A., Walker, W.A., Schindler, W.G., and Flores, C.M. (2001) An in vitro evaluation of the accuracy of the root ZX in the presence of various irrigants. *Journal of Endodontics*, 27, 209–211.

Kang, J.-A. and Kim, S.K. (2008) Accuracies of seven different apex locators under various conditions. *Oral Surgery, Oral Medicine, Oral Pathology, Oral Radiology, and Endodontics*, 106, e57–e62.

Kaufman, A.Y., Fuss, Z., Keila, S., and Waxenberg, S. (1997) Reliability of different electronic apex locators to detect root perforations in vitro. *International Endodontic Journal*, 30, 403–407.

Kim, E., Marmo, M., Lee, C.-Y., Oh, N.-S., and Kim, I.-K. (2008) An in vivo comparison of working length determination by only root-ZX apex locator versus combining root-ZX apex locator with radiographs using a new impression technique. *Oral Surgery, Oral Medicine, Oral Pathology, Oral Radiology, and Endodontics*, 105, e79–e83.

Kobayashi, C. (1995) Electronic canal length measurement. *Oral Surgery, Oral Medicine, Oral Pathology, Oral Radiology, and Endodontics*, 79, 226–231.

Kobayashi, C. (1997) The evolution of apex-locating devices. *The Alpha Omegan*, 90, 21–27.

Krajczar, K., Marada, G., Gyulai, G., and Toth, V. (2008) Comparison of radiographic and electronical working length determination on palatal and mesio-buccal root canals of extracted upper molars. *Oral Surgery, Oral Medicine, Oral Pathology, Oral Radiology, and Endodontics*, 106, e90–e93.

Kuttler, Y. (1955) Microscopic investigation of root apexes. *Journal of the American Dental Association (1939)*, 50, 544–552.

Kuttler, Y. (1958) A precision and biologic root canal filling technic. *Journal of the American Dental Association (1939)*, 56, 38–50.

Leonardo, M.R., da Silva, L.A.B., Nelson-Filho, P., da Silva, R.A.B., and Lucisano, M.P. (2009) Ex vivo accuracy of an apex locator using digital signal processing in primary teeth. *Pediatric Dentistry*, 31, 320–322.

Loushine, R.J., Weller, R.N., Kimbrough, W.F., and Potter, B.J. (2001) Measurement of endodontic file lengths: calibrated versus uncalibrated digital images. *Journal of Endodontics*, 27, 779–781.

Meares, W.A. and Steiman, H.R. (2002) The influence of sodium hypochlorite irrigation on the accuracy of the Root ZX electronic apex locator. *Journal of Endodontics*, 28, 595–598.

Mello-Moura, A.C.V., Moura-Netto, C., Araki, A.T., Guedes-Pinto, A.C., and Mendes, F.M. (2010) Ex vivo performance of five methods for root canal length determination in primary anterior teeth. *International Endodontic Journal*, 43, 142–147.

Nahmias, Y., Aurelio, J.A., and Gerstein, H. (1983) Expanded use of the electronic canal length measuring devices. *Journal of Endodontics*, 9, 347–349.

Nguyen, H.Q., Kaufman, A.Y., Komorowski, R.C., and Friedman, S. (1996) Electronic length measurement using small and large files in enlarged canals. *International Endodontic Journal*, 29, 359–364.

Odabas, M.E., Bodur, H., Tulunoglu, O., and Alacam, A. (2011) Accuracy of an electronic apex locator: a clinical evaluation in primary molars with and without resorption. *The Journal of Clinical Pediatric Dentistry*, 35, 255–258.

Pagavino, G., Pace, R., and Baccetti, T. (1998) A SEM study of in vivo accuracy of the Root ZX electronic apex locator. *Journal of Endodontics*, 24, 438–441.

Palmer, M.J., Weine, F.S., and Healey, H.J. (1971) Position of the apical foramen in relation to endodontic therapy. *Journal of the Canadian Dental Association*, 37, 305–308.

Patino-Marin, N., Zavala-Alonso, N.V., Martinez-Castanon, G.A., Sanchez-Benavides, N., Villanueva-Gordillo, M., Loyola-Rodriguez, J.P., and Medina-Solis, C.E. (2011) Clinical evaluation of the accuracy of conventional radiography and apex locators in primary teeth. *Pediatric Dentistry*, 33, 19–22.

Pilot, T.F. and Pitts, D.L. (1997) Determination of impedance changes at varying frequencies in relation to root canal file position and irrigant. *Journal of Endodontics*, 23, 719–724.

Pineda, F. and Kuttler, Y. (1972) Mesiodistal and bucco-lingual roentgenographic investigation of 7275 root canals. *Oral Surgery, Oral Medicine, and Oral Pathology*, 33, 101–110.

Plant, J.J. and Newman, R.F. (1976) Clinical evaluation of the Sono-Explorer. *Journal of Endodontics*, 2, 215–216.

Poyton, H.G. (1968) The effects of radiation on teeth. *Oral Surgery, Oral Medicine, and Oral Pathology*, 26, 639–646.

Real, D.G., Davidowicz, H., Moura-Netto, C., Zenkner, C.D.L.L., Pagliarin, C.M.L., Barletta, F.B., and de Moura, A.A.M. (2011) Accuracy of working length determination using 3 electronic apex locators and direct digital radiography. *Oral Surgery, Oral Medicine, Oral Pathology, Oral Radiology, and Endodontics*, 111, e44–e49.

Ricucci, D. (1998) Apical limit of root canal instrumentation and obturation: Part 1. Literature review. *International Endodontic Journal*, 31, 384–393.

Ricucci, D. and Langeland, K. (1998) Apical limit of root canal instrumentation and obturation: Part 2. A histological study. *International Endodontic Journal*, 31, 394–409.

Saad, A.Y. and al-Nazhan, S. (2000) Radiation dose reduction during endodontic therapy: a new technique combining an apex locator (Root ZX) and a digital imaging system (RadioVisioGraphy). *Journal of Endodontics*, 26, 144–147.

Schilder, H. (1967) Filling root canals in three dimensions. *Dental Clinics of North America*, 11, 723–744.

Seidberg, B.H., Alibrandi, B.V., Fine, H., and Logue, B. (1975) Clinical investigation of measuring working lengths of root canals with an electronic device and with digital-tactile sense. *Journal of the American Dental Association (1939)*, 90, 379–387.

Seltzer, S., Soltanoff, W., Sinai, I., and Smith, J. (1969) Biologic aspects of endodontics: IV. Periapical tissue reactions to root-filled teeth whose canals had been instrumented short of their apices. *Oral Surgery, Oral Medicine, and Oral Pathology*, 28, 724–738.

Shabahang, S., Goon, W.W., and Gluskin, A.H. (1996) An in vivo evaluation of Root ZX electronic apex locator. *Journal of Endodontics*, 22, 616–618.

Sunada, I. (1962) New method for measuring the length of the root canal. *Journal of Dental Research*, 41, 375–387.

Suzuki, K. (1942) Experimental study on iontophoresis. *Journal of Japanese Stomatology*, 16, 411–429.

Tamse, A., Kaffe, I., and Fishel, D. (1980) Zygomatic arch interference with correct radiographic diagnosis in maxillary molar endodontics. *Oral Surgery, Oral Medicine, and Oral Pathology*, 50, 563–566.

Thomas, A.S., Hartwell, G.R., and Moon, P.C. (2003) The accuracy of the Root ZX electronic apex locator using stainless-steel and nickel-titanium files. *Journal of Endodontics*, 29, 662–663.

Tosun, G., Erdemir, A., Eldeniz, A.U., Sermet, U., and Sener, Y. (2008) Accuracy of two electronic apex locators in primary teeth with and without apical resorption: a laboratory study. *International Endodontic Journal*, 41, 436–441.

Vande Voorde, H.E. and Bjorndahl, A.M. (1969) Estimating endodontic "working length" with paralleling radiographs. *Oral Surgery, Oral Medicine, and Oral Pathology*, 27, 106–110.

Vieyra, J.P., Acosta, J., and Mondaca, J.M. (2010) Comparison of working length determination with radiographs and two electronic apex locators. *International Endodontic Journal*, 43, 16–20.

Weine, F.S. (2004) *Endodontic Therapy*. Mosby, St. Louis, MO.

Woolley, L.H., Woodworth, J., and Dobbs, J.L. (1974) A preliminary evaluation of the effects of electrical pulp testers on dogs with artificial pacemakers. *Journal of the American Dental Association (1939)*, 89, 1099–1101.

15

Vertical Root Fractures: Radiological Diagnosis

Anil Kishen and Harold H. Messer

Introduction: Vertical root fracture (VRF) incidence and consequences

A true VRF is a longitudinal fracture confined to the root that usually initiates on the internal canal wall and extends toward the root surface (Figure 15.1). This is different from a cracked tooth, in which the tooth's structural discontinuity is incomplete in nature. A crack usually runs mesiodistally from the occlusal surface toward the cervical aspect of the tooth and eventually progresses apically to the root ("split root"). The incidence of VRF is more commonly found in endodontically treated teeth (Pitts et al., 1983; Yang et al., 1995), though it has been reported in nonendodontically treated teeth with intact crowns and no/minimal restoration (Chan et al., 1998; Yeh, 1997). Clinically, VRF in teeth is most commonly found in the buccolingual direction. The mesiodistal fractures of the root are considered less common. It may involve the whole length of the root or a portion of the root in the sagittal plane. Along the cross-sectional plane, it may be *complete* (extending from the facial/lingual surface and includes the root canal wall) or *incomplete* (initiating from the root canal or the external surface but not involving the opposite surface). Most VRFs are complete in nature (Walton et al., 1984).

The prevalence of VRF has not been well established to date. Different clinical surveys and follow-ups of endodontically treated teeth suggest a prevalence of 2% and 5% (Bergman et al., 1989; Morfis, 1990; Moule and Kahler, 1999; Testori et al., 1993; Torbjorner et al., 1995). However, determining the prevalence of VRF from studies primarily conducted to examine the causes of extraction of endodontically treated teeth may be erroneous. Some VRF cases in these studies could be diagnosed mistakenly as root canal treatment failure or progressive periodontal disease (Tamse et al., 2006). Interestingly, a prevalence of 11% and 20% was reported in root-filled teeth that were referred for extraction (Fuss et al., 1999; Coppens, 2003). This inconsistency in the reported prevalence may be attributed to the difficulty in diagnosing VRF. Diagnosis of VRF is a difficult and challenging experience for clinicians. The current methods used to diagnose VRF are transillumination, radiographs, periodontal probing, staining, surgical exploration, bite test, direct visual examination,

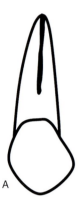

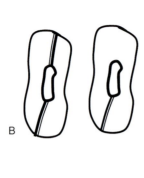

B

A

Figure 15.1 Schematic diagram showing the extension of vertical root fracture (a) in the apical to coronal direction on the buccal surface, and (b) complete and incomplete vertical root fracture in the cross-sectional plane.

and examination with operative-microscope. However, all these methods have limited success in clinical diagnosis. Evidence-based findings concerning the diagnostic accuracy and effectiveness of clinical and radiographic assessments for the diagnosis of VRF are lacking (Tsesis et al., 2010). There is often no single clinical feature that indicates the presence of VRF; and most of these signs/symptoms may be related with pulpal necrosis or failing root canal therapy. For that reason, those signs and symptoms, although helpful in arriving at a diagnosis of VRF, are generally not sufficient to diagnose VRF. In a study conducted on 92 endodontically treated teeth, it was concluded that general practitioners correctly diagnosed VRF in only 31% of the cases (Tamse et al., 1999a).

Identification of the teeth or roots that are susceptible to fracture is very important. A complete history and clinical examination of the susceptible tooth is mandatory. During clinical examination, periodontal probing is recommended to detect any osseous defects, especially on the buccal aspect of the root. Deep probing in two positions on opposite sides is almost pathognomonic for the presence of VRF. These sinus tracts are located close to the gingival margin in teeth associated with VRF, opposed to the sinus tracts in failed root canal-treated teeth that are generally located more apically. A sinogram may be useful to trace the sinus tract parallel to the periodontal space. The possibility of fracture is high if the pocket extends to the mid-root level rather than to the root apex. The presence of two sinus tracts at both buccal and lingual sides strongly suggests VRF (Moule and Kahler, 1999; Pitts et al., 1983). An in vitro study evaluated the accuracy of three electronic apex locators (Root ZX, Foramatron D10, and Apex NRG) for the detection of simulated horizontal and VRFs. Based on this study, it was concluded that the three electronic apex locators tested were accurate and acceptable in detecting horizontal root fractures. However, they were unreliable in detecting the positions of VRFs (Ebrahim et al., 2006). Inspection of VRF, either by nonsurgical or surgical procedures, is a useful step for the absolute confirmation of the diagnosis. Undiagnosed VRF may lead to perplexing clinical situations and inappropriate endodontic treatment.

Mechanisms and risk factors for VRF

VRF in teeth is unpredictable and is considered to be due to multifactorial causes. It is imperative to realize that most of the time, one factor does not always result in increased fracture susceptibility. Instead, many factors interact to influence the susceptibility of a tooth to fracture. Yet at a given time, any one factor can easily predominate over the rest. The factors that predispose teeth to VRF can be categorized as (1) non-iatrogenic and (2) iatrogenic causes (Kishen, 2006).

Non-iatrogenic causes

A tooth structure, during chewing, flexes and subsequently experiences bending stress distribution (Kishen and Asundi, 2002). Significant loss of healthy dentin structure due to the disease process or trauma and the presence of anatomical variations may significantly alter the functional stress distribution within the remaining tooth structure, increasing its predilection to VRF. Anatomical variations such as narrow mesiodistal root width and severe root curvature are reported to be risk factors for VRF in non-endodontically treated posterior teeth in a Chinese population (Chan et al., 1998; Yeh, 1997). Age changes in dentin are also considered as a risk factor that increases fracture predilection in teeth. Alteration of normal dentin to form transparent dentin is a common age-induced process. The dentinal tubules in transparent dentin are gradually filled up with minerals over time, beginning at the apical end of the root and often extending into the coronal dentin. The fracture toughness in transparent dentin is approximately 20% lower and their stress–strain response is characteristic of brittle material (Kinney et al., 2005). It has been reported that the tensile strength of aged dentin is lower than young dentin (Tonami and Takahashi, 1997). Hence, endodontic or restorative procedures in aged individuals might require modification to accommodate the reduced fracture toughness of dentin tissue. Abnormal parafunctional habits such as bruxisms, clenching of teeth, or chewing on hard objects, may generate large forces on the tooth surfaces. This may also contribute to microcracking in dentin and tooth fracture at a later date. Destructive parafunctional habits have been reported to be a cause of VRF in teeth with vital pulp (Cohen et al., 2003).

Iatrogenic factors

Root canal treatment procedures

The ultimate strength of a tooth is directly related to the amount of remaining tooth structure. Therefore, preservation of the tooth structure is very crucial in the successful management of structurally compromised teeth. The stress distribution pattern in post-core restored, root-filled teeth is distinctly dissimilar to that of an intact tooth. Excessive removal of healthy dentin during root canal enlargement, especially in curved and narrow roots, is one of the important predisposing factors for VRF (Kishen, 2006). Endodontic procedural errors that create sharp notches or crack(s) on the root canal wall would lead to a localized increase in stress concentrations, which could predispose the root to VRF. Unfortunately, access cavity preparation by itself compromises the mechanical integrity offered by the roof of the pulp chamber. Any compromise in the mechanical integrity offered by the roof of the pulp chamber would allow greater flexure of the tooth during function (Gutmann, 1992). Endodontic procedures have been shown to reduce the relative tooth stiffness by 5%. However, this value is less than that of an occlusal cavity

preparation, which reduces the relative tooth stiffness by 20%. The largest loss in stiffness was associated with the loss of marginal ridge integrity and mesio-occluso-distal cavity preparation, which resulted in 63% loss of relative tooth stiffness (Reeh et al., 1989).

Many studies have highlighted the deleterious effects of endodontic irrigants and medicaments on the mechanical properties of dentin. Sodium hypochlorite is a very reactive chemical, and when applied in high concentration for a long period, along with its desired therapeutic effects, produces undesired effects on the root dentin. There have been several reports of the adverse effects of sodium hypochlorite on the physical properties of dentin such as flexural strength, elastic modulus, and microhardness (Goldsmith et al., 2002; Grigoratos et al., 2001). Ethylenediaminetetraacetic acid (EDTA) is also an endodontic irrigant utilized to remove the smear layer formed after root canal preparation. The microhardness of root canal dentin irrigated with 5.25% NaOCl, 2.5% NaOCl, 3% H_2O_2, 17% EDTA, and 0.2% chlorhexidine gluconate for 15 minutes each was studied. Except for chlorhexidine, all irrigants were found to reduce the surface hardness of the dentin. Mechanical testing of dentin specimens treated with calcium hydroxide, mineral trioxide aggregate, and sodium hypochlorite for 5 weeks demonstrated a 32% mean decrease in the strength, while calcium hydroxide treatment produced a 33% decrease (Calt and Serper, 2002). The chemically affected radicular dentin can be a potential source for microcracking, and subsequent fatigue failures. Obturation techniques that generate heavy apical forces, such as lateral condensation, may also predispose the tooth to VRF (Holcomb et al., 1987). Clinically, it should be noted that the risk of VRF increases from the beginning of endodontic therapy. In endodontically treated teeth, the average time between root filling and the appearance of a VRF has been estimated to be between 39 months (Meister et al., 1980) and 52.5 months (Gher et al., 1987), with a range of 3 days to 14 years.

Restorative treatment procedures

In restored root-filled teeth, the mismatch between the elastic modulus of the post-core crown system and the remaining tooth structure would lead to altered stress distribution patterns, which in turn may predispose the tooth to fracture. Generally, the anatomy of the tooth, shape and stiffness of post, length of the post within the root canal, direction and magnitude of external forces, and the amount of remaining tooth structure will determine the nature and pattern of the final tooth fracture (Kishen, 2006). Excessive post space preparation leaving behind thin dentin walls, improper selection of post, excessive pressure application during intracanal restorations or cementation, and poor tooth selection as a fixed bridge abutment may all influence the susceptibility of teeth to VRF (Tjan and Whang, 1985).

Different studies have highlighted the dangers of using tapered cast-posts (Isidor and Brondum, 1992; Isidor et al., 1996). Although it is believed that the parallel-sided posts can distribute functional loads passively to the remaining tooth structure (Cooney et al., 1986; Sahafi et al., 2004), some studies have observed only minimal advantages with the parallel-sided posts when compared to the tapered posts (Freeman et al., 1998; Hu et al., 2003). However, the most important factor for preventing fractures is not the post design, but the final crown restoration (Hoag and Dwyer, 1982). Studies have also shown that the bonded posts resulted in less stresses within the dentin than non-bonded posts (Asmussen et al., 2005). There are many prefabricated post systems available in the market today. The disadvantage of the prefabricated posts is that the root canal is designed to receive the post rather than the post being designed to fit within the root canal. Active, threaded posts have the greatest retention; nonetheless, due to the threads indenting into the dentin, these posts can induce localized stress concentrations in the root dentin. This could lead to crack initiation and fatigue root fracture at a later time. Anatomical location of the tooth in the mouth influences predilection to fracture in root-filled teeth. Intact root-filled anterior teeth that have not lost further tooth structure beyond the endodontic access preparation are at minimal risk for fracture. On the other hand, posterior teeth bear greater occlusal loads than the anterior teeth during mastication, and adequate restorations must be planned to protect these teeth from VRF (Kishen, 2006).

Radiographic appearance of VRF

The radiographic appearance of VRF is highly variable and is influenced by the direction of fracture, whether or not a root filling and post are present, and the time since the crack was initiated. Unless separation of the root segments has occurred, the fracture line is generally very difficult to detect. An angle shift is not likely to resolve this difficulty despite recommendations for radiographs at different horizontal angles (Tamse, 2006). This is because the fracture line is obscured if the direction of the X-ray beam diverges from the line of fracture by more than 4° (Kositbwornchai et al., 2001). The superimposition of other anatomical structures further complicates the picture. Because the fracture line is visible on radiographs in only a minority of cases (25–45%), the appearance of the surrounding bone also needs to be evaluated carefully for signs consistent with root fracture (Tamse, 2006; Tsesis et al., 2010). Although the pattern of bone loss may be indicative of VRF, it is very variable and should not be considered pathognomonic. Diagnosis can only be confirmed by direct visual inspection of the root surface or unequivocal evidence from the radiograph.

Cracked/split tooth

The cracked and split teeth normally fracture in a mesiodistal direction. Therefore, the crack line is almost never visible on radiographs. The diagnosis is more likely made based on the patient's history, presenting signs, and clinical assessment, especially when the fracture is incomplete. The radiographic appearance of surrounding bone may provide supporting evidence, including a lateral lesion rather than a periapical lesion if the crack is incomplete (Figure 15.2). Sometimes an unusual and complex pattern of bone loss that includes the furcation area of molars may also be seen radiographically (Figures 15.3 and 15.4).

VRF

VRF in non-root-filled teeth, which is most commonly in a buccolingual direction, is readily

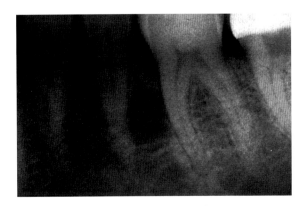

Figure 15.2   A mesiodistal crack in an otherwise intact mandibular molar. The crack is not visible on the radiograph because the direction of the crack is perpendicular to the direction of the X-ray beam. The localized periodontal defects at the alveolar crest and mid-root level on the mesial aspect are suggestive of an incomplete root fracture. Diagnosis must be confirmed based on clinical signs and symptoms, visual examination, and transillumination.

detected on radiographs (Figures 15.5 and 15.6). It is typically observed in severely worn dentitions and is associated with strong masticatory forces and habitual chewing of hard food (Chan et al., 1999). Surrounding bone loss may be minimal (Figure 15.5) or extensive depending on the separation of the root segments (Figure 15.6).

Fracture lines are less commonly visible in root-filled teeth because the radiopaque root filling or the post obscures the crack line unless the root segments are separated (Figure 15.7). If the fracture line is not visible, the pattern of surrounding bone loss may provide clues to the presence of a fracture. The pattern of bone loss is variable and is often complex in its distribution around the root (Kawamura-Hagiya et al., 2008). Despite the variability, two frequently occurring patterns of bone loss have been described: the "halo" lesion and the "periodontal" lesion type (Lustig et al., 2000; Tamse et al., 2006, 1999b). A "halo" lesion surrounds the root and extends further coronally than a typical periapical radiolucency of endodontic origin (Figure 15.7b). This type of lesion is found in approximately one-third to one-half of the confirmed cases of VRF (Tamse et al., 2006, 1999b). The "periodontal" lesion type, associated with up to 30% of VRF, is characterized by angular or more severe bone loss at the alveolar crest on one or both sides of the tooth, especially when a post is present (Figure 15.8) (Lustig et al., 2000; Tamse et al., 2006). In addition to these two distinctive patterns, bone loss may be indistinguishable from that of typical periapical radiolucency in certain cases (Figure 15.9). In its early stages, bone loss may be limited to the area immediately adjacent to the fracture (typically on the buccal or palatal/lingual surface), and not visible on a conventional radiograph (Figure 15.10). Among the more unusual presentations of VRF, a retrograde filling (perhaps inserted before VRF was diagnosed) may become loose and displaced into the surrounding tissues or completely lost (Figure 15.11).

Cone beam computed tomography (CBCT) as an aid in detecting VRF

Given the limitations of conventional radiography, it is not surprising that VRF is visible on radiographs in fewer than half of confirmed cases or in experimental studies only (Cohen et al., 2006; Hassan et al., 2010; Ozer, 2010; Tsesis et al., 2008, 2010). Recent technologies, specifically CBCT, are increasingly employed to aid the diagnosis of VRF. Surprisingly, the use of CBCT for the diagnosis of VRF was not specifically included in the recommended applications of CBCT in endodontics (other than in the evaluation of trauma cases) in the recent recommendations of the Joint Position Statement of the American Association of Endodontists and the American Academy of Oral and Maxillofacial Radiology (AAOMR, 2010).

CBCT offers the enhanced ability to detect fracture lines. The technical aspects of CBCT have already been described in some detail earlier in this textbook. While other types of computed tomography have been used, CBCT, particulary the smaller field of view (FoV) units, are by far the most commonly employed technology (AAOMR, 2010). CBCT offers several advantages over conventional radiography: it is three-dimensional; it eliminates superimposition of overlying structures; the voxel size can be small enough (less than 100 μm) to detect a small crack; the root can be examined systematically in different projections including axial

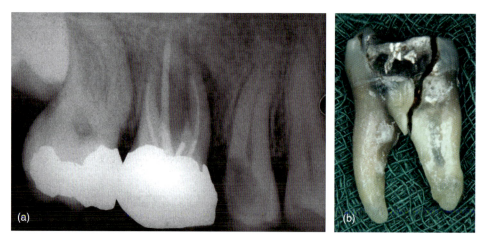

Figure 15.3 (a) Complex pattern of bone loss including the furcation area and a mesial periodontal defect, but little periapical spread. (b) Extracted tooth showing the complete fracture associated with a large amalgam restoration that does not provide any cuspal protection against such fracture.

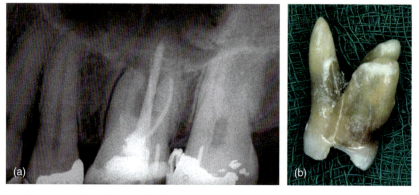

Figure 15.4 (a) Irregular pattern of bone loss in the furcation area, with widening of the periodontal ligament space on the mesial aspect of the mesiobuccal root. Removal of the resin composite restoration revealed a crack on the floor of the mesial proximal box, which after extraction was seen to extend onto the palatal root, where it terminated. (b) Extracted tooth showing the incomplete fracture.

plane (essentially cross sections of the root). At the time of writing, the use of CBCT for detecting VRF is still in its infancy, with only one clinical study (Edlund et al., 2011) correlating CBCT results with the direct visual (surgical) confirmation. Based on 32 suspected cases of VRF that were considered impossible to diagnose using conventional radiography, the overall accuracy in diagnosis using CBCT was 84%, with 88% sensitivity (or true positive rate, 21 of 24 with confirmed VRF) and 75% specificity (or true negative rate, 6 of 8 cases).

Numerous in vitro studies, usually involving artificially induced VRF in extracted teeth that were then inserted into tooth sockets of dry skulls, have reported substantially greater diagnostic accuracy with CBCT than with conventional radiography (Hassan et al., 2010; Ozer, 2010). In clinical practice, CBCT should permit the accurate diagnosis of VRF (or its absence) in approximately 80% of cases (Figure 15.12). It must be stressed that the diagnosis cannot be made based only on the pattern of bone loss or clinical signs/symptoms, and that skill

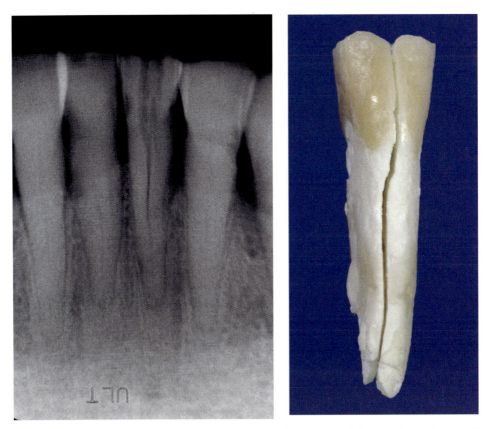

Figure 15.5 Vertical root fracture in an intact, non-root filled mandibular incisor, with little evidence of surrounding bone loss. The incisors all had substantial incisal wear.

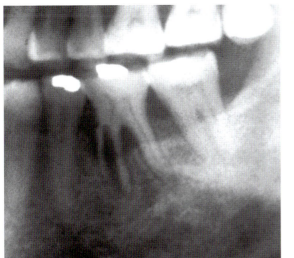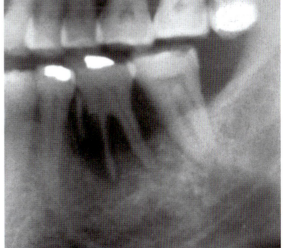

Figure 15.6 Two radiographs taken 1 year apart demonstrating a fractured mesial root of a mandibular first molar. (The views are taken from OPG radiographs and are of low resolution.) The root segment has become completely dislodged and migrated into the interproximal area, where it caused minor clinical symptoms. The tooth had only a small occlusal amalgam restoration, but the dentition is extensively worn.

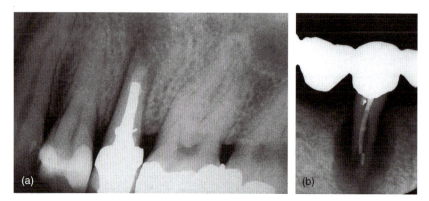

Figure 15.7 (a) VRF is obscured by the large post present in the canal. The tooth had been subjected to periapical surgery for a persistent lesion, and VRF was not detected at the time of surgery. (b) Mandibular premolar showing a clearly visible VRF, with the root segments widely separated. An extensive "halo" lesion embraces the root. As a bridge abutment, the mandibular premolar was subjected to excessive occlusal forces which resulted in fracture. The lesion extends more than halfway to the alveolar crest on the mesial aspect and embraces the root surface rather than spreading away from the root apex.

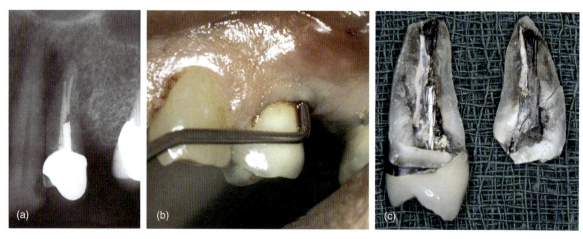

Figure 15.8 (a) Typical "periodontal" lesion associated with vertical root fracture. (b) The lesion is associated with a narrow, deep periodontal defect on the buccal aspect. (c) A complete bucco-palatal root fracture has occurred despite the conservative size and length of the prefabricated metal post placed in the tooth, plus full coronal coverage.

in interpreting CBCT scans is essential. Several factors will assist in maximizing the diagnostic potential of CBCT.

FoV

CBCT systems are categorized based on FoV into large, medium, and small volume, which influ-ences the voxel size and hence the resolution and contrast of the images. Given the relatively narrow dimensions of a fracture line, small FoV and high resolution are desirable to detect VRF. A small FoV also reduces the radiation exposure compared to medium volume (both jaws and adjacent struc-tures) or large volume (entire maxillofacial region). A small FoV should be used whenever VRF is suspected.

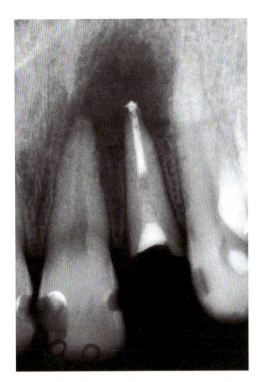

Figure 15.9 Periapical radiolucency associated with vertical root fracture but similar in location and appearance to a typical radiolucency of endodontic origin. A history of repeated loosening of the post is suggestive of VRF, which could be confirmed by visual inspection.

Resolution

Voxel sizes of less than 100 µm per side are available with contemporary CBCT systems, which should be sufficient to detect even partial fractures without separation of the root segments. Ex vivo studies have indicated that a voxel size of 200 µm provides sufficient resolution and permits lower radiation exposure than with smaller voxel size (Ozer et al., 2011). However, more recent CBCT systems with 80 µm voxel size (Edlund et al., 2011) may provide much sharper images (Figure 15.13).

Projections

Standard software permits systematic examination of the image in three planes (axial, coronal, and sagittal). Axial slices, which are perpendicular to the direction of the fracture line, offer the best orientation for crack detection (Hassan et al., 2010; Ozer et al., 2011) (Figure 15.14). Systematic paging through the stacks of images is necessary to confirm the presence of a fracture line running longitudinally through the root. Because the patterns of root fracture are well documented, examination should focus on buccolingual areas for VRF and mesiodistal areas for split root. Training and experience are necessary to develop a facility for interpreting CBCT images.

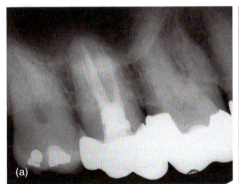
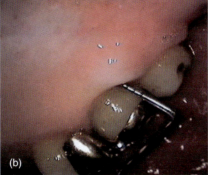
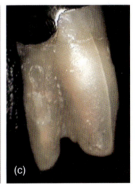

Figure 15.10   (a) Maxillary second molar showing little evidence of periradicular bone loss. (b) Clinically, a narrow periodontal defect plus gingival swelling was noted on the palatal aspect. (c) VRF was evident throughout the full length of the palatal root. The tooth had been root filled 2 years previously and restored without a post but with complete occlusal coverage. Symptoms were vague until the acute palatal swelling occurred.

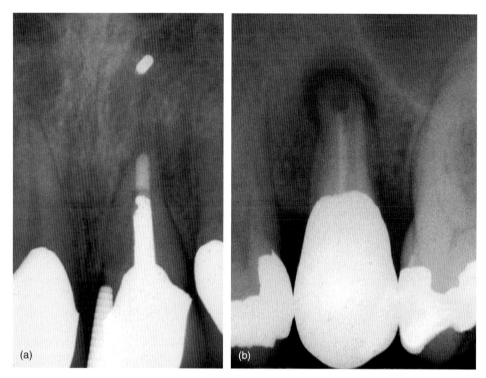

Figure 15.11 (a) Maxillary central incisor with a displaced retrograde amalgam filling lodged within a periapical lesion some distance from the root tip. VRF was confirmed during surgery. (b) Maxillary premolar with an empty retrograde cavity preparation. The tooth had a narrow periodontal defect on the buccal aspect and a sinus tract. The patient could recall finding a small metallic object in her mouth without knowing where it had come from. In both cases, the patients had undergone periapical surgery for persistent lesions, without a fracture line being detected.

Limitations and disadvantages

CBCT involves a longer exposure time and a higher radiation dose than conventional radiography, and images have lower resolution. Hence, its use should be limited to challenging diagnostic cases that justify the additional radiation (AAOMR, 2010). Image artifacts may also compromise diagnostic ability. Although much reduced in comparison with medical CT images, beam hardening and streak artifacts occur in the presence of radiopaque materials (Bernardes et al., 2009; Melo et al., 2010; Patel, 2009) (Figure 15.15). Since most cases of VRF have been root filled and many involve the presence of a metallic post, these artifacts can interfere with the identification of a crack.

Recommendations

A definite diagnosis of VRF (or its absence) from clinical and radiographic features would preclude the need for exploratory surgery. Hence, CBCT should be used whenever VRF or split tooth is suspected but cannot be observed directly. The diagnosis, however, requires the correlation of radiographic features with the clinical picture and should not be made on the basis of a CBCT scan alone. Accuracy of diagnosis is currently reported to be better than 80% and is likely to increase as systems undergo further development. Systems that permit limited field of view (preferably 4 cm) and high resolution (voxel size of 0.2 mm and preferably less) should be used if possible, but a larger

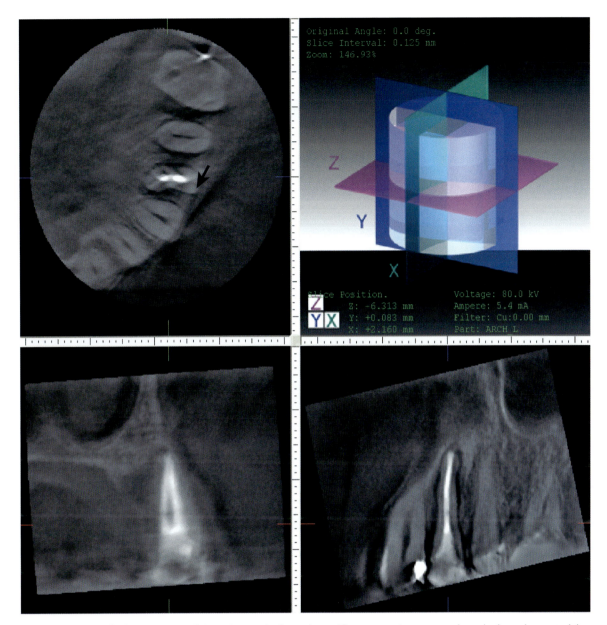

Figure 15.12 Standard presentation of CBCT images in three planes. The arrow points to a crack on the buccal aspect of the maxillary first premolar in the axial slice.

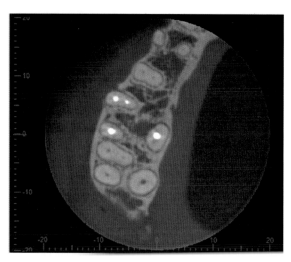

Figure 15.13 Image taken with 80 μm voxel size. The sharpness of the image is enhanced and beam hardening is minimal. Nonetheless, detection of a crack requires careful scrutiny of multiple image slices before the crack can be reliably distinguished.

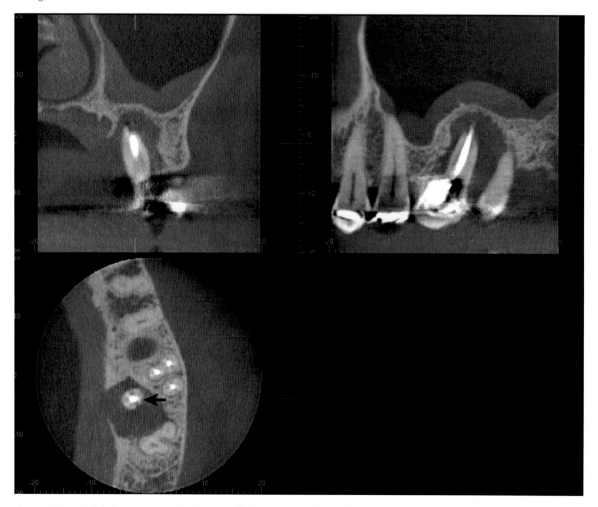

Figure 15.14 Axial slices are most likely to reveal the presence of a crack, since the crack will be perpendicular to the slice. Scrolling through slices in all three planes is required before a fracture line (or its absence) can be determined reliably.

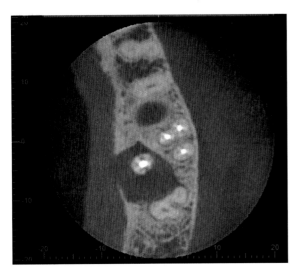

Figure 15.15   Beam hardening and streak artifacts associated with the more radiodense root filling make it difficult to identify the radiolucent line of the fracture.

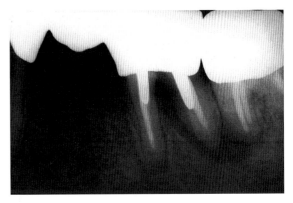

Figure 15.16   Mandibular molar with a large post in the distal canal. A periapical radiolucency surrounds the distal root and extends into the furcation area. A deep periodontal pocket was present in the buccal furcation area. Differential diagnosis requires considerable skill, to decide between a persistent lesion of endodontic origin associated with either the first or second molar, a furcation defect of periodontal origin, or VRF.

field of view and larger voxel size may still be useful. Images should be examined in multiple planes, but scrolling through axial slices (cross sections of the root) is most likely to reveal the presence of a fracture line. Considerable skill is required in interpreting CBCT images, and training/experience are essential.

Diagnosis of VRF: The integration of clinical and radiographic signs

VRF must be distinguished from a persistent periapical lesion of endodontic origin and from localized periodontal disease (Figure 15.16). The poor prognosis for VRF and the consequences of severe bone loss make it important to diagnose VRF as promptly as possible. Diagnosis has been described in detail (Cohen et al., 2003; Meister et al., 1980; Tamse, 2006) and will be considered more briefly in this section. Clinical signs and symptoms are often vague, with mild-to-moderate pain and tenderness on biting or percussion in only about 50–60% of cases. The single most distinguishing sign of VRF is a narrow, deep periodontal pocket, typically on the buccal aspect, which is present in a large majority of cases (Tsesis et al., 2010) (Figure 15.8). Thus, careful periodontal probing is an essential part of the evaluation of every case where VRF is suspected. A sinus tract, often located close to the gingival margin, is less frequent (30–40%), but in association with a narrow periodontal defect, it is a strong indication of the presence of VRF. When present, these two clinical features plus the radiographic appearance of a "halo" lesion are essentially diagnostic of VRF. Definitive diagnosis may require surgical exposure to allow direct visual observation of the root surface.

Incomplete fractures will be more difficult to detect, and their diagnosis may be further complicated by the absence of clinical signs such as a narrow periodontal defect (Figure 15.17). Time is an important element in the progression of VRF, and the fracture often becomes symptomatic only years after the crack is initiated.

Conclusions

Longitudinal root fractures are characterized by their variability and are difficult to diagnose from radiographic appearance alone. Both the tooth root and surrounding bone may provide clues to the presence of a fracture, but definitive diagnosis requires the correlation of radiographic features with clinical signs. CBCT may be a valuable aid in

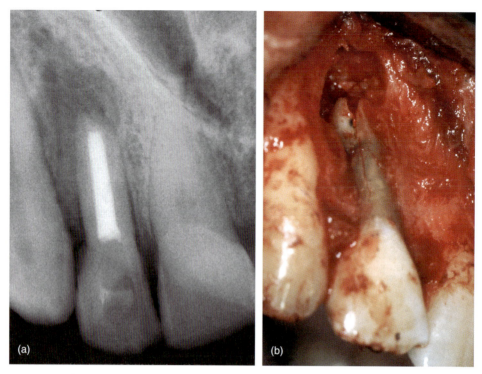

Figure 15.17 (a) Incomplete VRF of a maxillary lateral incisor, not visible on the radiograph. A persistent periapical radiolucency did not resolve following orthograde retreatment. No probing defect could be detected. (b) Surgical exposure revealed a buccal fracture line.

enhancing diagnosis, but surgical exposure will often be required to confirm the diagnosis visually. Because of their poor prognosis, it is important to differentiate between VRF and a persistent periapical lesion of endodontic origin or a lesion of periodontal origin.

References

American Association of Endodontists; American Academy of Oral and Maxillofacial Radiology. (2010) Use of cone-beam computed tomography in endodontics Joint Position Statement of the American Association of Endodontists and the American Academy of Oral and Maxillofacial Radiology. *Oral Surg Oral Med Oral Pathol Oral Radiol Endod*, 111, 234–237.

Asmussen, E., Peutzfeldt, A., and Sahafi, A. (2005) Finite element analysis of stresses in endodontically treated, dowel-restored teeth. *J Prosthet Dent*, 94(4), 321–329.

Bergman, B., et al. (1989) Restorative and endodontic results after treatment with cast posts and cores. *J Prosthet Dent*, 61(1), 10–15.

Bernardes, R.A., et al. (2009) Use of cone-beam volumetric tomography in the diagnosis of root fractures. *Oral Surg Oral Med Oral Pathol Oral Radiol Endod*, 108(2), 270–277.

Calt, S. and Serper, A. (2002) Time-dependent effects of EDTA on dentin structures. *J Endod*, 28(1), 17–19.

Chan, C.P., et al. (1998) Vertical root fracture in non-endodontically treated teeth—a clinical report of 64 cases in Chinese patients. *J Endod*, 24(10), 678–681.

Chan, C.P., et al. (1999) Vertical root fracture in endodontically versus nonendodontically treated teeth: a survey of 315 cases in Chinese patients. *Oral Surg Oral Med Oral Pathol Oral Radiol Endod*, 87(4), 504–507.

Cohen, S., Blanco, L., and Berman, L. (2003) Vertical root fractures: clinical and radiographic diagnosis. *J Am Dent Assoc*, 134(4), 434–441.

Cohen, S., et al. (2006) A demographic analysis of vertical root fractures. *J Endod*, 32(12), 1160–1163.

Cooney, J.P., Caputo, A.A., and Trabert, K.C. (1986) Retention and stress-distribution of tapered-end endodontic posts. *J Prosthet Dent*, 55(5), 540–546.

Coppens, C.R.M.D. and DeMoor, R.J.G. (2003) Prevalence of vertical root fractures in extracted endodontically treated teeth. *Int Endod J*, 36, 926.

Ebrahim, A.K., Wadachi, R., and Suda, H. (2006) Ex vivo evaluation of the ability of four different electronic apex locators to determine the working length in teeth with various foramen diameters. *Aust Dent J*, 51(3), 258–262.

Edlund, M., Nair, M.K., and Nair, U.P. (2011) Detection of vertical root fractures by using cone-beam computed tomography: a clinical study. *J Endod*, 37(6), 768–772.

Freeman, M.A., et al. (1998) Leakage associated with load fatigue-induced preliminary failure of full crowns placed over three different post and core systems. *J Endod*, 24(1), 26–32.

Fuss, Z., Lustig, J., and Tamse, A. (1999) Prevalence of vertical root fractures in extracted endodontically treated teeth. *Int Endod J*, 32(4), 283–286.

Gher, M.E., Jr., et al. (1987) Clinical survey of fractured teeth. *J Am Dent Assoc*, 114(2), 174–177.

Goldsmith, M., Gulabivala, K., and Knowles, J.C. (2002) The effect of sodium hypochlorite irrigant concentration on tooth surface strain. *J Endod*, 28(8), 575–579.

Grigoratos, D., et al. (2001) Effect of exposing dentine to sodium hypochlorite and calcium hydroxide on its flexural strength and elastic modulus. *Int Endod J*, 34(2), 113–119.

Gutmann, J.L. (1992) The dentin-root complex: anatomic and biologic considerations in restoring endodontically treated teeth. *J Prosthet Dent*, 67(4), 458–467.

Hassan, B., et al. (2010) Comparison of five cone beam computed tomography systems for the detection of vertical root fractures. *J Endod*, 36(1), 126–129.

Hoag, E.P. and Dwyer, T.G. (1982) A comparative evaluation of three post and core techniques. *J Prosthet Dent*, 47(2), 177–181.

Holcomb, J.Q., Pitts, D.L., and Nicholls, J.I. (1987) Further investigation of spreader loads required to cause vertical root fracture during lateral condensation. *J Endod*, 13(6), 277–284.

Hu, Y.H., et al. (2003) Fracture resistance of endodontically treated anterior teeth restored with four post-and-core systems. *Quintessence Int*, 34(5), 349–353.

Isidor, F. and Brondum, K. (1992) Intermittent loading of teeth with tapered, individually cast or prefabricated, parallel-sided posts. *Int J Prosthodont*, 5(3), 257–261.

Isidor, F., Odman, P., and Brondum, K. (1996) Intermittent loading of teeth restored using prefabricated carbon fiber posts. *Int J Prosthodont*, 9(2), 131–136.

Kawamura-Hagiya, Y., Yoshioka, T., and Suda, H. (2008) Logistic regression equation to screen for vertical root fractures using periapical radiographs. *Dentomaxillofac Radiol*, 37(1), 28–33.

Kinney, J.H., et al. (2005) Age-related transparent root dentin: mineral concentration, crystallite size, and mechanical properties. *Biomaterials*, 26(16), 3363–3376.

Kishen, A. (2006) Mechanisms and risk factors for fracture predilection in endodontically treated teeth. *Endod Top*, 13, 57–83.

Kishen, A. and Asundi, A. (2002) Photomechanical investigations on post endodontically rehabilitated teeth. *J Biomed Opt*, 7(2), 262–270.

Kositbowornchai, S., et al. (2001) Root fracture detection: a comparison of direct digital radiography with conventional radiography. *Dentomaxillofac Radiol*, 30(2), 106–109.

Lustig, J.P., Tamse, A., and Fuss, Z. (2000) Pattern of bone resorption in vertically fractured, endodontically treated teeth. *Oral Surg Oral Med Oral Pathol Oral Radiol Endod*, 90(2), 224–227.

Meister, F., Jr., Lommel, T.J., and Gerstein, H. (1980) Diagnosis and possible causes of vertical root fractures. *Oral Surg Oral Med Oral Pathol*, 49(3), 243–253.

Melo, S.L., et al. (2010) Diagnostic ability of a cone-beam computed tomography scan to assess longitudinal root fractures in prosthetically treated teeth. *J Endod*, 36(11), 1879–1882.

Morfis, A.S. (1990) Vertical root fractures. *Oral Surg Oral Med Oral Pathol*, 69(5), 631–635.

Moule, A.J. and Kahler, B. (1999) Diagnosis and management of teeth with vertical root fractures. *Aust Dent J*, 44(2), 75–87.

Ozer, S.Y. (2010) Detection of vertical root fractures of different thicknesses in endodontically enlarged teeth by cone beam computed tomography versus digital radiography. *J Endod*, 36(7), 1245–1249.

Ozer, S.Y., Unlu, G., and Deger, Y. (2011) Diagnosis and treatment of endodontically treated teeth with vertical root fracture: three case reports with two-year follow-up. *J Endod*, 37(1), 97–102.

Patel, S. (2009) New dimensions in endodontic imaging: Part 2. Cone beam computed tomography. *Int Endod J*, 42(6), 463–475.

Pitts, D.L., Matheny, H.E., and Nicholls, J.I. (1983) An in vitro study of spreader loads required to cause vertical root fracture during lateral condensation. *J Endod*, 9(12), 544–550.

Reeh, E.S., Douglas, W.H., and Messer, H.H. (1989) Stiffness of endodontically-treated teeth related to restoration technique. *J Dent Res*, 68(11), 1540–1544.

Sahafi, A., et al. (2004) Retention and failure morphology of prefabricated posts. *Int J Prosthodont*, 17(3), 307–312.

Tamse, A. (2006) Vertical root fractures in endodontically treated teeth: diagnostic signs and clinical management. *Endod Top*, 13, 84–94.

Tamse, A., et al. (1999a) An evaluation of endodontically treated vertically fractured teeth. *J Endod*, 25(7), 506–508.

Tamse, A., et al. (1999b) Radiographic features of vertically fractured, endodontically treated maxillary premolars. *Oral Surg Oral Med Oral Pathol Oral Radiol Endod*, 88(3), 348–352.

Tamse, A., et al. (2006) Radiographic features of vertically fractured endodontically treated mesial roots of mandibular molars. *Oral Surg Oral Med Oral Pathol Oral Radiol Endod*, 101(6), 797–802.

Testori, T., Badino, M., and Castagnola, M. (1993) Vertical root fractures in endodontically treated teeth: a clinical survey of 36 cases. *J Endod*, 19(2), 87–91.

Tjan, A.H.L. and Whang, S.B. (1985) Resistance to root fracture of dowel channels with various thicknesses of buccal dentin walls. *J Prosthet Dent*, 53(4), 496–500.

Tonami, K. and Takahashi, H. (1997) Effects of aging on tensile fatigue strength of bovine dentin. *Dent Mater J*, 16(2), 156–169.

Torbjorner, A., Karlsson, S., and Odman, P.A. (1995) Survival rate and failure characteristics for two post designs. *J Prosthet Dent*, 73(5), 439–444.

Tsesis, I., et al. (2008) Comparison of digital with conventional radiography in detection of vertical root fractures in endodontically treated maxillary premolars: an ex vivo study. *Oral Surg Oral Med Oral Pathol Oral Radiol Endod*, 106(1), 124–128.

Tsesis, I., et al. (2010) Diagnosis of vertical root fractures in endodontically treated teeth based on clinical and radiographic indices: a systematic review. *J Endod*, 36(9), 1455–1458.

Walton, R.E., Michelich, R.J., and Smith, G.N. (1984) The histopathogenesis of vertical root fractures. *J Endod*, 10(2), 48–56.

Yang, S.F., Rivera, E.M., and Walton, R.E. (1995) Vertical root fracture in nonendodontically treated teeth. *J Endod*, 21(6), 337–339.

Yeh, C.J. (1997) Fatigue root fracture: a spontaneous root fracture in non-endodontically treated teeth. *Br Dent J*, 182(7), 261–266.

16 Healing of Chronic Apical Periodontitis

Dag Ørstavik

Introduction

Modern maxillofacial radiology has several advanced methodologies for diagnostic assessment of endodontically related diseases and conditions. Some of these are used mainly in hospitals and universities; others are gradually being employed by expansive public and private clinics. Cone beam computed tomography (CBCT) has become extremely useful in selected endodontic cases. However, cost and, particularly, radiation concerns limit the general applicability of this and other relatively advanced methods.

The periapical radiograph therefore remains the primary source of diagnostic insight beyond clinical examination in endodontic practice. It has a history of approximately one century, during which time the whole dental profession has accumulated and shared information derived from its application, especially information related to endodontics. In fact, the concepts that have developed regarding the three-dimensional features of apical periodontitis are based and rely on the two-dimensional renderings of the periapical radiograph.

Aspects of cost and radiation concern also dictate that for large-scale epidemiological studies and in clinical research, the periapical radiograph (or the orthopanthomogram) often is the only method available that can give sufficiently precise data.

So while the amount of information that is potentially available through the use of CBCT, it is imperative that we systematize and maximize the information that can be obtained with the conventional, periapical radiograph.

Radiographic features of apical periodontitis

Chronic apical periodontitis

Periodontitis resulting from pulp infection usually locates to the area of the apical entrance of vessels and nerves to the pulp, hence the conventional term apical periodontitis. Periodontal inflammation from pulp infection may also occur in lateral and furcal infection, with optional nomenclatures such as lateral, furcal, and periradicular periodontitis. The pathognomonic, radiographic features

Endodontic Radiology, Second Edition. Edited by Bettina Basrani.
© 2012 John Wiley & Sons, Inc. Published 2012 by John Wiley & Sons, Inc.

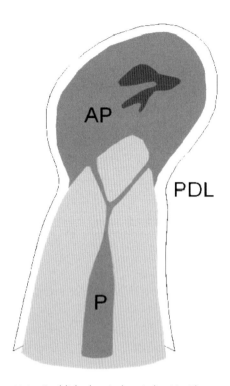

Figure 16.1   Established, apical periodontitis. The radiolucent lesion has a droplet-shaped appearance; the PDL tapers off toward the outer periphery of the lesion; and the lamina dura is absent at the apex. The lesion itself starts from the infected contents of the root canal (Reprinted from Ørstavik and Larheim, 2008, with permission from John Wiley & Sons).

are the same: the apical lesion has a droplet-shaped, radiolucent appearance, the periodontal ligament (PDL) tapers off into the outer periphery of the lesion, and the lamina dura is absent at the apex and/or other portals of pulp entry. The size of the lesion varies from but a few millimeters to several centimeters (Figure 16.1).

Incipient and acute apical periodontitis

These may show minimal or no changes detectable in radiographs. In humans, little is known about the speed and dynamics of the initial changes in bone mineral content and structural changes occurring in the initial stages of infection. In some cases, a diffuse reduction in mineral content may be detectable; in others, incipient or low-grade infec-

tion may be associated with structural disorganization of bone in the periapical area (Brynolf, 1967) (Figure 16.2).

More is known from animal studies. Within a period of weeks to several months prior to the establishment of a periapical granuloma or cyst, tissue changes occur which may be detectable as a reorganization of the area to become occupied by the lesion (Friedman et al., 1997; Ørstavik & Larheim, 2008).

Periapical cyst

Periapical cysts are traditionally divided into two categories: the bay or pocket cyst and the "true" periapical cyst (Nair et al., 1996; Simon, 1980). The lumen of the former is in continuity with the root canal lumen; the "true" cyst is dissociated from the root and may therefore be resistant to conventional root canal treatment (RCT) and need surgical extirpation. It is debatable whether the radiographic appearance holds features helpful in differentiating between a cyst and a granuloma (Shrout et al., 1993; White et al., 1994). The traditional belief that a radiopaque rim is indicative of a cyst has been challenged (Ricucci et al., 2006). What is more generally agreed is that with increasing size, possibly also age, of the lesion, the greater the likelihood of finding cystic elements in the lesion (Carrillo et al., 2008; Kizil and Energin, 1990).

Tissue responses to materials and procedures

Responses to foreign objects and endodontic filling materials

While extruded root filling material may have a negative prognostic influence on healing in the treatment of chronic apical periodontitis (Sjögren et al., 1990), the materials themselves seem to have little influence on bone mineral content or structure. It is traditionally accepted, though, that a small radiolucent zone may persist around such surplus material at the root canal orifice (Strindberg, 1956). With some materials, such as resins and mineral trioxide aggregate, one may hope for better tissue integration with no or smaller radio-

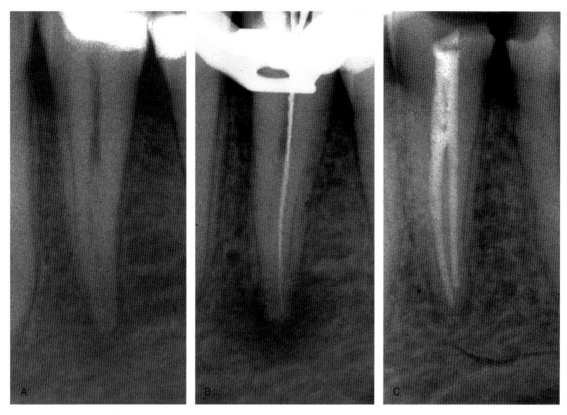

Figure 16.2   Incipient or low-grade infection may be associated with structural disorganization of bone in the periapical area. (A) Symptomatic with acute apical periodontitis. (B) 2 weeks later the lesion is entering a chronic phase. (C) Control after 1 year.

lucent zone peripheral to the material (Rud et al., 1991; Torabinejad et al., 1995).

Treatment and filling procedures may cause a transient loss of mineral (increased radiolucency) at the periapex (Benfica e Silva et al., 2010; Ørstavik, 1991), but this is reversible and does not normally initiate or sustain either acute or chronic apical periodontitis (Sjögren et al., 1990) (Figure 16.3). However, extruded material has been associated with granuloma and cyst formation (Koppang et al., 1989; Love and Firth, 2009).

Responses to surgical procedures

Radiographic analyses of jaw bones after apical surgery present particular problems. The cavity created during surgery becomes the starting point for follow-up controls of healing. Two processes may now be operating: on the one hand, the blood clot will become organized and start to mineralize. On the other, residual infection may in part or totally interfere with the healing of the surgical site. The ensuing radiographic image may be difficult to interpret, and special caution must be exercised when assessing the healing (Figure 16.4).

Thus, in a classic study comparing the radiographic healing of chronic apical periodontitis treated conventionally or surgically, it was found that short-term observation periods (6 months) tended to favor surgical treatment, whereas the results were considered just as good or better for conventional retreatment after 1–2 years of observation (Kvist and Reit, 1999).

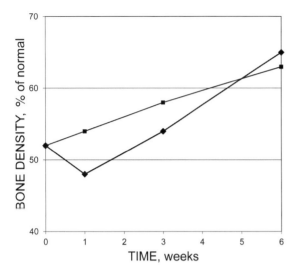

Figure 16.3   Average change in bone density (ratio of diseased area vs. normal peripheral bone in percent) after treatment of apical periodontitis with Sealapex (squares) or ProcoSol (diamonds) (Modified from Ørstavik, 1991, with permission from John Wiley & Sons).

Characteristics of healing of chronic apical periodontitis

Dynamics of the healing process and its reflection in radiographic changes

The biological processes leading to the clearing of an apical granuloma or cystic lesion are poorly understood. The fibrous character of most lesions makes it likely that healing requires a substantial amount of time in all cases. Furthermore, factors related to lesion size and location, the patient's general health and constitution, and residual infection in the area, (Brummer and van Wyk 1987, Fouad and Burleson, 2003; Segura-Egea et al., 2005) may contribute to variations in the healing pattern. While it may be tempting to look at bony healing as a balloon which shrinks in size, mineralization may also start irregularly from within the lesion, and as spicules penetrating from the periphery toward the central area. Such different patterns of healing are likely to produce different radiographic

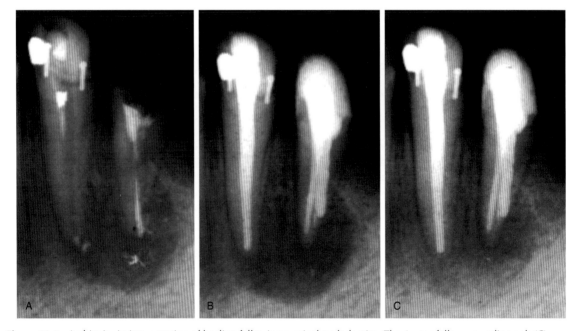

Figure 16.4   Ambiguity in interpretation of healing following surgical endodontics. The 1-year follow-up radiograph (C) shows clear sign of healing, but residual infection of the first premolar cannot be ruled out. (A) Case on admission. (B) Immediate postoperative radiograph.

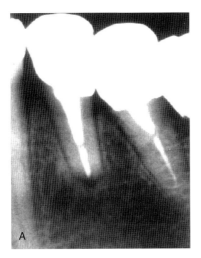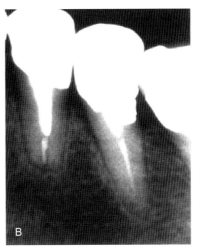

Figure 16.5   For observation of so-called "complete" healing, individual cases may have to be followed for several years, with "late" healing observed decades after treatment. (a) Lesion at 17 years after treatment; (b) healing after 27 years (Reprinted from Molven et al., 2002, with permission from John Wiley & Sons).

appearances. For observation of so-called "complete" healing, individual cases may have to be followed for several years, with "late" healing observed as much as 17–27 years postoperatively (Molven et al., 2002) (Figure 16.5).

Time course of healing processes

Computer-assisted means of radiographic analysis have indicated that in many, if not most cases, increased radiographic density may often be seen after a few weeks and quite regularly at 3–6 months (Kerosuo and Ørstavik, 1997). Also, by conventional radiographic analyses, changes may be detected early (Figure 16.6).

However, a period of 1 year may be necessary to assess the overall outcome after treatment of chronic apical periodontitis; even those cases that require longer time for complete healing generally improve sufficiently to be classified as clinically successful after 1 year (Cvek, 1972; Ørstavik, 1996; Reit, 1987) (Figure 16.7).

Assessment of healing in clinical practice

The radiographic control of healing is usually done by comparing a recall radiograph with one taken

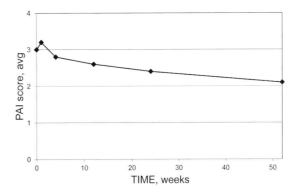

Figure 16.6   In many, if not most cases, signs of healing may often be seen after a few weeks and quite regularly at 12–26 weeks (Modified from Trope et al., 1999, with permission from Elsevier Ltd.).

at the time of treatment. Teaching and clinical practices vary with regard to the criteria used to make a diagnosis of posttreatment disease (Friedman, 2008). Computer-assisted, automated means of analyzing and comparing periapical radiographs are available, but documentation of precision and accuracy is weak. Methods for determination of healing of apical periodontitis include ratio measurements of bone density in the lesion versus normal bone surrounding it; digital subtraction of densities in corresponding areas in two

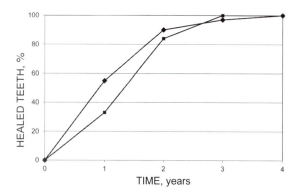

Figure 16.7 Cumulative percentage of teeth that will eventually heal at yearly intervals from endodontic treatment of teeth with apical periodontitis (Modified from Ørstavik, 1996, with permission from John Wiley & Sons: Solid squares, data from Cvek et al. (1976); solid diamonds, data from Ørstavik et al., 1987).

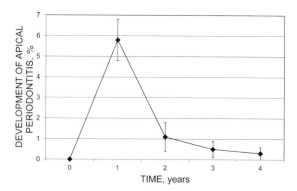

Figure 16.8 Some 90% of teeth that develop a lesion (secondary apical periodontitis) can be detected with conventional radiographs after 1 year. Bars are standard deviations (Reprinted from Ørstavik, 1996, with permission from John Wiley & Sons).

radiographs; and measurement of the lesion size (see below).

Clinical experiments and epidemiology

Prevention and treatment

The fundamental difference between RCT of infected and noninfected teeth should be recognized. The prognosis of RCT after vital pulp extirpation is clearly superior to that of RCT on infected teeth with chronic apical periodontitis (Kerekes and Tronstad, 1979; Ng et al., 2011; Ørstavik et al., 1987). With the application of more sensitive means of detection (CBCT), it is likely that even more teeth may show residual infection than has currently been assumed (de Paula-Silva et al., 2009). It is most unfortunate that clinical and experimental studies are still carried out where the two preoperative diagnoses are mixed in the design. The situation is more or less unavoidable in epidemiology, which makes the interpretation of such data very complex (see below).

Treatment of teeth with no preoperative lesion

The development of a granuloma is usually asymptomatic, and primary chronic apical periodontitis

(CAP) is often detected in a radiograph taken for other reasons. A time course for its development in humans is hard to establish for primary apical periodontitis. However, after root filling of vital teeth, many studies have monitored the outcome of treatment by repeated and regular radiographic follow-ups. It has been found that some 90% of teeth that develop a lesion (secondary apical periodontitis) can be detected with conventional radiographs after 1 year (Ørstavik, 1996) (Figure 16.8).

The success/failure concept in everyday practice and clinical research

Endodontic success is usually described as the absence, clinically and radiographically, of signs of apical periodontitis. In practice, the radiographic analysis is carried out by comparison of recall radiographs with preoperative or immediate postoperative radiographs of the tooth in question. For teeth without a preoperative lesion, a failure is recorded when the periapical area becomes more radiolucent; otherwise, it is a success. For teeth with a lesion, the comparison looks for healing, which may be recorded when the change is clearly in favor of the recall X-ray (Figure 16.9).

Otherwise it is a failure. With this scoring method, success rates are generally recorded as very high for both diagnostic categories. In the

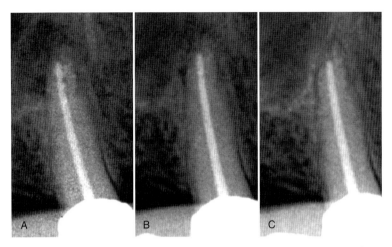

Figure 16.9   Conventional monitoring of healing of apical periodontitis. Compared with the immediate postoperative radiograph (A), bone is forming after 3 months (B), and complete healing is observed after 12 months (C).

individual case, the assessment of success/failure is further blended with the patient's and operator's predefined goal of the procedure (Friedman, 2008). The problems with such assessment in scientific studies are lack of agreement on what constitutes "appearance of a lesion" for vital tooth treatment, and when an increase in bone density at the apex of a tooth with a preoperative lesion is large enough to be termed "normal," "healing," or "healed." It is difficult if not impossible to harmonize observers using a system based on verbal descriptors of subjective parameters (Goldman et al., 1972; Reit and Hollender, 1983). In clinical practice, however, such comparison of radiographs over time is an important aid in treatment planning, even though consensus does not exist also at this level (Reit and Gröndahl, 1984).

Reproducibility and quantification of treatment outcome assessments in endodontics

Computer-based analyses

Computer-assisted means of monitoring healing may provide numerical and reproducible data. They need standardized radiographic exposures for reduction of changes introduced by variations in angulation of the beam.

Area measurements

For follow-up of large, well-defined lesions, simple recording of the area or width of the lesion can be used and may provide some quantitative measure of progress (Heling et al., 2001; Ortega-Sánchez et al., 2009). Lack of precise knowledge of the healing pattern of cysts and granulomas may introduce errors in assessment (Rózyło-Kalinowska, 2007).

Gray value measurement

Simple measurement of gray value levels within the lesion has been attempted and may give sensitive detection of changes in mineral content over time (Camps et al., 2004).

Digital subtraction

Since the late 1980s, digital subtraction techniques have been proposed and used for monitoring periapical healing (Gröndahl et al., 1983; Ørstavik et al., 1990; Pascon et al., 1987; Tyndall et al., 1990). The analysis as such can be automated, but they require careful, usually manually assisted alignment of radiographs for precise recordings. However, quantitative data with high sensitivity may be obtained. Thus, indications of healing may be seen as early as a few weeks after treatment

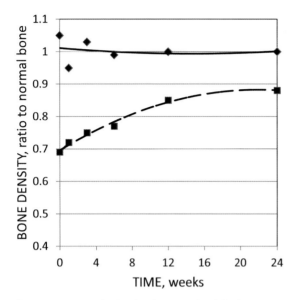

Figure 16.10 Monitoring the density ratio of the lesion in a tooth with healing apical periodontitis (dotted line) in comparison with the density ratio around a sound tooth (solid line) (Adapted from Kerosuo and Ørstavik, 1997, with kind permission from the British Institute of Radiology).

Table 16.1 Advantages and drawbacks of the Periapical Index (PAI).

Advantages	Drawbacks
Related to a gold standard	Molars and premolars have no histological reference
Visual reference dissociated from local interpretation	Sensitivity is (probably) low
Subject to quantifiable harmonization of observers	Cut-off for presence/absence of disease arbitrary
Calibration kit provided	

(Kerosuo and Ørstavik, 1997; Ørstavik, 1997; Trope et al., 1999).

Ratio

A more robust, digital technique has been proposed that may also provide good precision and sensitivity. Here a ratio of the density within the lesion compared with the density in a stable, healthy area of bone in the vicinity is computed for each radiograph in a follow-up series. Changes in this ratio is followed over time, and healing is recorded as the ratio approaches unity. This approach has been used successfully with good discrimination among groups of cases (Delano et al., 2001; Ørstavik et al., 1990; Pettiette et al., 2001) (Figure 16.10).

Visual analyses of periapical healing

A common feature of computerized approaches for assessment of healing is that they are often cumbersome and require time and effort. No method has shown advantages that have made them a standard in either clinical practice or research, although subtraction and density measurements are now integral to many commercial programs for acquisition and analysis of digital radiographs.

Conventional methods

Classic methods for assessing "success" and "failure" in endodontics have been used since the introduction of radiology. A well-known set of criteria for healing are those proposed by Strindberg (1956), which have been used in several clinical studies that have provided scientific support for many current clinical practices (Bystrom et al., 1987; Sjögren et al., 1991). Drawbacks of conventional success/failure analyses are that they are difficult to standardize and that the verbal descriptors used may be subject to differential interpretation (Table 16.1). When used in research, it is certainly imperative that calibration procedures are described and implemented (Friedman, 2008).

Healing after surgery

Landmark publications by Rud et al. (1972) and Molven et al. (1987) have led to improved standardization of postoperative monitoring of healing after apicoectomies. The use of visual references introduced by Molven et al. (1987) allows for effective harmonization and calibration, with possible

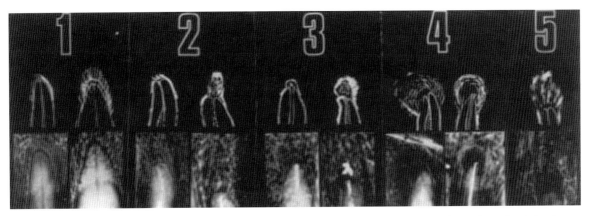

Figure 16.11   The periapical index (PAI) (Reprinted from Ørstavik et al., 1986, with permission from John Wiley & Sons).

comparisons across studies by different observers and in different locations. The complex interaction of surgical wound healing and the possible negative influence of residual or recurrent infection make observation periods of 2 years or more desirable (Kvist and Reit, 1999)

Indices

The use of indices with reproducible scoring characteristics has been hugely successful in cariology (the Decayed, Missing, Filled [DMF] index) and in periodontology (gingival and periodontal indices). In fact, their application in clinical and not least epidemiological studies may be seen as a prerequisite for the acceptance of these diseases as objects of scientific studies that in turn could be used to assess the efficacy of clinical procedures and of public health interventions.

The periapical index (PAI)

The PAI (Ørstavik et al. 1986) was developed based on the format of such indices in related clinical disciplines. The PAI makes use of a 5-step scale of increasing levels of periapical inflammation. The unique material and report of Brynolf (1967) were available and made a relationship to the histologic appearance of type lesions possible. Her "golden standard" (correlation of radiography with histol-

ogy) thus formed the basis for the extrapolations into the PAI scoring system. The PAI has several advantages, but also a few drawbacks, the latter shared by most or all other visual assessments of periapical radiographs. Table 16.1 lists some properties of the PAI scoring system (Figure 16.11).

The 5-category scale allows for rather sensitive statistical methods to be applied, which is useful in comparative clinical studies. For epidemiology and for the sake of relating to conventional success/failure analyses, a cutoff for health and disease between 2 and 3 may be applied. While a score of 2 in principle detects disease, it comprises many, if not most, cases classified as success in conventional studies. And the cutoff point above 2 ensures that there is no overscoring of disease, which is important in epidemiological research.

The index may be used to categorize teeth at the start of treatment, and large-scale studies have shown that this is highly relevant for prognostic evaluations (Figure 16.12).

The index has been used in more than 60 peer-reviewed articles and may now be seen as a standard for studies where more sophisticated radiographic techniques are not applicable. It has been used with film and digital images, and with periapical as well as orthopantomographic exposures. Detection of periapical lesions may be as effective in orthopantomograms as in periapical radiographs (Molander et al., 1993).

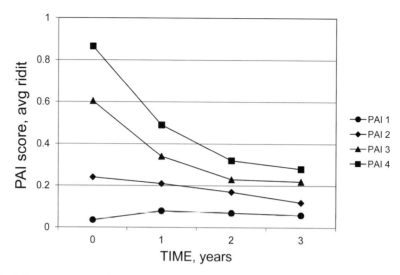

Figure 16.12   Periapical status (average ridits) in groups of teeth with similar periapical situation (identical PAI scores) at start (Adapted from Ørstavik et al., 1987, with permission from John Wiley & Sons).

The PAI in clinical studies

The index was primarily developed for use in clinical, comparative studies of endodontic materials and techniques (Huumonen et al., 2003; Ørstavik et al., 1987; Ørstavik and Hørsted-Bindslev, 1993; Waltimo et al., 2001). Here, focus is on the comparison of products rather than assessment of the final outcome in all cases. As sufficient information on treatment prognosis both for vital pulps and for treatment of apical periodontitis is available after 1 year, this has become the norm in such studies of clinical variables. There is little evidence to suggest that one needs 4 or 5 years for detection of differences between groups of teeth, even though complete healing in individual cases may take that long or longer (Molven et al., 2002; Ørstavik, 1996; Reit, 1987).

Using the PAI and setting failure at PAI > 2, the data from clinical studies have uniformly shown a failure rate (definite presence of apical periododontitis) at 1 year of some 5–10% for root filling of vital teeth, whereas root filling of teeth with apical periodontitis routinely carries a failure rate of 20–30%, even in specialist practices (Conner et al., 2007; Cotton et al., 2008; Eriksen et al., 1988).

It follows that it is very hard indeed to carry out such studies on vital teeth and document improve-

ments of one product or technique over another. Simple mathematical calculations tell us that to detect an improvement of 5% down from 10 with a power of 20%, one needs at least 342 cases in each group for chi square analyses to document the difference. Three per cent down from 5% brings the number up to 462. With such a high success rate to start with, and with the moderate probability that any material or technique will override the operator influence or other factors as a source of at least some failures, it is rather questionable whether clinical studies addressing this issue can be ethically or financially defensible.

Treatment of apical periodontitis, on the other hand, has a much larger window for improvement. Given the infectious nature of the underlying disease, there is also a much higher probability that at least some materials or aspects of procedures may improve results substantially. In statistical terms, one could hope for an improvement in the order of 10–15% which, compared to a reference of 75% success, would require sample sizes of 78 and 197, respectively. Individual and public health benefits should outweigh the human and financial cost of carrying out such a study. However, with few exceptions, even modern materials and techniques, when tested in radiographic follow-up studies, have not so far shown dramatic improvements in performance in relation to standard products and methods (Cotton et al., 2008; Penesis et al., 2008; Peters et al., 2004).

Epidemiology of apical periodontitis

For proper application to epidemiologic studies, the use of PAI2 to PAI3 as the cutoff point for determination of disease was a necessary adaptation. In these studies, orthopantomograms have been a major source of data, with the possible further reduction in sensitivity. It should also be realized that cross-sectional, epidemiological studies do not provide information of the diagnosis that initiated the RCT. Therefore, the presence of apical periodontitis in a root-filled tooth cannot distinguish

as to whether it is a failure to cure or to prevent disease.

Epidemiological studies have focused on two particular aspects (Eriksen, 2008; Kirkevang, 2008): (1) the prevalence in cross-sectional studies of CAP irrespective of prior treatment, and (2) the occurrence of CAP in relation to root-filled teeth. Figure 16.13 shows an overview of some salient results from such studies. Briefly, one may generalize the findings to state that in 40-year-olds in Sweden (Western Europe), 2–4% of teeth have radiographically detectable CAP, increasing to some 15% in the seventh decade of life. Given that many teeth will have been extracted, not least for endodontic reasons, in older age, the proportion of teeth that develops CAP must be higher (Figure 16.13).

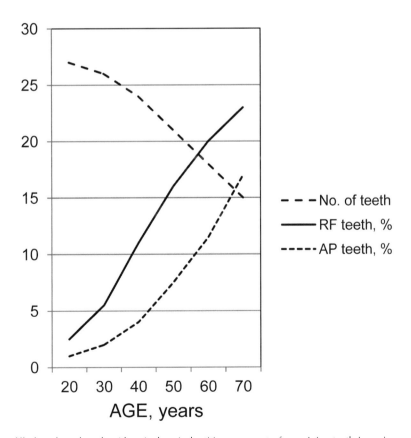

Figure 16.13 Root-filled teeth and teeth with apical periodontitis as percent of remaining teeth in various age groups (Adapted from Eriksen, 2008, with permission from John Wiley & Sons).

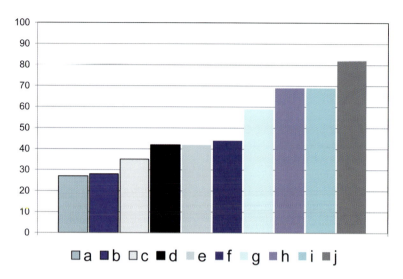

Figure 16.14 The prevalence of apical periodontitis in different populations measured with the PAI scoring system. Use of identical methodology for scoring makes direct comparison of populations possible (Courtesy of HM Eriksen). (a) Dugas et al., 2003; (b) Marques et al., 1998; (c) Loftus et al., 2005; (d) Eriksen and Bjertness 1991; (e) Dugas et al., 2003; (f) Kirkevang et al., 2000; (g) Jiménez-Pinzón et al., 2004; (h) Sidaravicius et al., 1999; (i) Tsuneishi et al., 2005; (j) Segura-Egea et al., 2005.

The proportion of root-filled teeth that has CAP is in the order of 30–50%, consistently around 35% for Western Europe and North America. This is a remarkably high proportion of teeth, considering that institution-based studies show figures from 5% to 30%, with the higher numbers reflecting treated teeth that had CAP at the onset. The inescapable conclusion is that endodontic treatment as it is generally carried out today does not provide adequate protection from, or cure of, apical periodontitis, at least when radiographic criteria are applied. While some of this data have been collected with various methods, the use of PAI in many of them makes direct comparisons possible (Figure 16.14).

These relatively poor results in practice are underscored by the poor sensitivity of the radiographic detection method. When endodontic treatment results are assessed by both periapical images and CBCT, it is a consistent finding that more lesions are detected by the latter method (de Paula-Silva et al., 2009; Liang et al., 2011).

Speculating further that treatment results are generally better for initially vital teeth, which by most accounts make up a majority of teeth that are selected for endodontic treatment, the low success percentage is probably reflecting an even poorer result for the group of teeth with preoperative CAP.

Concluding remarks

The periapical radiograph remains a most important tool for monitoring healing of periapical lesions. While other techniques provide more detailed information, it is essential that we systematize and extract as much information as possible from conventional exposures.

Direct digital images and digitization of conventional films make possible computer-based analyses of changes in bone density by a variety of methods. These analyses are valuable in research and are part of many programs for chairside assessment of periapical healing. Standardization of procedures and relationship to biological processes may be difficult.

For clinical experiments and epidemiological research, the periapical index scoring system has been widely used, especially during the past decade. Its relationship to histologically verified cases and the possibility of calibration and unbiased scoring make the system particularly valuable for clinical long-term studies. By its adoption in various centers for endodontic research, it may aid in the production of solid data from a much larger patient base than can be obtained by other methods.

Radiographic survey projects utilizing the PAI scoring system have facilitated collection of comparable data on a global scale and have permitted assessments of the prevalence and distribution of apical periodontitis from Australia to Portugal and Canada.

More extensive knowledge and use of CBCT may further improve our diagnostic abilities of the periapical status during healing.

References

Benfica e Silva, J., Leles, C.R., Alencar, A.H., Nunes, C.A., and Mendonça, E.F. (2010) Digital subtraction radiography evaluation of the bone repair process of chronic apical periodontitis after root canal treatment. *Int Endod J*, 43, 673–680.

Brummer, H.J. and van Wyk, P.J. (1987) The correlation between systemic allergies and radiologically visible periapical pathosis. *J Endod*, 13, 396–399.

Brynolf, I. (1967) Histological and roentgenological study of periapical region of human upper incisors. *Odontol Revy*, 18(Suppl. 11), 1–176.

Byström, A., Happonen, R.P., Sjögren, U., and Sundqvist, G. (1987) Healing of periapical lesions of pulpless teeth after endodontic treatment with controlled asepsis. *Dent Traumatol*, 3, 58–63.

Camps, J., Pommel, L., and Bukiet, F. (2004) Evaluation of periapical lesion healing by correction of gray values. *J Endod*, 30, 762.

Carrillo, C., Penarrocha, M., Ortega, B., Martí, E., Bagán, J.V., and Vera, F. (2008) Correlation of radiographic size and the presence of radiopaque lamina with histological findings in 70 periapical lesions. *J Oral Maxillofac Surg*, 66, 1600–1605.

Conner, D.A., Caplan, D.J., Teixeira, F.B., and Trope, M. (2007) Clinical outcome of teeth treated endodontically with a nonstandardized protocol and root filled with resilon. *J Endod*, 33(11), 1290–1292.

Cotton, T.P., Schindler, W.G., Schwartz, S.A., Watson, W.R., and Hargreaves, K.M. (2008) A retrospective study comparing clinical outcomes after obturation with Resilon/Epiphany or Gutta-Percha/Kerr sealer. *J Endod*, 34, 789–797.

Cvek, M. (1972) Treatment of non-vital permanent incisors with calcium hydroxide. *Odontol Revy*, 23, 27–44.

Cvek, M., Hollender, L., and Nord, C.-E. (1976) Treatment of non-vital permanent incisors with calcium hydroxide. *Odontol Revy*, 27, 93–108.

Delano, E.O., Ludlow, J.B., Ørstavik, D., Tyndall, D., and Trope, M. (2001) Comparison between PAI and quantitative digital radiographic assessment of apical healing after endodontic treatment. *Oral Surg Oral Med Oral Pathol Oral Radiol Endod*, 92, 108–115.

de Paula-Silva, F.W., Wu, M.K., Leonardo, M.R., da Silva, L.A., and Wesselink, P.R. (2009) Accuracy of periapical radiography and cone-beam computed tomography scans in diagnosing apical periodontitis using histopathological findings as a gold standard. *J Endod*, 35, 1009–1012.

Dugas, N.N., Lawrence, H.P., Teplitsky, P.E., and Pharoah, M.J., Friedman, S. (2003) Periapical health and treatment quality assessment of root-filled teeth in two Canadian populations. *Int Endod J*, 36, 181–192.

Eriksen, H. (2008) Epidemiology of apical periodontitis. In: D. Ørstavik and T. Pitt Ford, eds., *Essential Endodontology*, Blackwell Munksgaard, Oxford.

Eriksen, H.M. and Bjertness, E. (1991) Prevalence of apical periodontitis and results of endodontic treatment in middle-aged adults in Norway. *Dent Traumatol*, 7, 1–4.

Eriksen, H.M., Ørstavik, D., and Kerekes, K. (1988) Healing of apical periodontitis after endodontic treatment using three different root canal sealers. *Dent Traumatol*, 4, 114–117.

Fouad, A.F. and Burleson, J. (2003) The effect of diabetes mellitus on endodontic treatment outcome: data from an electronic patient record. *J Am Dent Assoc*, 134, 43–51.

Friedman, S. (2008) Expected outcomes in the prevention and treatment of apical periodontitis. In: D. Ørstavik and T. Pitt Ford, eds., *Essential Endodontology*, Blackwell Munksgaard, Oxford.

Friedman, S., Torneck, C.D., Komorowski, R., Ouzounian, Z., Syrtash, P., and Kaufman, A. (1997) In vivo model for assessing the functional efficacy of endodontic filling materials and techniques. *J Endod*, 23, 557–561.

Goldman, M., Pearson, A.H., and Darzenta, N. (1972) Endodontic success—who's reading the radiograph? *Oral Surg Oral Med Oral Pathol*, 33, 432–437.

Gröndahl, H.G., Gröndahl, K., and Webber, R.J. (1983) A digital subtraction technique for dental radiography. *Oral Surg Oral Med Oral Pathol*, 55, 96–102.

Heling, I., Bialla-Shenkman, S., Turetzky, A., Horwitz, J., and Sela, J. (2001) The outcome of teeth with periapical periodontitis treated with nonsurgical endodontic treatment: a computerized morphometric study. *Quintessence Int*, 32, 397–400.

Huumonen, S., Lenander-Lumikari, M., Sigurdsson, A., and Ørstavik, D. (2003) Healing of apical periodontitis after endodontic treatment: a comparison between a silicone-based and a zinc oxide-eugenol-based sealer. *Int Endod J*, 36, 296–301.

Jiménez-Pinzón, A., Segura-Egea, J.J., Poyato-Ferrera, M., Velasco-Ortega, E., and Ríos-Santos, J.V. (2004) Prevalence of apical periodontitis and frequency of root-filled teeth in an adult Spanish population. *Int Endod J*, 37, 167–173.

Kerekes, K. and Tronstad, L. (1979) Long-term results of endodontic treatment performed with a standardized technique. *J Endod*, 5, 83–90.

Kerosuo, E. and Ørstavik, D. (1997) Application of computerised image analysis to monitoring endodontic therapy: reproducibility and comparison with visual assessment. *Dentomaxillofac Radiol*, 26, 79–84.

Kirkevang, L.L. (2008) Root canal treatment and apical periodontitis: what can be learned from observational studies? *Endod Top*, 18, 51–61.

Kirkevang, L.L., Ørstavik, D., Hørsted-Bindslev, P., and Wenzel, A. (2000) Periapical status and quality of root fillings and coronal restorations in a Danish population. *Int Endod J*, 33, 509–515.

Kizil, Z. and Energin, K. (1990) An evaluation of radiographic and histopathological findings in periapical lesions. *J Marmara Univ Dent Fac*, 1, 16–23.

Koppang, H.S., Koppang, R., Solheim, T., Aarnes, H., and Stølen, S.O. (1989) Cellulose fibers from endodontic paper points as an etiological factor in post-endodontic periapical granulomas and cysts. *J Endod*, 15, 369–372.

Kvist, T. and Reit, C. (1999) Results of endodontic retreatment: a randomized clinical study comparing surgical and nonsurgical procedures. *J Endod*, 25(12), 814–817.

Liang, Y.H., Li, G., Wesselink, P.R., and Wu, M.K. (2011) Endodontic outcome predictors identified with periapical radiographs and cone-beam computed tomography scans. *J Endod*, 37, 326–331.

Loftus, J.J., Keating, A.P., and McCartan, B.E. (2005) Periapical status and quality of endodontic treatment in an adult Irish population. *Int Endod J*, 38, 81–86.

Love, R.M. and Firth, N. (2009) Histopathological profile of surgically removed persistent periapical radiolucent lesions of endodontic origin. *Int Endod J*, 42, 198–202.

Marques, M.D., Moreira, B., and Eriksen, H.M. (1998) Prevalence of apical periodontitis and results of endodontic treatment in an adult, Portuguese population. *Int Endod J*, 31, 161–165.

Molander, B., Ahlqwist, M., Gröndahl, H.G., and Hollender, L. (1993) Comparison of panoramic and intra-oral radiography for the diagnosis of caries and periapical pathology. *Dentomaxillofac Radiol*, 22(1), 28–32.

Molven, O., Halse, A., and Grung, B. (1987) Observer strategy and the radiographic classification of healing after endodontic surgery. *Int J Oral Maxillofac Surg*, 16, 432–439.

Molven, O., Halse, A., Fristad, I., and MacDonald-Jankowski, D. (2002) Periapical changes following root-canal treatment observed 20–27 years postoperatively. *Int Endod J*, 35, 784–790.

Nair, P.N.R., Pajarola, G., and Schroeder, H.E. (1996) Types and incidence of human periapical lesions obtained with extracted teeth. *Oral Surg Oral Med Oral Pathol*, 81, 93–102.

Ng, Y.L., Mann, V., and Gulabivala, K. (2011) A prospective study of the factors affecting outcomes of nonsurgical root canal treatment: Part 1: Periapical health. *Int Endod J*, 44, 583–609.

Ørstavik, D. (1991) Radiographic evaluation of apical periodontitis and endodontic treatment results: a computer approach. *Int Dent J*, 41, 89–98.

Ørstavik, D. (1996) Time-course and risk analyses of the development and healing of chronic apical periodontitis in man. *Int Endod J*, 29, 150–155.

Ørstavik, D. and Larheim, T.A. (2008) Radiology of apical periodontitis. In: D. Ørstavik and T. Pitt Ford, eds., *Essential Endodontology*, Blackwell Munksgaard, Oxford.

Ørstavik, D., Kerekes, K., and Eriksen, H.M. (1986) The periapical index: a scoring system for radiographic assessment of apical periodontitis. *Dent Traumatol*, 2, 20–34.

Ørstavik, D., Kerekes, K., and Eriksen, H.M. (1987) Clinical performance of three endodontic sealers. *Dent Traumatol*, 3, 178–186.

Ørstavik, D., Farrants, G., Wahl, T., and Kerekes, K. (1990) Image analysis of endodontic radiographs: digital subtraction and quantitative densitometry. *Dent Traumatol*, 6, 6–11.

Ørstavik, D. and Hørsted-Bindslev, P. (1993) A comparison of endodontic treatment results at two dental schools. *Int Endod J*, 26, 348–354.

Ortega-Sánchez, B., Peñarrocha-Diago, M., Rubio-Martínez, L.A., and Vera-Sempere, J.F. (2009) Radiographic morphometric study of 37 periapical lesions in 30 patients: validation of success criteria. *J Oral Maxillofac Surg*, 67, 846–849.

Pascon, E.A., Introcaso, J.H., and Langeland, K. (1987) Development of predictable periapical lesion monitored by subtraction radiography. *Dent Traumatol*, 3, 192–208.

Penesis, V.A., Fitzgerald, P.I., Fayad, M.I., Wenckus, C.S., BeGole, E.A., and Johnson, B.R. (2008) Outcome of one-visit and two-visit endodontic treatment of necrotic teeth with apical periodontitis: a randomized controlled trial with one-year evaluation. *J Endod*, 34, 251–257.

Peters, O.A., Barbakow, F., and Peters, C.I. (2004) An analysis of endodontic treatment with three nickel-titanium rotary root canal preparation techniques. *Int Endod J*, 37(12), 849–859.

Pettiette, M.T., Delano, E.O., and Trope, M. (2001) Evaluation of success rate of endodontic treatment performed by students with stainless-steel K-files nickel-titanium hand files. *J Endod*, 27, 124–127.

Reit, C. (1987) Decision strategies in endodontics: on the design of a recall program. *Endod Dent Traumatol*, 3, 233–239.

Reit, C. and Gröndahl, H.G. (1984) Management of periapical lesions in endodontically treated teeth. A study on clinical decision making. *Swed Dent J*, 8, 1–7.

Reit, C. and Hollender, L. (1983) Radiographic evaluation of endodontic therapy and the influence of observer variation. *Scand J Dent Res*, 91, 205–212.

Ricucci, D., Mannocci, F., and Ford, T.R. (2006) A study of periapical lesions correlating the presence of a radiopaque lamina with histological findings. *Oral Surg Oral Med Oral Pathol Oral Radiol Endod*, 101, 389–394.

Rózyło-Kalinowska, I. (2007) Digital radiography density measurements in differentiation between periapical granulomas and radicular cysts. *Med Sci Monit*, 13(Suppl. 1), 129–136.

Rud, J., Andreasen, J.O., and Jensen, J.E. (1972) Radiographic criteria for the assessment of healing after endodontic surgery. *Int J Oral Surg*, 1, 195–214.

Rud, J., Munksgaard, E.C., Andreasen, J.O., Rud, V., and Asmussen, E. (1991) Retrograde root filling with composite and a dentin-bonding agent. 1. *Endod Dent Traumatol*, 7, 118–125.

Segura-Egea, J.J., Jiménez-Pinzón, A., Ríos-Santos, J.V., Velasco-Ortega, E., Cisneros-Cabello, R., and Poyato-Ferrera, M. (2005) High prevalence of apical periodontitis amongst type 2 diabetic patients. *Int Endod J*, 38, 564–569.

Shrout, M.K., Hall, J.M., and Hildebolt, C.E. (1993) Differentiation of periapical granulomas and radicular cysts by digital radiometric analysis. *Oral Surg Oral Med Oral Pathol*, 76, 356–361.

Sidaravicius, B., Aleksejuniene, J., and Eriksen, H.M. (1999) Endodontic treatment and prevalence of apical periodontitis in an adult population of Vilnius, Lithuania. *Dent Traumatol*, 15, 210–215.

Incidence of periapical cysts in relation to the root canal. *J Endod*, 6(11), 845–848.

Sjögren, U., Hägglund, B., Sundqvist, G., and Wing, K. (1990) Factors affecting the long-term results of endodontic treatment. *J Endod*, 16(10), 498–504.

Sjögren, U., Figdor, D., Spångberg, L., and Sundqvist, G. (1991) The antimicrobial effect of calcium hydroxide as a short-term intracanal dressing. *Int Endod J*, 24, 119–125.

Strindberg, L.Z. (1956) The dependence of the results of pulp therapy on certain factors. An analytic study based on radiographic and clinical follow-up examination. *Acta Odontol Scand*, 14(Suppl. 21), 1–175.

Torabinejad, M., Hong, C.U., Lee, S.J., Monsef, M., and Pitt Ford, T.R. (1995) Investigation of mineral trioxide aggregate for root end filling in dogs. *J Endod*, 21, 603–608.

Trope, M., Delano, E.O., and Ørstavik, D. (1999) Endodontic treatment of apical periodontitis: single vs. multivisit treatment. *J Endod*, 25, 345–350.

Tsuneishi, M., Yamamoto, T., Yamanaka, R., Tamaki, N., Sakamoto, T., Tsuji, K., and Watanabe, T. (2005) Radiographic evaluation of periapical status and prevalence of endodontic treatment in an adult Japanese population. *Oral Surg Oral Med Oral Pathol Oral Radiol Endod*, 100, 631–635.

Tyndall, D.A., Kapa, S.F., and Bagnell, C.P. (1990) Digital subtraction radiography for detecting cortical and cancellous bone changes in the periapical region. *J Endod*, 16, 173–178.

Waltimo, T.M., Boiesen, J., Eriksen, H.M., and Ørstavik, D. (2001) Clinical performance of 3 endodontic sealers. *Oral Surg Oral Med Oral Pathol Oral Radiol Endod*, 92, 89–92.

White, S.C., Sapp, J.P., Seto, B.G., and Mankovich, N.J. (1994) Absence of radiometric differentiation between periapical cysts and granulomas. *Oral Surg Oral Med Oral Pathol*, 78(5), 650–654.

Part 4

Teaching and Research

Chapter 17   Radiographic Consideration for Endodontic Teaching
Chapter 18   Micro-Computed Tomography in Endodontic Research

17 Radiographic Consideration for Endodontic Teaching

Preclinical Exercises

Bettina Basrani

Tell me and I'll forget;
Show me and I may remember;
Involve me and I'll understand.

Chinese proverb

Preclinical endodontics

Preclinical exercises increase the knowledge of endodontic procedures. Therefore, enough time should be provided for this part of the student's education. The knowledge and understanding of the "hidden" view in endodontics will increase confidence of the dental students. With the use of the operative microscope, cone beam computed tomography (CBCT), and micro computed tomography (CT) scan, the complex dental anatomy can be predictably evaluated. Unfortunately, these sophisticated technologies are not universally available in all teaching facilities.

One of the challenges in contemporary dental education is to achieve a smooth transition from preclinical teaching environments to patient-care clinics in a cost-effective manner. Preclinical endodontic courses should provide a unique learning environment that enables the student to perform

endodontic treatment on extracted teeth, mounted in a typodont, and to be involved in diagnosis and treatment-planning discussions. The typodonts should have a special design to allow radiographic examination, rubber dam placement, endodontic instrumentation, and obturation (Pileggi and Glickman, 2004).

Initially, the student should become familiarized with endodontic treatment by first working in transparent teeth and then extracted natural teeth.

The student should then progress using the typodont and simulating the clinical environment (Basrani, 1988).

Internal anatomy

One way to understand the internal anatomy of teeth is by taking radiographs of the extracted teeth with two different angulations (buccal-lingual and mesial-distal) and then seeing the discrepancies that exist with these two views. If conventional radiographs are used, it is possible to take the two views in one film. The technique allows two images of the same tooth. The technique uses a conventional film which is folded in two with lead foil

Endodontic Radiology, Second Edition. Edited by Bettina Basrani.
© 2012 John Wiley & Sons, Inc. Published 2012 by John Wiley & Sons, Inc.

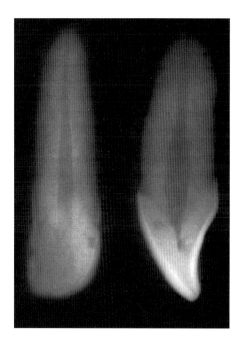

Figure 17.1　Two images of the same tooth appear side by side on the same film.

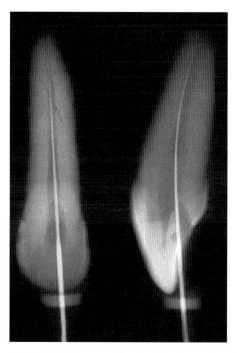

Figure 17.2　Trial file or working length radiograph and postaccess radiograph.

secured between the two halves. The extracted tooth is placed on the film and the radiograph is taken. With careful positioning of the film and thoughtful beam angulation, the first image is exposed, and the film is then turned so that the unexposed side is adjacent to the tooth and a second exposure is taken at a different angulation. Following conventional processing, the two images of the same tooth appear side by side on the same film (Figure 17.1).

Radiographic series of endodontic treatment in a preclinical setting

1. *Preoperative radiograph*: The preoperative radiograph in a preclinical setting will help in identifying the outline of the roots, studying the anatomical structures of the pulp chamber and the root canals, and calculating the estimated working length.
2. *Trial file or working length radiograph and post access radiograph*: This is taken to confirm the estimated working length. It is recommended that for optimal visualization and identifica-

tion, files # 15 or higher should be used inside the canals. This radiograph with the two views will also help to define the access as well (Figure 17.2).

When rectification of the access cavity needs to be done, a new radiograph can then be taken (Figures 17.3 and 17.4).

These views can also be useful aids to show that on many occasions, the radiographic apex and the apical foramen do not coincide (Figure 17.5).

3. *Master apical file radiograph*: This radiograph is taken once the final apical enlargement has been accomplished. It is used to determine the final shape and length of the canals before obturation. It can also help to identify if an accident during instrumentation has occurred, such as transportation, creation of a ledge, and separation of an instrument (Figure 17.6A,B).
4. *Master gutta-percha cone radiograph*: This radiograph is taken after placement of the master cone(s) and once tug-back has been confirmed prior to cementation. It allows the student to

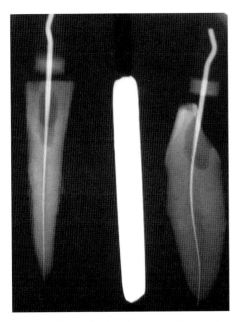

Figure 17.3   Radiographs showing access that needs rectification.

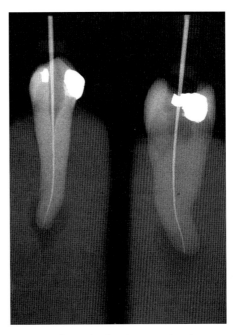

Figure 17.5   Radiographs showing apex that do not coincide with the anatomic apex.

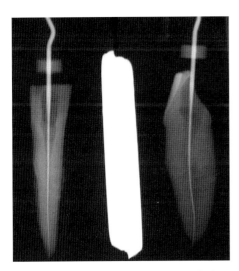

Figure 17.4   Radiographs showing access rectified.

technique is used. This allows one to confirm checking the quality of the obturation in the apical one-third of the canal, which is important in order to obtain an appropriate apical seal. If any mistake is observed, this is the appropriate time to remove the maser cone and the accessory cones and make the necessary adjustments (Figure 17.8A,B).

6. *Final obturation radiograph*: This radiograph is taken after the canals have been obturated, the access cavity sealed with a temporary restorative material (e.g., Cavit, IRM, glass ionomer) and the rubber dam removed (Figure 17.9A,B) (Figure 17.10).

Didactic approaches to learn the correct position of the access cavity can be done during this learning process. Some examples of these exercises are listed below:

check the length of the master cone(s) and the shape of the prepared canal (Figure 17.7).

5. *Mid-obturation radiograph*: This radiograph is taken after cementing the master apical cone in place and after adding two or three accessory cones in each canal when lateral condensation

1. *Coronal access*: The student requires a preoperative radiograph of the tooth in question. He/she is asked to make a drawing of the tooth and design the correct access preparation. A

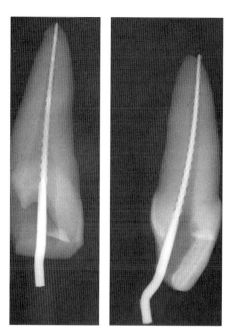

Figure 17.6   Master apical file radiograph.

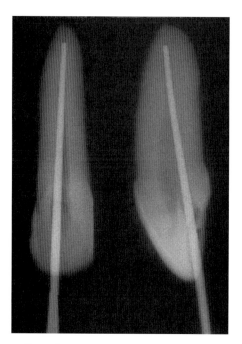

Figure 17.7   Master gutta-percha cone radiograph.

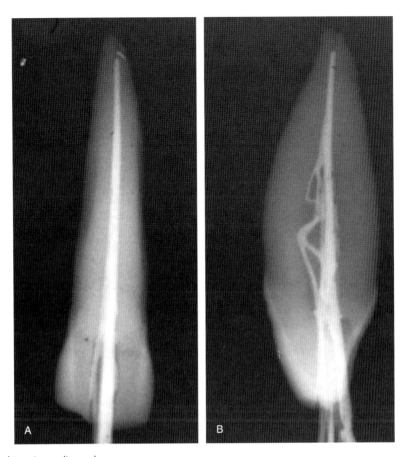

Figure 17.8   Mid-obturation radiograph.

form to be completed by the student is prepared. In this form, the participant needs to
have the preoperative radiograph and he/she
needs to make a drawing of the contour of the
tooth and design the correct access preparation.
After the access cavity is completed on the
tooth, a radiograph with the two views is taken
which will demonstrate if the access should be
modified or not (Figure 17.11).
2. *Chamber analysis*: The teeth are sectioned at the
cemento–enamel junction (CEJ). Radiopaque
material (Cavit) will be placed in the chamber
and a radiograph is taken. This image will
show the student the location of the chamber and the relationship between the pulp
chamber and occlusal wall of the tooth (Figure
17.12A,B).
3. *Postobturaion analysis*: After the root canal procedure is completed, other analysis can be
made. For example, the teeth can be sectioned
or made transparent to evaluate the quality of
the obturation (Figure 17.13).

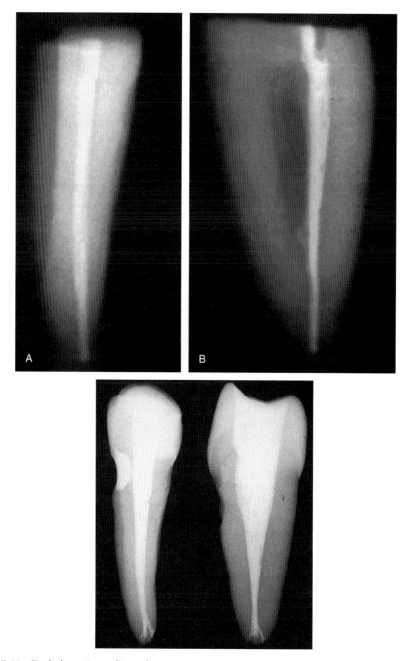

Figure 17.9 and 17.10   Final obturation radiograph.

FORM #3.A.:
CORONAL ACCESS

RADIOGRAPH

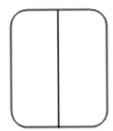

DRA WING OF THE TOOTH

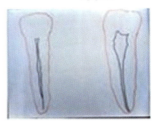

DIAGRAM OF THE ACCESS

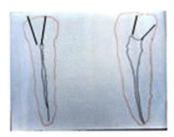

RX POST ACCESS

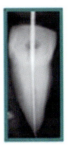 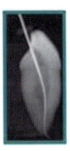

Figure 17.11 Coronal access form.

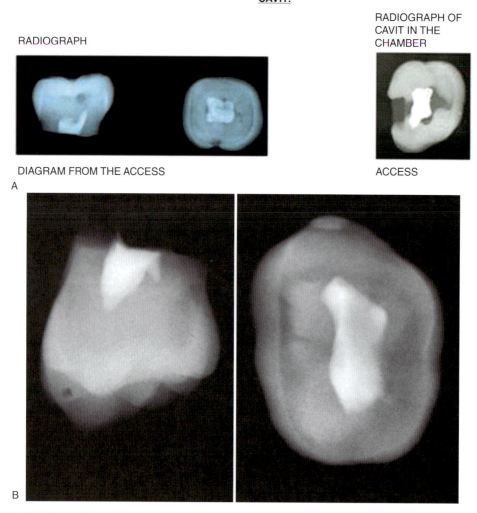

RADIOGRAPH OF
CAVIT IN THE
CHAMBER

RADIOGRAPH

DIAGRAM FROM THE ACCESS

ACCESS

A

B

Figure 17.12   Chamber analysis.

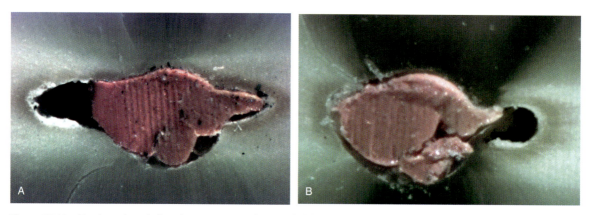

A

B

Figure 17.13   Tooth sectioned after obturation. Note the gaps left by the instruments and by the obturation material.

Concluding remark

Preclinical exercises are a great opportunity to teach students the hidden third dimension in endodontics. For those who think that endodontics is the art of working in a blind field, working on extracted teeth can be a means to overcoming this problem. There is no doubt that the use of the operative microscopes and CBCT are a great aid in seeing the endodontic field. Unfortunately, most schools do not have access to these technologies during preclinical training.

References

Basrani, E. (1988) Endodoncia: Tecnicas en Preclinical y Clinica. Ed Medica Panamericana.
Pileggi, R. and Glickman, G.N. (2004) A cost-effective simulation curriculum for preclinical endodontics. *Eur J Dent Educ*, 8(1), 12–17.

18 Micro-Computed Tomography in Endodontic Research

Mana Mirfendereski and Ove Peters

Introduction

High-resolution micro-computed tomography is an innovative technology with several applications in endodontic research and education. Conventional X-ray computed tomography (CT) is an imaging modality that was first described by Hounsfield (1973). This technique produces a series of images through tomography or imaging by sections, which are then reconstructed three-dimensionally using computer software programs (Hounsfield, 1973).

The possibility of traditional CT application in endodontics to three-dimensionally reconstruct teeth was first explored by Tachibana and Matsumoto (1990). While these investigators were able to demonstrate anatomical configuration of teeth using CT, the spatial resolution of 0.6 mm was found to be insufficient to allow for detailed analysis of root anatomy and structures. The authors concluded that conventional CT offered only limited application in endodontics due to its high radiation dose, time consumption, cost, insufficient resolution, and inadequate computer software capability. However, some investigators (Velvart et al., 2001) still found traditional CT useful compared to peri-

apical radiographs when planning for periapical surgery of mandibular molars and premolars. These authors concluded that CT imaging provided beneficial information on mandibular canals and their proximity to the lesion or root apex that is not available from dental radiographs. Further advancements in technology resulted in the development of newer versions of CT scanning such as cone beam computed tomography (CBCT). In clinical settings, CBCT imaging has surpassed conventional CT and has become increasingly popular for endodontic presurgical treatment planning and diagnosis. Detailed discussion of CBCT technology and its applications in clinical practice are beyond the scope of this chapter.

Other technological advancements allowed for the introduction of a miniaturized form of tradiional CT, the micro-CT (Kak and Stanley, 1988) for use in nonclinical settings. Micro-CT applies comparable principles to those of conventional CT, but the three-dimensional reconstructions of small objects, such as teeth, are developed to a resolution of within a few microns (<2 μm for Scanco μCT50, SCANCO Medical, Switzerland). While initial investigations using micro-CT technology were hampered by limited vertical resolution capacity of

Endodontic Radiology, Second Edition. Edited by Bettina Basrani.
© 2012 John Wiley & Sons, Inc. Published 2012 by John Wiley & Sons, Inc.

1–2 mm (Dowker et al., 1997; Nielsen et al., 1995), improvements in the micro-CT machinery and computer software employed in reconstruction of images have allowed for significantly more accurate analysis of root canal systems (Dowker et al., 1997; Peters et al., 2000, 2001).

How does micro-CT work?

Micro-CT scanners employ a micro-focus X-ray source that enables high-resolution detectors to collect magnified projection images of a small object. The first generation machines were equipped with a line detector. As the object rotated around the z-axis, differences in radiodensity were detected and a slice could then be reconstructed. With advancements along the z-axis, the acquisition of numerous two-dimensional views became possible, which were then processed by computer softwares to produce three-dimensional images (De Santis et al., 2005). The reconstructed three-dimensional images generated could then be sliced along any plane to further analyze the external and internal structures of the scanned object.

Other commercial units (e.g., SkyScan 1172, SkyScan, Belgium) use miniaturized cone beam geometry that scans the entire object in one rotation. This mode of acquiring images results in a data volume rather than individual slices. However, the data block can be resliced at selected angles and slice thicknesses. The latest generation of micro-CT units, such as newer Scanco units (SCANCO Medical), use a stacked fan beam geometry that with a special collimator are able to acquire 256 slices with one rotation. The main practical difference between fan beam and cone beam geometry is faster data acquisition (with a reliance on accurate reconstruction algorithms) with cone beam and slightly better perceived data quality (with a much longer acquisition time) with fan beam machines.

Independent of the data acquisition mode, three-dimensional reconstruction of objects with any micro-CT data sets requires segmentation. This relies on threshold values that differentiate a particular structure of interest from its surrounding material. The three-dimensional reconstruction can then be executed on these thresholds based on calculation of data slices or a data volume from the individual projections. This allows for outlines of enamel, dentine, and the root canal as well as its content to be segmented and assessed.

Applications in endodontics

As a nondestructive imaging tool, micro-CT may be applied to assess an object many times, allowing it to remain unaltered for further experimentation and future scans. The three-dimensional images gather considerable data, allowing for both qualitative and quantitative evaluation of the sample (Rhodes et al., 1999). These characteristics make micro-CT a desirable tool for in vitro studies that evaluate root canal morphology and procedures of root canal preparation and obturation. Thus, a scanned tooth can be analyzed along its length to acquire data for calculating areas and volumes before and after endodontic procedures. The data offered by micro-CT technology can lead to clinical applications such as development of new techniques, comparative analysis of existing approaches in endodontic treatment, and enhancement of dental education in preclinical and clinical stages.

The development of the micro-CT technology has allowed for better assessment of the anatomy of the root canal system with unprecedented accuracy, which in turn has resulted in the adoption of this technology in endodontic research. Using micro-CT with a resolution of 127 µm, Nielsen et al. (1995) demonstrated accurate three-dimensional rendering of external and internal morphologies of root canals in extracted calcified human maxillary molars. They concluded that it was possible to reproduce tooth anatomy nondestructively and to assess area and volume changes after root canal instrumentation and obturation procedures (Nielsen et al., 1995). Dowker et al. (1997) improved on the work of Nielsen et al. (1995) by presenting micro-CT images of root canals in extracted teeth at approximately 40 µm resolution. These investigators were able to display significant details, such as unfilled canal areas and the presence of dentinal debris. Jung et al. (2005) evaluated the accuracy of micro-CT for imaging of filled root canals when compared to histological examination. These authors demonstrated that micro-CT was a highly accurate and nondestructive method for assessing root canal fillings and their content. Its use for assessing the intricacies of C-shaped canals (Cheung and Cheung, 2008; Cheung et al., 2007; Fan et al., 2004a, 2004b) and morphology of pulp chamber floor (Min et al., 2006) have also been reported. More recently, further advancements in micro-CT technology and improvements in imaging software have tremendously increased the vertical resolution capacity. The ability to accurately reconstruct the root canal system using micro-CT has provided researchers with an advanced nondestructive tool and has led to its increasing popularity in experimental endodontology (Guillaume et al., 2006; Hammad et al., 2009; Jung et al., 2005; Mirfendereski et al., 2009; Peters et al., 2001, 2003; Rigolone et al., 2003).

Another application of micro-CT is in comparative research of different endodontic approaches, such as various instrumentation and root filling procedures. Micro-CT has been used to compare the performance of different rotary instruments in preparing root canals and to assist with characterization of morphological changes associated with each technique (Peters et al., 2001) (Figure 18.1a–c). The micro-CT-generated images from this study also displayed that approximately 35–40% of root canals' surface areas remain unchanged after mechanical preparation (Peters et al., 2001).

Relative performance of a rotary instrument system in shaping root canals of varying preoperative root canal geometry has also been investigated using micro-CT imaging (Peters et al., 2001, 2003). Furthermore, micro-CT-generated images have revealed the extent of root canal transportation that occurs after instrumentation with different rotary files (Paque et al., 2005).

Micro-CT technology has further been used to compare and measure the adaptation of different root filling techniques to the root canal walls (Hammad et al., 2009; Mirfendereski et al., 2009). In one study, micro-CT was employed to evaluate the effectiveness of hand and rotary instrumentation for retreatment of root canals filled with different root filling materials (Hammad et al., 2008). It concluded that none of the tested root filling materials was completely removed during retreatment using hand or rotary files and that gutta-percha was more effectively removed by hand files (Hammad et al., 2008). Micro-CT has been shown to be a promising tool in its application for educational purposes. In separate studies to evaluate the skills of novice dental students in performing root canal preparation and fillings, micro-CT imaging was utilized to assess the adequacy of canal preparations (Gekelman et al., 2009) and root fillings (Mirfendereski et al., 2009). It appeared that novice operators were able to instrument mesial root canals in mandibular molars adequately with two rotary instrumentation techniques (Gekelman et al., 2009). Moreover, the micro-CT reconstruction of the root-filled teeth showed that in the hands of inexperienced dental students, carrier-based root filling technique had significantly less void volume when compared to warm vertical compaction technique (Mirfendereski et al., 2009) (Figure 18.2a,b).

Micro-CT-generated imaging can also serve in computer-assisted learning in preclinical dental training (Dowker et al., 1997a, 1997b; Swain and Xue, 2009). Future directions with micro-CT may involve use in virtual reality techniques of endodontic teaching (Dowker et al., 1997).

Limitations

The limitations of the earlier versions of the micro-CT technology were mainly length of time required for the scanning and reconstruction processes, and the need for advanced computer expertise (Rhodes et al., 1999). These factors continue to limit the utility of micro-CT despite improvements in the technology over the last decade. Additionally, micro-CT equipment continues to be expensive and is thus not universally available. The high radiation doses also preclude micro-CT from use in clinical settings.

Conclusions

Micro-CT technology has shown to be a promising tool in endodontic research as a nondestructive method that maintains the integrity of tooth samples throughout the analysis process. It provides highly accurate three-dimensional images of the samples. Its use in in vitro research may advance the development of new techniques of instrumentation and obturation, and the emergence of new approaches to endodontics treatment options available to dental practitioners. The

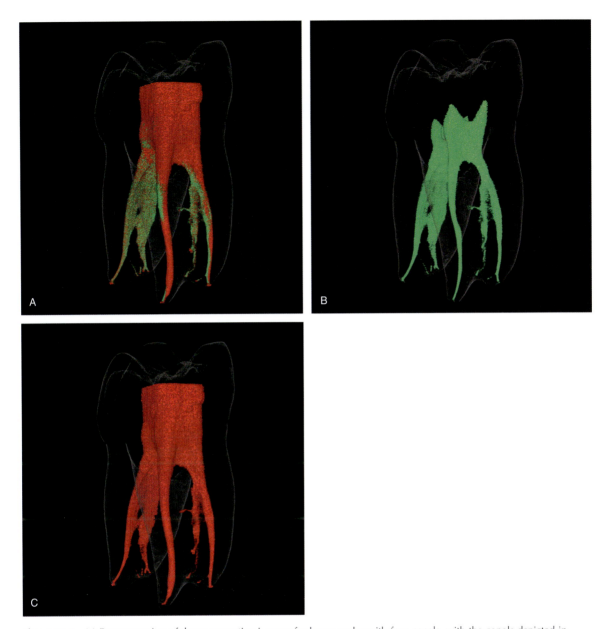

Figure 18.1 (a) Reconstruction of the preoperative image of a lower molar with four canals, with the canals depicted in green and the tooth structure shaded. (b) The merged images show the uninstrumented distal canals in red/green and the instrumented areas of mesial canals and the access cavity in red. Initially, the mesial canals were instrumented using Lightspeed size 30 and ProTaper F1 instruments. (c) The instrumentation was then completed with Lightspeed size 50 and step back as well as with ProTaper F3 instruments. The areas of the canals that were not touched during instrumentation can be seen in green.

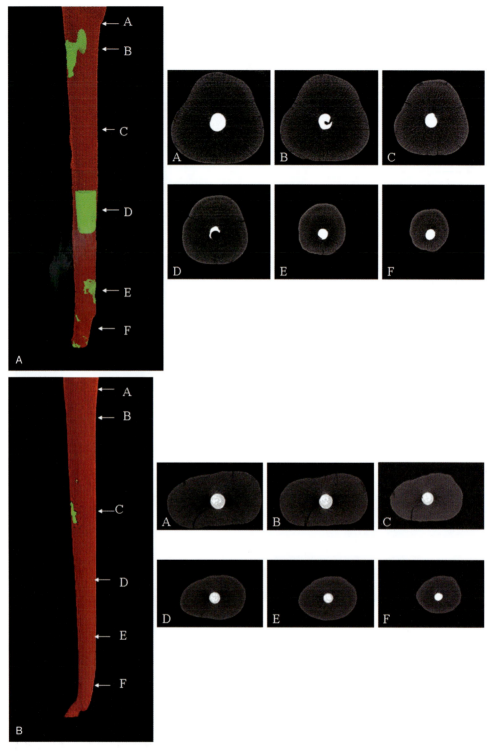

Figure 18.2 (a) Micro-CT horizontal cross sections and 3D reconstruction of apical 9 mm of a root canal filled by System B down-pack and Calamus backfill. Filled areas are red and voids are green. Section D demonstrates void at junction of gutta-percha down-pack mass and backfill (Courtesy of Dr Fan Bing). (b) Micro-CT horizontal cross sections and 3D reconstruction of apical 9 mm of a root canal filled by ProTaper Obturator System. Filled areas are red and voids are green (Courtesy of Dr Fan Bing).

utilization of micro-CT in comparative research can also provide insights in determining the relative superiority of current treatment techniques and the emergence of best practices and clinical treatment guidelines. Finally, micro-CT analysis can help enhance the development of novel educational approaches for dental students at all levels of training by providing detailed analysis of root canal anatomy, preparation, and filling volumes. While the current technology still has many limitations, its continued adoption in research and education promises to be an important tool in enhancing our understanding of the field of endodontics.

References

Cheung, G.S., Yang, J., and Fan, B. (2007) Morphometric study of the apical anatomy of C-shaped root canal systems in mandibular second molars. *Int Endod J*, 40, 239–246.

Cheung, L.H. and Cheung, G.S. (2008) Evaluation of a rotary instrumentation method for C-shaped canals with micro-computed tomography. *J Endod*, 34, 1233–1238.

De Santis, R., Mollica, F., Prisco, D., Rengo, S., Ambrosio, L., and Nicolais, L. (2005) A 3D analysis of mechanically stressed dentin-adhesive-composite interfaces using X-ray micro-CT. *Biomaterials*, 26, 257–270.

Dowker, S.E., Davis, G.R., and Elliott, J.C. (1997a) X-ray microtomography: nondestructive three-dimensional imaging for in vitro endodontic studies. *Oral Surg Oral Med Oral Pathol Oral Radiol Endod*, 83, 510–516.

Dowker, S.E., Davis, G.R., Elliott, J.C., and Wong, F.S. (1997b) X-ray microtomography: 3-dimensional imaging of teeth for computer-assisted learning. *Eur J Dent Educ*, 1, 61–65.

Fan, B., Cheung, G.S., Fan, M., Gutmann, J.L., and Bian, Z. (2004a) C-shaped canal system in mandibular second molars: Part I. Anatomical features. *J Endod*, 30, 899–903.

Fan, B., Cheung, G.S., Fan, M., Gutmann, J.L., and Fan, W. (2004b) C-shaped canal system in mandibular second molars: Part II. Radiographic features. *J Endod*, 30, 904–908.

Gekelman, D., Ramamurthy, R., Mirfarsi, S., Paqué, F., and Peters, O.A. (2009) Rotary nickel titanium GT and ProTaper files for root canal shaping by novice operators: a radiographic and micro-computed tomography evaluation. *J Endod*, 35, 1584–1588.

Guillaume, B., Lacoste, J.P., Gaborit, N., et al. (2006) Microcomputed tomography used in the analysis of the morphology of root canals in extracted wisdom teeth. *Br J Oral Maxillofac Surg*, 44, 240–244.

Hammad, M., Qualtrough, A., and Silikas, N. (2008) Three-dimensional evaluation of effectiveness of hand and rotary instrumentation for retreatment of canals filled with different materials. *J Endod*, 34, 1370–1373.

Hammad, M., Qualtrough, A., and Silikas, N. (2009) Evaluation of root canal obturation: a three-dimensional in vitro study. *J Endod*, 35, 541–544.

Hounsfield, G.N. (1973) Computerized transverse axial scanning (tomography): 1. Description of system. *Br J Radiol*, 46, 1016–1022.

Jung, M., Lommel, D., and Klimek, J. (2005) The imaging of root canal obturation using micro-CT. *Int Endod J*, 38, 617–626.

Kak, A.C. and Stanley, M. (1988) *Principles of Computerized Tomographic Imaging*. IEEE Press, New York.

Min, Y., Fan, B., Cheung, G.S., Gutmann, J.L., and Fan, M. (2006) C-shaped canal system in mandibular second molars. Part III: The morphology of the pulp chamber floor. *J Endod*, 32, 1155–1159.

Mirfendereski, M., Roth, K., Fan, B., et al. (2009) Technique acquisition in the use of two thermoplasticized root filling methods by inexperienced dental students: a microcomputed tomography analysis. *J Endod*, 35, 1512–1517.

Nielsen, R.B., Alyassin, A.M., Peters, D.D., Carnes, D.L., and Lancaster, J. (1995) Microcomputed tomography: an advanced system for detailed endodontic research. *J Endod*, 21, 561–568.

Paque, F., Barbakow, F., and Peters, O.A. (2005) Root canal preparation with Endo-Eze AET: changes in root canal shape assessed by micro-computed tomography. *Int Endod J*, 38, 456–464.

Peters, O.A., Laib, A., Rüegsegger, P., and Barbakow, F. (2000) Three-dimensional analysis of root canal geometry by high-resolution computed tomography. *J Dent Res*, 79, 1405–1409.

Peters, O.A., Schönenberger, K., and Laib, A. (2001) Effects of four Ni-Ti preparation techniques on root canal geometry assessed by micro computed tomography. *Int Endod J*, 34, 221–230.

Peters, O.A., Peters, C.I., Schönenberger, K., and Barbakow, F. (2003) ProTaper rotary root canal preparation: effects of canal anatomy on final shape analysed by micro CT. *Int Endod J*, 36, 86–92.

Rhodes, J.S., Ford, T.R., Lynch, J.A., Liepins, P.J., and Curtis, R.V. (1999) Micro-computed tomography: a new tool for experimental endodontology. *Int Endod J*, 32, 165–170.

Rigolone, M., Pasqualini, D., Bianchi, L., Berutti, E., and Bianchi, S.D. (2003) Vestibular surgical access to the palatine root of the superior first molar: "low-dose cone-beam" CT analysis of the pathway and its anatomic variations. *J Endod*, 29, 773–775.

Swain, M.V. and Xue, J. (2009) State of the art of micro-CT applications in dental research. *Int J Oral Sci*, 1, 177–188.

Tachibana, H. and Matsumoto, K. (1990) Applicability of X-ray computerized tomography in endodontics. *Endod Dent Traumatol*, 6, 16–20.

Velvart, P., Hecker, H., and Tillinger, G. (2001) Detection of the apical lesion and the mandibular canal in conventional radiography and computed tomography. *Oral Surg Oral Med Oral Pathol Oral Radiol Endod*, 92(6), 682–688.

Part 5

Advanced Techniques

Chapter 19   Alternative Imaging Systems in Endodontics

Chapter 20   Introduction to Cone Beam Computed Tomography

Chapter 21   Interpretation of Periapical Lesions Using Cone Beam Computed Tomography

19

Alternative Imaging Systems in Endodontics

Elisabetta Cotti and Girolamo Campisi

The primary objective of any alternative technique for morphological imaging of the maxillary bones and of the teeth, which is of importance to the endodontic field, is to detect the pathologic structures. It is also important to ascertain the exact anatomical relations of a pathologic structure with the surrounding tissues. Furthermore, the imaging procedure should yield information (if possible) on the histopathology of a lesion in order to enable a differential diagnosis and the selection of adequate therapeutic measures (Cotti, 2010; Patel et al., 2009).

The development of noninvasive and therefore safer (Berrington de Gonzalez and Darby, 2004) imaging technology (which does not use ionizing radiation) such as ultrasound real-time echotomography and magnetic resonance imaging (MRI) have revolutionized pathomorphological diagnosis in many cases, permitting precise location and delineation of a lesion (Cotti and Campisi, 2004).

Ultrasound real-time echotomography

General concepts on ultrasound real-time echotomography

The first application of acoustic echoes for object localization took place under water in search for the wreck of the Titanic in 1912. Seventy years ago Dussik introduced the use of ultrasounds as a diagnostic tool in the medical field to evaluate a cerebral pathosis (Auer and Van Velthoven, 1990).

Since that far, 1942 diagnostic ultrasounds have gained more and more importance, and nowadays, there is no diagnostic field in medicine in which ultrasonic imaging does not find a specific indication.

Ultrasound real-time echotomography is also called echography: the exam is based on the *piezoelectric effect* and on the *reflection* of ultrasound (US) waves called "echos." When a synthetic ceramic crystal is placed into an electric field, the electrons

Endodontic Radiology, Second Edition. Edited by Bettina Basrani.
© 2012 John Wiley & Sons, Inc. Published 2012 by John Wiley & Sons, Inc.

cause a sudden change in the structure of its grid: growth or shrinkage. This structural change emits mechanical energy in the form of sound waves. Each crystal distributes waves at one frequency depending on the alternating current it is exposed to (i.e., a crystal exposed to a 5 MHz alternating current will create sound waves oscillating at a frequency of 5 MHz). US waves for diagnostic purposes are mostly generated employing frequencies ranging from 1.6 to 20 MHz.

The synthetic crystal can also transform a US wave back to an electromagnetic wave. The crystal sends the US waves in all directions; therefore, they are bundled to a focal zone by means of an acoustic lens. The US waves oscillating at the same frequency are sent toward the biologic tissues via the ultrasonic probe (transducer) which contains the crystals. When the US waves hit the interface between two tissues (which possess different acoustic impedance), they undergo both *reflection* and *refraction*. The echo is the part of the US wave that is reflected back to the crystal. The echoes reflected back to the crystal are transformed by the crystal into electrical energy which is again transformed into light signals in a computer built into the US machine.

The US image we see on the monitor is produced by the movement of the crystal over a tissue plane. Each movement of the crystal over a plane of tissue gives one image of this tissue: a frequency of 30–50 movements per second will produce an average of 30 images per second. When the US probe is moved and oriented by hand, the sector plane is changed, and a real-time image is produced. The US exam appears in the monitor like a movie. The intensity of the echoes depends on the difference in acoustic properties of two adjacent tissues, which is the result of the density of the tissues and the velocity of the US waves through them: the greater the difference, the greater the reflected US energy. The resolution of the US image depends on the distance between the focus and the tissue section imaged.

The interpretation of the gray values of the images is based on the comparison with those of normal tissues: *low echo signals* appear as *dark spots*, and *high echo signals* appear as *bright/white spots* (Auer and Van Velthoven, 1990).

An acoustically homogeneous area displays a low-echo intensity (*hypoechoic*) while tissues with different densities exhibit high-echo intensity (*hyperechoic*).

The presence of air in the field of observation acts as a barrier because total reflection of US waves occurs at the interface between tissue and air; it is therefore important to use a gel as an interface between the probe and the tissue.

Total reflection also occurs at the surface of bone (*hyperechoic*).

In the presence of fluids, no reflection occurs because there is no echo intensity (*transonic/anechoic*).

We distinguish the echographic appearance of the tissues as follows:

- *Liquid structures*: "transonic" with reinforced walls and lateral acoustic shadows.
  Within this category we find fluid tissues which can be (1) liquid corpuscolated (containing solid or liquid aggregates); (2) liquid with septa; (3) liquid with parietal echogenic vegetations.
- *Solid structures*: "echogenic," reflecting the echoes in a variety of ways (hypo and hyperechoic), within this group we find: (1) solid homogeneous structures; (2) solid dishomogeneous structures; (3) solid structures with colliquations; (4) solid structures with posterior shadow (as for calcific formations).

The latest US imaging systems use multifrequency, wide-band transducers with multiple, low-impedance linear crystals (up to 256) organized in 3–5 layers and electronically connected in a variable sequence.

The transducers that are best suited for the field of dentistry are linear probes, and allow the formation of a high-frequency (7.5–15 MHz) rectangular or trapezoidal image, which exhibit both optimal lateral resolution and optimal contrast of the superficial structures (Ghorayeb et al., 2008).

The dynamic focalization gives a precise resolution in structures smaller than 2 mm by varying the frequencies within 5–10 MHz. Furthermore, the digital era has made possible to reduce most of the artifacts which are built in the high-resolution systems.

To better evaluate bone lesions in the jaws, and especially to reduce the artifacts in fluid structures (cysts), these are simultaneously insonated with

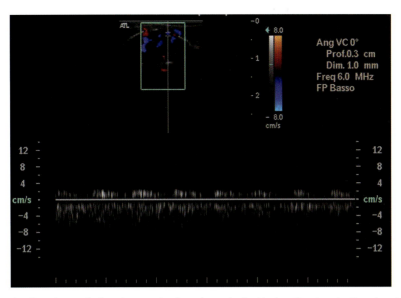

Figure 19.1 Echo-color Doppler applied to the examination of a periapical lesion showing the Doppler signal in the lower portion of the figure, and the color Dopper in the format of colored spots superimposed on the lesion, in the upper part of the figure (framed).

converging boundless US waves sent from different directions (*compound technique*) (Hofer, 2005b)

The color-power Doppler (CPD) flowmetry applied to the US examination allows the accurate evaluation of the blood flow within a given tissue, and it is based on the "Doppler effect" discovered in 1842 (Fleischer and Emerson, 1993) as a consequence of the frequency shift that occurs in the reflected sound waves when the US waves are directed toward the moving blood cells. The Doppler signal is in the audible range (2–4 MHz) and is represented on a graph with its changes in real time: the spectra obtained are plotted as a function of time (horizontal axis) and frequency shifts (vertical axis). The signal is influenced by the insonation angle of the US and by the changes in frequency (Hofer, 2005a).

The color Doppler is the technique used for visualizing the presence and velocity of the blood flow within an image plane. It measures the Doppler shifts in the volumes located in an image plane and shows the flow in the form of color spots superimposed on the gray-scale image. Blood vessels moving toward the transducer appear as red (*positive Doppler shifts*), while vessels moving away from the transducer appear as blue (*negative Doppler shifts*). The higher velocities of the

flow are represented in brighter shades of the same colors (red and blue); the scheme of the color which encodes the frequency shifts is indicated by the color bar to the side of the screen/image (Figure 19.1).

Color Doppler images are updated several times per second.

The *power Doppler*, based on the *integrated power spectrum*, adds sensitivity to the exam and discloses the presence of the network of minor vessels and slower flows within the tissue of interest; it is less influenced by the insonation angle (Fleischer and Emerson, 1993; Hofer, 2005b; Wolf and Fobbe, 1995).

The intensity of the echo-CPD signal is strengthened by the intravenous (IV) injection of *contrast media* that increase the echogenicity of the blood. The use of second-generation *contrast media*, which reach the lumen of the smaller vessels, allows the evaluation of the blood flow in its wash-in and wash-out phases and the study of the microvascular system (Hofer, 2005a).

In the field of endodontics, the echo-CDP discloses the vascular map around and within a lesion and shows the direction of blood flow (Cotti, 2008).

US real-time imaging does not use ionizing radiations, and it is therefore considered a much safer

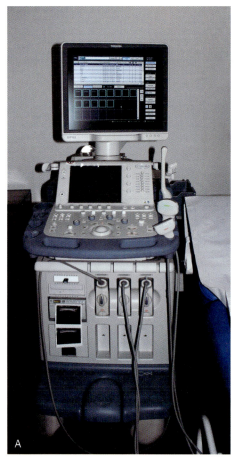
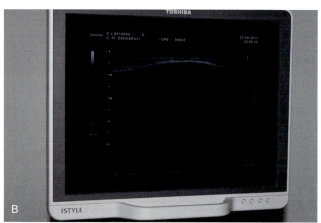
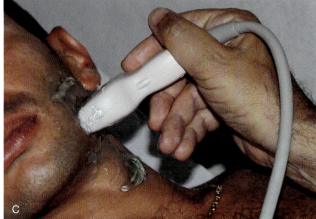

Figure 19.2 Ultrasound imaging of last-generation apparatus (A), details of the monitor (B), extra-oral examination of the mandible with a linear probe (C).

technique than radiographic examinations (Barnett et al., 1997, 2000; Martin, 1984). The only potential adverse effects of the system is the consequence of the cavitation and vibration effects created by the transfer of heat and mechanical energy into biological tissues. These phenomena depend on the time of application of the sound energy: it is therefore important to limit the repetitions of the exams (Auer and Van Velthoven, 1990).

Use of US imaging in endodontics

US real-time imaging has been applied to the endodontic field for the diagnosis, evaluation, and

follow-up of bone lesions in the jaws (Cotti, 2008, 2010; Cotti et al., 2002, 2003, 2006; Gundappa et al., 2006; Sumer et al., 2009).

The technique is relatively easy to perform: the patient is sitting on the echographic bed, and the operator moves the probe (protected with a latex/plastic cover and topped with the echographic gel) inside the buccal area of the mandible or the maxilla which corresponds to the periapical area of the tooth of interest (as previously assessed with a radiograph). The same examination can also be performed extra-orally, by placing the probe on the external surface of the skin (Figure 19.2). The operator is facing the computer, while gently moving the probe around the area of interest to obtain an

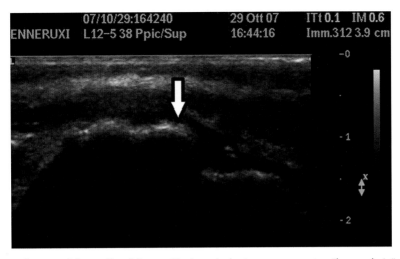

Figure 19.3   Ultrasound image of the profile of the maxilla (arrow); the image represents a "hyperechoic" area where total reflection occurs.

adequate number of scans to define the lesion in real time.

Each moving sequence or single image can be selected and stored in the computer.

The probes that are used to investigate bone lesions in the jaws are multifrequency high-resolution transducers either in the format of linear probes or in the format of intraoperatory probes (smaller probes useful for intraoral examination), and support a digital US apparatus.

Based on the studies reported on the application of US real-time echotomography to the endodontic field (Cotti, 2008, 2010; Cotti et al., 2002, 2003, 2006; Gundappa et al., 2006; Rajendran and Sundaresan, 2007; Sumer et al., 2009), the healthy and pathologic tissues within the maxillary bones appear as follows in the echographic images:

1. Alveolar bone: total reflecting surface (*hyperechoic*) = white (Figure 19.3).
2. Roots of the teeth: total reflecting surfaces (*hyperechoic*) = white (Figure 19.4).
3. Bone cavities filled with fluid (i.e., cystic cavity):
   a. nonreflecting surface (*anechoic/transonic*) = dark, if filled with clear fluid, without inclusions (Figure 19.5);
   b. scarcely reflecting surface (*hypoechoic*) = dark with some echogenic shades if

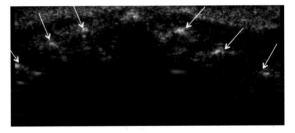

Figure 19.4   Ultrasound image of the maxilla showing the contours of the roots of the teeth (arrows); the contours are hyperechoic.

filled with fluid containing inclusions (Figure 19.6).

The sensitivity of the technique makes possible the distinction between serous and inflammatory exudates.

4. Solid lesions in the bone: reflect the echoes with various intensities (*echogenic*) = light grey (Figure 19.7).
5. Mandibular canal, mental canal, and maxillary sinus = these anatomic landmarks are visible and are mostly transonic (Cotti, 2008).

The study of periapical lesions is still one of the hot issues in endodontics (Cotti et al., 2006).

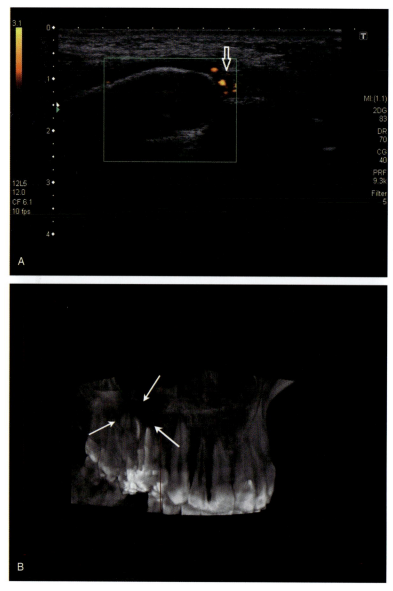

Figure 19.5 Cystic lesion as seen in the ultrasound image (squared): it is an "anechoic" cavity where no reflection occurs: it exhibits reinforced bony contours which are hyperechoic; at the CPD it shows only perilesional vascular supply (arrow) (A). The same lesion (periapical lesion on tooth # 16) as it appears in the cone beam computed tomography: volume (B),

The possibility of diagnosing a periapical lesion and to make a distinction between a cyst and a granuloma, and between other bone lesions of non-endodontic origin, may help in predicting and understanding their healing potential (Nair, 1998; Simon, 1980). This differential diagnosis cannot be

made using traditional radiographic techniques (Cotti, 2010).

Trope et al. (1989) correlated the computed tomography (CT) scan evaluations of 8 periapical lesions from human cadavers to the histopathology and concluded that cysts could be differentiated

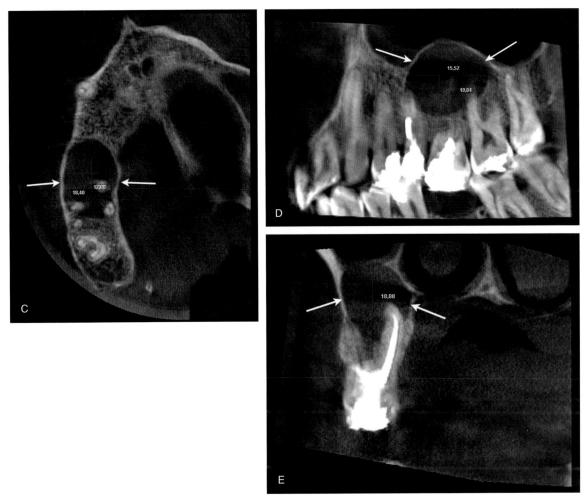

Figure 19.5 *(Continued)*   axial (C), sagittal (D), and coronal (E). The histopathologic report confirmed it was a cyst.

form granulomas based on their CT appearance. On axial CT scans, a cyst would display an area with a density reading similar to the background (darker than a granuloma), while the granuloma would show a cloudy appearance and a density similar to that of the surrounding soft tissues.

On the other hand, controversial results come from the application of CBCT to the differential diagnosis of cystic lesions from granulomas as reported from Simon et al. (2006) and Rosenberg et al. (2010).

Few studies published in the last 10 years have focused on the possibility of addressing a differential diagnosis between cystic lesions and periapical granulomas, based on the interpretation of the US images with the application of the echo-CPD exam.

Three different studies (Cotti et al., 2003, 2006; Gundappa et al., 2006) were conducted on a total of 24 cases diagnosed as periapical lesions of endodontic origin and validated by the histopathological reports obtained following the surgical excision of the lesions. They all concluded that a periapical cyst can be diagnostically differentiated from a granuloma as follows:

Cystic lesion: well-contoured transonic lesion filled with fluid, with reinforced walls (hyperechoic/ bright white contour) and a lateral acoustic shadow, with no perfusion inside, may have

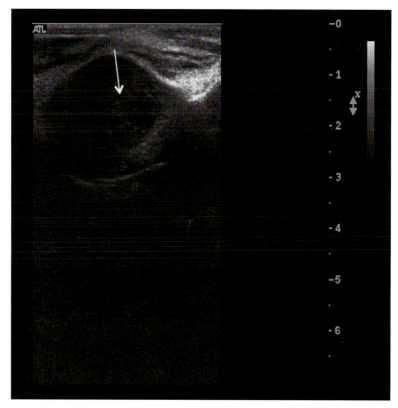

Figure 19.6 Ultrasound image of a cystic lesion of the upper maxillary bone: the lesion appears filled with fluid containing inclusions (arrow).

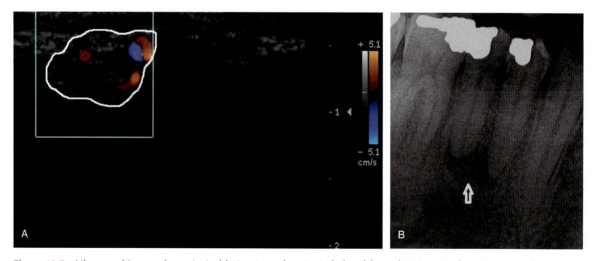

Figure 19.7 Ultrasound image of a periapical lesion (granuloma) (circled and framed): it is an "echogenic" area where echoes are reflected at different intensities: The colored spots represent the vascularization within the lesion (A). The lesion was periapical to teeth # 44 and # 45 as shown in the radiograph (B), and the diagnosis of granuloma was confirmed following the biopsy.

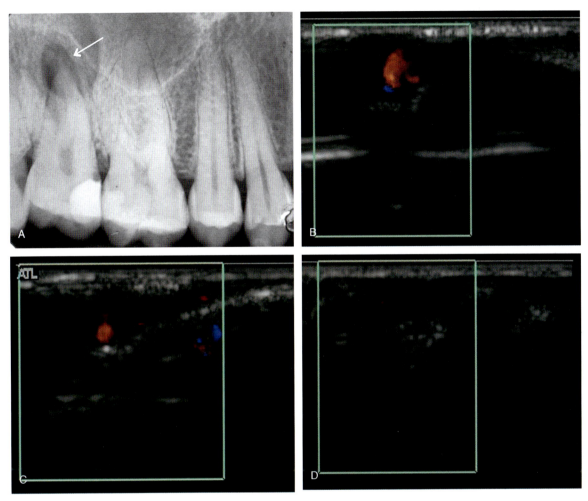

Figure 19.8 Periapical radiograph showing a lesion in tooth #17 (A). Ultrasound imaging with echo-CPD of the lesion before the treatment was initiated (B). The vascular supply is extensive. The echo-CPD of the same lesion 1 week after endodontic treatment was started (cleaning, shaping, and disinfection of the root canals + intermediate medication) shows a reduction of the blood flow within the lesion (C). The echo-CPD of the same lesion 1 month after completion of treatment shows a drastic reduction in the perfusion within the lesion (D).

vascular supply on the outside (Figures 19.5 and 19.6).

Periapical granuloma: lesion with less regular contours, which can be echogenic, or may show mixed echogenic and hypoechoic areas, exhibiting a vascular supply within its tissue at the color-power Doppler (Figures 19.7 and 19.8).

If the bone contour is irregular or resorbed in proximity of the lesion, this can be seen as a *dishomogeneous echo*.

In a later study (Sumer et al., 2009), 22 lesions of the jaws were examined using the US real-time imaging with the echo-CPD. Unlike what was done in the previous studies, in this investigation, the sample group comprised several different kinds of lesions, not only from endodontic origin. The results showed that the diagnosis of periapical granulomas were consistent with the biopsy reports while the lesions diagnosed as cysts with the histopathological examination (4 keratocysts, 2 dentigerous cysts, 4 residual cysts, 7 radicular cysts) showed a more composite US appearance. Some of them were transonic, others had a mixed internal content, and all were without vascularization, but one which had a vascular supply: this unusual observation was explained with the presence of a very thick perilesional capsule.

The authors concluded that the US diagnosis of periapical granuloma is reliable, while the diagnosis of periapical cyst is less precise and depends mostly on the type of cyst and the thickness of its capsule.

The sensitivity of US has been useful to detect the early stage of bone thinning and expansion, associated with the sun-ray erosion of the cortical bone and with growth of soft tissue mass, which were early features of an osteosarcoma (Ng et al., 2001).

The US examination associated to CPD can also be used both for the short- and long-term follow-up of the endodontic lesions. With regard to the short-term outcome of endodontic treatment in clinical cases of apical periodontitis (AP), the various degrees of inflammation of a given lesion can be assumed by evaluating the perfusion within or/and around the lesion with the CPD which has also the sensitivity to detect the presence of newly formed vessels. This type of follow-up has been assessed in a clinical pilot project conducted on 6 teeth with AP examined with US and CPD before treatment (to assess the content of the lesion and its blood supply): 1 week after root canal cleaning and disinfection; 1 month after the completion of treatment. The preliminary data obtained by comparing the US/CPD examinations of the same cases showed changes in the perfusion around and/or within the lesions both after the first appointment and after the completion of treatment. In most cases, a gradual reduction of the vascular supply was noticed as to indicate a progressive reduction in the inflammation in the area. These observations open to a new possibility to assess the behaviour of AP in the different stages (and types) of treatment (Figure 19.8) (Cotti, 2008).

As for the long-term follow up, US examination with CPD has been used to monitor AP in the mandible and maxilla 6 months after endodontic treatment was completed (Rajendran and Sundaresan, 2007). The report showed that as the healing process started within a lesion, there was an increase in the Doppler signal which slowly decreased and disappeared as the healing of the lesion progressed and was completed.

In conclusion, the US imaging offers a safe diagnostic tool, and it is the only exam that possesses the sensitivity to detect bone lesions in the jaws while assessing their solid or fluid content and their internal and external blood supply at the same time.

It also permits the follow-up of treatment based on the changes in vascular perfusion.

It does not perform a precise differential diagnosis between different kinds of cystic conditions, but it allows changes in their shape and fluid/solid content to be observed.

As an opening to the near future, US has promise for study and early diagnosis of a variety of dental diseases: (1) caries, cracks, and fractures by measuring enamel thickness and track changes in enamel thickness over space and time, (2) periodontal disease, by qualitatively assessing the periodontium, (3) bone characterization for implant treatment plan and osteoporosis, via noninvasive measurements during routine visits (Ghorayeb et al., 2008).

New dedicated high-frequency probes are currently being tested (Salmon and Le Denmat, 2011).

MRI

General concepts on MRI

MRI has been available since 1984. The production of MRI images is made possible because of the hydrogen content in the organic compounds. The nuclei of the hydrogen atom have an uneven number of protons and in the presence of a stable external magnetic field, they are set into a spinning motion. When a high-frequency electromagnetic field, perpendicular to the stationary magnet, is created, the protons are tipped on their axes and absorb energy. When the high-frequency electromagnetic field is shut off, they return to their original position (*relaxation*) releasing a signal of the same frequency (*resonance*) (Pasler and Visser, 2007). During the MRI exam, a strong magnetic field is created around the body of the patient: this causes the protons in the atoms of water within the tissues to line up. Then high-frequency pulses of radio waves are sent toward the tissue, perpendicular to the magnetic field, from a scanner. Many of the protons are moved out of alignment (transversal): this generates a weak radio signal (resonance). As the nuclei realign back into their original position (longitudinal), they send out the resonance. The signals are captured by a radio antenna and then received and measured from a computer system that converts them into an image of the tissue being explored.

The tissue-specific *relaxation time* is primarily responsible for the great soft tissue contrast provided by the MRI. The images from MRI are tomograms (Whaites, 2007).

Magnetic resonance is a noninvasive technique since it uses radio waves; it also allows the acquisition of direct views of the body in almost all orientations. Its best performance is in showing soft tissues and vessels whereas it does not provide great details of the bony structures. The strength of the MRI system magnetic field is measured in metric units called Tesla.

In MRI, bright means *high signal intensity*, dark means *low signal intensity*, with all the intermediate shades: bone: *low signal* = dark; air: *low signal* = dark; fat: *strong signal* = bright; soft tissues: *strong signal* = bright.

Using a special program, STIR (*short tau inversion recovery, fat annulling sequences*), water and blood will appear bright.

Disadvantages of MRI are a longer scanning time compared to CT, and the generation of the strong magnetic field that cannot be used in patients carrying a pacemaker or metal pieces in the areas to be investigated (Patel et al., 2009). Furthermore, MRI is an expensive examination, and some of the systems available still use narrow tubes (Gahleitner et al., 1999; Gray et al., 1996; Tutton and Goddard, 2002; Uberoi et al., 1996).

Use of MRI in endodontics

The application of MRI to dentistry has more often involved the temporomandibular joints (Uberoi et al., 1996) and salivary glands (Bornstein et al., 2011). Its use has also been reported on the assessment of the jaw bones prior to implant surgery (Gray et al., 1996), and on the differential diagnosis of lesions in the mandibula and maxillary bones (Minami et al., 1996; Rodrigues et al., 2011)

When MRI has been applied to the study of the dental tissues (Gahleitner et al., 1999), an adequate imaging of the maxillary bones, of the teeth, and periapical tissues were obtained; it was also noticed that the pulp space could be better observed using a contrast medium and that edema in the periapical region was detectable. In a comprehensive review on MRI and its relationship with the teeth and periapical tissues (Tutton and Goddard, 2002), an open MRI system was used to examine the dental and periapical status in normal patients and in patients with AP. Three millimeter slices were undertaken in the transverse, coronal, and oblique sagittal planes using T1-weighted spin echo, STIR, and fast low-angle shot, and these are the conclusions drawn:

1. In MRI, enamel and dentin appear *black*, the pulp chamber and root canal are either *white* or *light grey*, root fillings are dark. The cortical bone is a *black area* outlined by lighter, soft external tissues and internal *bright* fatty marrow (Figure 19.9). On STIR scans, fatty marrow has a low signal and appears dark grey.
2. Periapical lesions are clearly visualized as well as any interruption of the cortical bone.
   a. On T1 shots, they have a moderate signal (grey) as opposed to the medullary marrow, which appears white. This is probably due to the replacement of bone

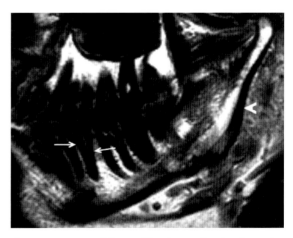

Figure 19.9 MRI of the maxillary bones showing the teeth (long arrows), the mandible (short arrow), and the surrounding soft tissue (bright signal).

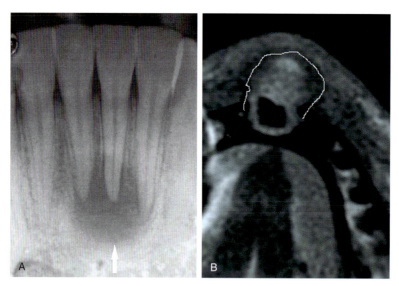

Figure 19.10   Mandibular lesion (arrowed) corresponding to the periapical area of teeth # 31-32-41-42 (A), the lesion was not endodontic in origin. MRI examination (axial slice) of the same lesion showing a solid lesion in the center of the mandible extending through the buccal cortical plate and involving the soft tissues (circle) (B). The MRI diagnosis was of a fibromatous lesion.

marrow by inflammatory exudate. Areas of bone sclerosis, which usually surround the lesion, have a low signal (black) (Figure 19.10).

b. The same lesions seen on STIR shots, on the contrary, appear as low-grey to bright white areas. This indicates that the area has a high water content and may be edematous in nature.

3. The lesions as seen on MRI are more extensive than the same areas when observed in the panoramic or intraoral radiographs. If the signal is low on T1 and high on STIR, it may be deduced that the lesion is cystic in nature (more water content). If the signal is mixed on both, then the lesion is more likely to be a granuloma or an infected cyst.

Furthermore, different MRI signal intensities characterize pulp tissue from older and younger patients (Kress et al., 2007), and contrast-enhanced MRI exams underline the difference between vital and nonvital teeth (Kress et al., 2004). MRI is also feasible for looking at dental carious lesions in three dimensions and no artifacts are created by metallic restorations within this exam (Tymofiyeva et al., 2009), but it is difficult to distinguish the

hard tissues of the tooth within the MRI scans because of their scarce water content. To overcome these problems, a new MRI technique has been developed very recently: the SWIFT (*Sweep Imaging with Fourier Transformation*) imaging. With this system, while the cancellous bone, the gingival, and the oral mucosa all appear bright, the dentin of the whole tooth is well distinguished. The presence of newly calcified tooth structure (reparative dentin), pulp tissue with lateral canals, the presence and extension of a carious lesion, and the status of the periapical tissues can also be seen in detail. This newly designed exam seems to be very promising for the evaluation of the status of the pulp tissue within the tooth. The method was shown to be extremely effective in ex vivo evaluations, while it still needs to be perfected for its in vivo application (Idiyatullin et al., 2011) (Figure 19.11).

When an infective lesion of the jaws spreads out to the bone and to the corresponding soft tissues, degenerating into osteomyelitis, MRI becomes an elective diagnostic technique (Del Balso, 1995). Stafne's bone cyst is another lesion of the jaws which can represent a diagnostic challenge (Katz et al., 2001) for which MRI is indicated. It is a depression in the lingual surface of the mandible usually located below the level of the mandibular canal in the area between the first molar and the angle of the mandible, and it results from aberrant tissue of the submandibular gland. In some cases, it may be found apical to lower anterior teeth, and it results from an accessory part of the sublingual gland. Surgical exploration in these cases can be avoided by using CBCT which shows a well-corticated defect in the lingual aspect of the mandible, in conjunction with MRI which discloses the continuity of the glandular tissue within the bone lesion and allows to compare the signal intensity

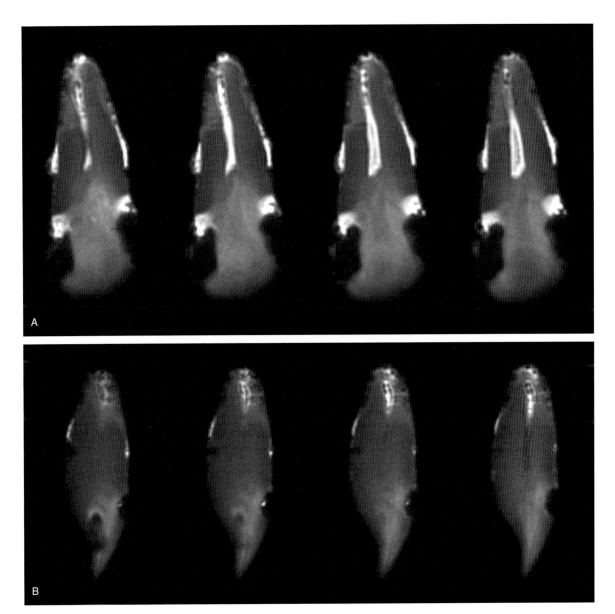

Figure 19.11 MRI images of an incisor obtained using the new SWIFT technique: the white signal represents the root canal and the carious lesions on the cervical portion of the tooth in a mesiodistal view (A) and in the buccolingual view (B). (Reprinted from Idiyatullin et al., 2011, "Dental MRI: making the invisible visible." *Journal of Endodontics*, 37(6), 745–752, with permission from Elsevier Ltd.)

of the lesion's tissue with that of the salivary gland (Bornstein et al., 2011) (Figure 19.12).

MRI is an expensive exam that has several advantages over CT/CBCT in the diagnosis of soft tissue lesions and should be left to differential diagnostic problems when abnormal spreading of lesions occurs in the bones and when there is the involvement of soft tissues, nerves, and vascular supply.

Its future applications will be probably in the three-dimensional investigation of the pulp space, the periapical tissues, and the diffusion of caries.

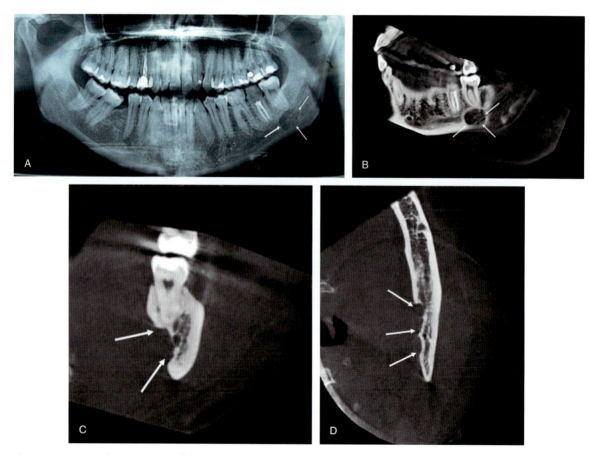

Figure 19.12 Bone lesion (arrows) of the posterior mandible as seen in the panoramic radiograph taken during a routine examination (A). The patient was a 35-year-old woman. The same lesion represented in the CBCT in (B) the sagittal (arrow), (C) coronal (arrows), and (D) axial scans (arrows). The CBCT scans show a well-corticated lesion open to the floor of the mouth (C and D), apical to the lower left third molar (B and C), lingual to the mandibular canal (C). This exam does not offer information on the kind of tissue within the lesion. The MRI of the same lesion (E) in the axial slice, reveals a lesion (arrows) arising from the left submandibular gland (star) with the homogeneous contrast uptake. The signal of the invaginated tissue had the same intensity of the tissue from the salivary gland (axial contrast enhanced T1-weighted imaging, TR 507 ms, TE, 17 ms, slice thickness 3 mm). The ultrasound image of the same lesion (F), displays a solid lesion with an intense vascularization typical of a glandular tissue (squared). The diagnosis is of Stafne's bone cyst.

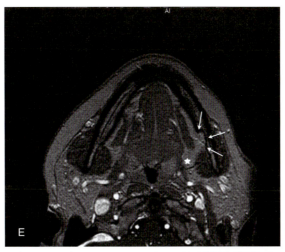

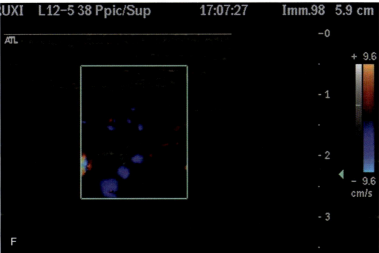

Figure 19.12   (Continued)

References

Auer, L.M. and Van Velthoven, V. (1990) *Intraoperative Ultrasound Imaging in Neurosurgery*, 1st ed. Springer Verlag, Berlin.

Barnett, S.B., Rott, H.D., Ter Haar, G.R., Ziskin, M.C., and Maeda, K. (1997) The sensitivity of biological tissue to ultrasound. *Ultrasound in Medicine and Biology*, 23, 805–812.

Barnett, S.B., Ter Haar, G.R., Ziskin, M.C., Rott, H.D., Duck, F.A., and Maeda, K. (2000) International recommendations and guidelines for the safe use of diagnostic ultrasound in medicine. *Ultrasound in Medicine and Biology*, 20, 355–366.

Berrington De Gonzalez, A. and Darby, S. (2004) Risk of cancer from diagnostic X-rays: estimates for the UK and 14 other countries. *Lancet*, 363(9406), 345–351.

Bornstein, M.M., Wiest, R., Balsiger, R., and Reichart, P.A. (2011) Anterior Stafne's bone cavity mimicking a periapical lesion of endodontic origin: report of two cases. *Journal of Endodontics*, 35, 1598–1602.

Cotti, E. (2008) Ultrasonic imaging. In: J.I. Ingle, L.K. Bakland, and J.C. Baumgartner, eds., *Ingle's Endodontics*, 6th ed., pp. 590–599. BC Decker Inc, Hamilton, Ontario.

Cotti, E. (2010) Advanced techniques for detecting lesions in bone. *Dental Clinics of North America*, 54, 215–235.

Cotti, E. and Campisi, G. (2004) Advanced radiographic techniques for the detection of lesions in bone. *Endodontic Topics*, 7, 52–72.

Cotti, E., Campisi, G., Garau, V., and Puddu, G. (2002) A new technique for the study of periapical bone lesions: ultrasound real time imaging. *International Endodontic Journal*, 35, 148–152.

Cotti, E., Campisi, G., Ambu, R., and Dettori, C. (2003) Ultrasound real-time imaging in the differential diagnosis of periapical lesions. *International Endodontic Journal*, 36, 556–564.

Cotti, E., Simbola, V., Dettori, C., and Campisi, G. (2006) Echographic evaluation of bone lesions of endodontic origin: report of two cases in the same patient. *Journal of Endodontics*, 32, 901–905.

Del Balso, A.M. (1995) Lesions of the Jaws. *Seminars in ultrasound, CT, and MRI*, 6, 487–512.

Fleischer, A. and Emerson, D.S. (1993) *Color Doppler Sonography in Obstetrics and Gynaecology*, 1st ed. Churchill Livingstone Inc, New York.

Gahleitner, A., Solar, P., Nasel, C., et al. (1999) Magnetic resonance tomography in dental radiology. *Der Radiologe*, 39, 1044–1050.

Ghorayeb, S.R., Bertoncini, C.A., and Hinders, M.K. (2008) Ultrasonography in dentistry. *IEEE Transactions on Ultrasonics, Ferroelectrics, and Frequency Control*, 55, 1256–1266.

Gray, C.F., Redpath, T.W., and Smith, F.W. (1996) Pre-surgical dental implant assessment by magnetic resonance imaging. *Journal of Oral Implantology*, 22, 147–153.

Gundappa, M., Ng, S.Y., and Whaites, E.J. (2006) Comparison of ultrasounds, digital and conventional radiography in differentiating periapical lesions. *Dentomaxillofacial Radiology*, 35, 326–333.

Hofer, M. (2005a) *Teaching Manual of Color Duplex Sonography*. Medidak Publishing GmbH, Bern.

Hofer, M. (2005b) *Ultrasound Teaching Manual: The Basic of Performing and Interpreting Ultrasound Scans*, 2nd ed. Thieme Ed, Stuttgart, Germany.

Idiyatullin, D., Corum, C., Moeller, S., et al. (2011) Dental magnetic resonance imaging: making the invisible visible. *Journal of Endodontics*, 37, 745–752.

Katz, J., Chaushu, G., and Rotstein, I. (2001) Stafne's bone cavity in the anterior mandible: a possible diagnostic challenge. *Journal of Endodontics*, 27, 304–307.

Kress, B., Buhl, Y., Anders, L., et al. (2004) Quantitative analysis of MRI signal intensity as a tool for evaluating tooth pulp vitality. *Dentomaxillofacial Radiology*, 33, 241–244.

Kress, B., Buhl, Y., Hahnel, S., et al. (2007) Age- and tooth-related pulp cavity signal intensity changes in healthy teeth: a comparative magnetic resonance imaging analysis. *Oral Surgery, Oral Medicine, Oral Pathology, Oral Radiology, and Endodontics*, 103, 134–137.

Martin, A.O. (1984) Can ultrasound cause genetic damage? *Journal of Clinical Ultrasound*, 12, 11–20.

Minami, M., Kaneda, T., Ozawa, K., Yamamoto, H., Itai, Y., Ozawa, M., Yoshikwa, K., and Sasaki, Y. (1996) Cystic lesions of the maxillomandibular region: MR imaging distinction of odontogenic keratocysts and ameloblastomas from other cysts. *American Journal of Roentgenology*, 166, 943–949.

Nair, P.N.R. (1998) New perspective on radicular cysts: do they heal? *International Endodontic Journal*, 31, 155–160.

Ng, S.Y., Songra, A., Nayeem, A., and Carter, J.L.B. (2001) Ultrasound features of osteosarcoma of the mandible: a first report. *Oral Surgery, Oral Medicine, Oral Pathology, Oral Radiology, and Endodontics*, 92, 582–586.

Pasler, F.A. and Visser, H. (2007) Magnetic resonance imaging. In: F.A. Pasler and H. Visser, eds., *Pocket Atlas of Dental Radiology*, pp. 108–109. Thieme Ed, Stuttgart, Germany.

Patel, S., Dawood, A., Whaites, E., et al. (2009) New dimensions in endodontic imaging: Part 1. Conventional and alternative radiographic systems. *International Endodontic Journal*, 42, 447–462.

Rajendran, N. and Sundaresan, B. (2007) Efficacy of ultrasound and color power Doppler as a monitoring tool in the healing of endodontic periapical lesions. *Journal of Endodontics*, 33, 181–186.

Rodrigues, C.D., Villar-Neto, M.J., Sobral, A.P., et al. (2011) Lymphangioma mimicking apical periodontitis. *Journal of Endodontics*, 37, 91–96.

Rosenberg, P.A., Frisbie, J., Lee, J., et al. (2010) Evaluation of pathologists (histopathology) and radiologists (cone beam computed tomography) differentiating radicular cysts from granulomas. *Journal of Endodontics*, 36, 423–428.

Salmon, B. and Le Denmat, D. (2011) Intraoral ultrasonography: development of a specific high frequency probe and clinical pilot study. *Clinical Oral Investigations*, 5, 643–649. [Epub].

Simon, J.H. (1980) Incidence of periapical cysts in relation to the root canal. *Journal of Endodontics*, 6, 845–848.

Simon, J.H.S., Enciso, R., Malfaz, J.M., et al. (2006) Differential diagnosis of large periapical lesions using cone beam computed tomography measurements and biopsy. *Journal of Endodontics*, 32, 833–837.

Sumer, A.P., Danaci, M., Ozen Sandikci, E., Sumer, M., and Celenk, P. (2009) Ultrasonography and Doppler ultrasonography in the evaluation of intraosseous lesions in the jaws. *Dentomaxillofacial Radiology*, 38, 23–27.

Trope, M., Pettigrew, J., Petras, J., Barnett, F., and Tronstad, L. (1989) Differentiation of periapical granulomas and radicular cysts by digital radiometric analysis. *Endodontics and Dental Traumatology*, 5, 69–72.

Tutton, L.M. and Goddard, P.L. (2002) MRI of the teeth. *British Journal of Radiology*, 75, 552–562.

Tymofiyeva, O., Boldt, K., Rottner, K., et al. (2009) High resolution 3D magnetic resonance imaging and quantification of carious lesions and dental pulp in vivo. *MAGMA*, 22, 365–374.

Uberoi, R., Goddard, P., Ward-Booth, P., and Kabala, J. (1996) TMJ function and dysfunction. *Developments in Magnetic Resonance*, 2, 9–15.

Whaites, E. (2007) *Essentials of Dental Radiology and Radiography*, 4th ed. Elsevier, Oxford, UK.

Wolf, K.J. and Fobbe, F. (1995) *Color Duplex Sonography. Principles and Clinical Application*. Thieme, New York.

20 Introduction to Cone Beam Computed Tomography

Ernest W. N. Lam

This technology, first described in 1998 for applications in dentistry (Mozzo et al., 1998), employs a cone-shaped X-ray beam emanating from a point source coupled with a planar digital sensor. During image acquisition, both the radiation source and sensor rotate around the patient, who is stationary. There are two classes of cone beam systems currently, ones that employ small fields of view with dimensions of less than 8 cm, and large fields of view with dimensions of greater than 8 cm upward to 30 cm.

Unlike intraoral digital imaging, the anatomy of the area imaged is recreated in three dimensions rather than two. The three-dimensional (3D) elements that recreate the anatomy are referred to as cube-shaped volume elements or voxels. Small field of view systems (Figure 20.1) employ pixel dimensions as low as 0.076 mm while the larger field machines employ pixel dimensions of between 0.20 mm and 0.40 mm.

For endodontic applications (Nurbakhsh et al., 2011; Wang et al., 2011), which often require imaging resolutions at the level of the tooth and/ or their supporting structures, the smaller field, higher resolution machines may be of greater value.

Prior to image acquisition, the area of interest is centered within the imaging volume. The center of the field determines what tissues may potentially be irradiated, and this has a bearing on patient radiation doses. Although radiation dose considerations are of particular concern in 3D imaging, they are less for small volume cone beam computed tomography (CBCT) than large volume CBCT or medical CT. For these systems, the effective radiation doses have been reported to range from approximately 5.3 to 38.3 microSievert (μSv) (Ludlow and Ivanovic, 2008). For context, the effective dose from panoramic radiography has been reported to be up to 24.3 μSv and for a full mouth series of intraoral radiographs using American National Standards Institute (ANSI) D speed film and round collimation, 388 μSv. Since radiation-effective dose calculations are based on the volume and sensitivity of a tissue contained within the imaging volume, dose variations from region-to-region are normal. For large field CBCT systems, depending on the system, the effective dose may range from 74 μSv to 1073 μSv. The large range can be attributed to the operating peak kilovoltage and milliamperes of the different machines, different field of view sizes, and the mode in which the radiation is delivered (pulsed or constant output).

Once acquisition is complete, the volume of information contained within the volume is reviewed in two-dimensioinal (2D) images formatted in one of three orthogonal planes: axial, coronal, and sagittal (Figure 20.2).

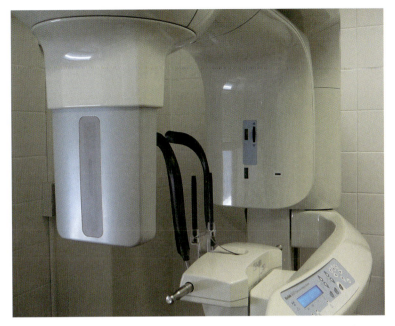

Figure 20.1   Small field of view CBCT system (Kodak 9000 3D, Carestream, Rochester, New York).

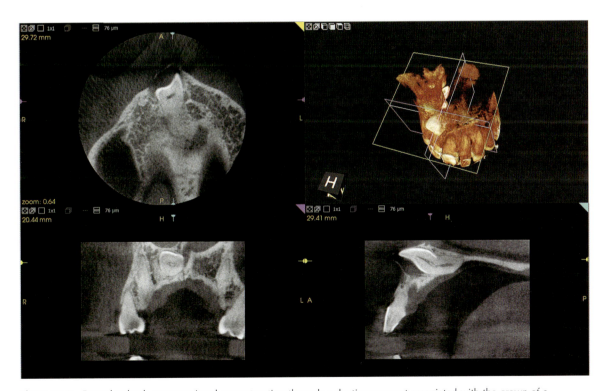

Figure 20.2   Buccal-palatal, cross-sectional reconstruction through a dentigerous cyst associated with the crown of a maxillary right permanent central incisor (lower right). Axial (upper left) and three-dimensional surface renderings of the volume (upper right) are shown, as is a coronal (lower left) image.

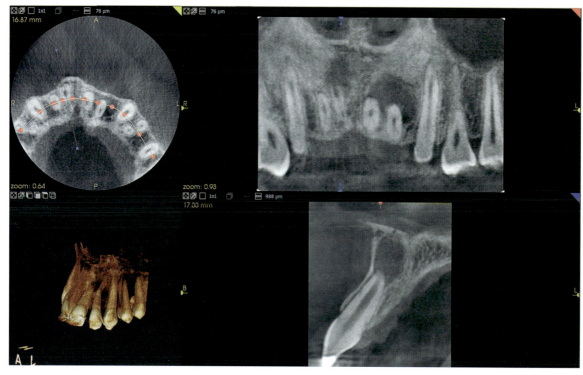

Figure 20.3 Buccal-palatal, cross-sectional reconstruction through an area of rarefying osteitis associated with the apex of a maxillary left permanent lateral incisor (lower right). Axial (upper left) and three-dimensional surface renderings of the volume (lower left) are shown, as is a panoramic reconstruction (upper right).

Should an abnormality be identified in one plane, it can be colocalized in either of the other two planes by noting the positions of bony anatomical landmarks, adjacent teeth, or a combination of the two. As well, oblique 2D reconstructions of the data set can also be made (e.g., buccal-lingual/palatal cross sections, tangential to the body of the mandible), and these may offer additional information to the clinician (Figure 20.3).

And finally, 3D renderings of the area of interest can be made to highlight either the teeth or the bone, and these can be manipulated in 3D virtual space so that the clinician can view spatial relationships of different structures within the image volume. Understanding how an image volume can be manipulated and viewed may have significant bearing on how an abnormality is visualized. This, in turn, may ultimately affect image interpretation and patient diagnosis.

References

Ludlow, J.B. and Ivanovic, M. (2008) Comparative dosimetry of dental CBCT devices and 64-slice CT for oral and maxillofacial radiology. *Oral Surg Oral Med Oral Pathol Oral Radiol Endod*, 106, 106–114.

Mozzo, P., Procacci, C., Tacconi, A., Martini, P.T., and Andreis, I.A. (1998) A new volumetric CT machine for dental imaging based on the cone-beam technique: preliminary results. *Eur Radiol*, 8, 1558–1564.

Nurbakhsh, B., Friedman, S., Kulkarni, G.V., Basrani, B., and Lam, E. (2011) Resolution of maxillary sinus mucositis after endodontic treatment of maxillary teeth with apical periodontitis: a cone-beam computed tomography pilot study. *J Endod*, 37, 1504–1511.

Wang, P., Yan, X.B., Lui, D.G., Zhang, W.L., Zhang, Y., and Ma, X.C. (2011) Detection of dental root fractures by using cone-beam computed tomography. *Dentomaxillofac Radiol*, 40, 290–298.

21 Interpretation of Periapical Lesions Using Cone Beam Computed Tomography

Carlos Estrela, Mike Reis Bueno, and Ana Helena Gonçalves Alencar

Introduction

Diagnostic accuracy is essential for endodontic treatment success, and the correct management of information obtained from the patient's history, clinical examinations, and complementary test results poses a great challenge (Kerr et al., 1978).

Radiolucent images in the mandibular or maxillary area surrounding the root apices might be a sign of endodontic disease or nonendodontic disease, and might lead to a misdiagnosis of apical periodontitis, particularly when the radiolucency is associated with an endodontically treated tooth. Thus, a diagnosis involves the establishment of a differential diagnosis (Wood and Goaz, 1991), which should distinguish periapical diseases which have been misdiagnosed as apical periodontitis (Bueno et al., 2008; Estrela et al., 2009c; Faitaroni et al., 2008; Rodrigues and Estrela, 2008).

The periapical inflammation represents a biological answer of natural defense, caused by several etiologic agents (microbial, chemical, physical, and others). The model of the inflammatory response is similar to other parts of the organism.

Several studies have discussed factors related to the etiology of posttreatment disease in endodontics: microbial etiologic factors (intraradicular and extraradicular infection—bacteria, fungi) and nonmicrobial etiologic factors (endogenous—true cysts; exogenous—foreign-body reaction) (Nair, 2004, 2006, 2009; Nair et al., 1996, 1999).

Apical periodontitis often appears as a response to endodontic infection, which may lead to inflammatory and immunologic changes of periapical tissues seen on radiographs as bone radiolucencies (Nair, 2004).

The analysis of types and incidence of human periapical lesions in 256 extracted teeth revealed that 35% were periapical abscess, 50%, granulomas, and 15% cysts (9% apical true cysts, 6% apical pocket cysts) (Nair et al., 1996). Radiographic features of the cysts may be similar, with some exceptions (Yoshiura et al., 2003). The location, shape, peripheral sclerosis, expansion, and contents of the lesion are important radiographic features that may help to determine an initial diagnostic hypothesis (Weber, 1993).

The acceptance of endodontic therapeutic protocol to treat a disease has usually been based

Endodontic Radiology, Second Edition. Edited by Bettina Basrani.
© 2012 John Wiley & Sons, Inc. Published 2012 by John Wiley & Sons, Inc.

on pathological and clinical characteristics aided frequently by radiographic exam (Nair, 2004). The periapical reaction is observed by the apical extension of the pulpal aggressor agents. After pulpal necrosis, the environment of the pulpal cavity becomes propitious and ideal to the factors that influence microbial growth and colonization (nutrients, low tension of oxygen, carbonic gas, and the existent interactions). These factors are connected to aggressions and responses, and are related to the microbial pathogenicity and virulence.

The presence and distribution of the microorganisms in infected root canals and their influence as expressive precursors of the inflammatory reactions of the dental pulp and periapical tissues established an important association of cause and effect, better defining some parameters of responses to different aggressor agents (Nair, 2004, 2009; Nair et al., 1996, 1999). The dynamic existent between microorganism, virulence, and organic response led to further research that resulted in more comprehensible and convincing explanations and definitions about the intimate relation between microbiology and pathology. The microorganisms represent an important role in the establishment of the periapical lesion (Estrela and Bueno, 2009).

The inflammatory diseases of the periapical region are influenced by the pathogenic characteristics, by the number of aggressor microorganisms (gifted with the respective virulence armory) that invade this area, associated with the dynamic of responses of the host. This interaction between microorganisms and host's responses determines the different types of periapical alterations.

Considering that the diagnostic hypothesis of periapical alterations have been made on the basis of the clinical evidences and the difficulties of correlation with possible histopathological events, the classification adopted was based on the clinical context and structured according to the treatment (Estrela and Bueno, 2009) (Figure 21.1). Periapical bone radiolucencies might be a sign of endodontic or nonendodontic lesion. In this chapter, several aspects related with periapical radiolucencies from endodontic origin based on cone beam computed tomography (CBCT) technology will be analyzed.

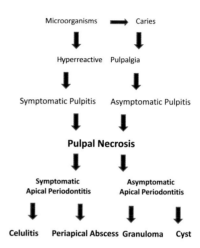

Figure 21.1   Sequence of pulpal and periapical pathological events.

Apical periodontitis detected using CBCT images

The diagnosis of apical periodontitis represents an essential strategy to determine the selection of an effective therapeutic protocol for endodontic infection control. Apical periodontitis is a consequence of root canal system infection, which can involve progressive stages of inflammation and changes of periapical bone structure, resulting in resorption identified as radiolucencies in radiographs (Nair et al., 1993). Some studies have shown that a periapical lesion from endodontic infection might be present without being radiographically visible (Bender, 1982; Bender and Seltzer, 1961a, 1961b).

The radiographic image corresponds to a two-dimensional (2D) aspect of a three-dimensional (3D) structure (Bender, 1982; Bender and Seltzer, 1961a, 1961b; Van der Stelt, 1985; White et al., 1995). Artificial lesions produced in cadavers can be detected by conventional radiography only if perforation, extensive destruction of the bone cortex on the outer surface, or erosion of the cortical bone from the inner surface is present. Lesions confined within the cancellous bone cannot be detected, whereas lesions with buccal and lingual cortical involvement produce distinct radiographic areas of rarefaction. To be visible radiographically, a periapical radiolucency should reach nearly 30–50% of bone mineral loss (Bender, 1982). Other conditions, such as apical morphologic variations, surrounding bone density, X-ray angulations, and radiographic contrast, also influence radiographic interpretation (Halse et al., 2002). An experimentally induced lesion might or might not be detected, depending on its location. A periapical lesion of a certain size can be detected in a region covered by a thin cortex, whereas the same size lesion will not be seen in a region covered by a thicker cortex. Lesion location in different types of bone influences the radiographic visualization (Huumonen and Ørstavik, 2002). Studies with different diagnostic methods have evaluated the type and incidence of periapical lesions (Laux et al., 2000; Nair et al., 1996). Scientific consensus has been reached to the fact that apical periodontitis is accurately identified by histologic analysis (Laux et al., 2000).

It is important to be aware of the limitations of radiographic assessment as a study method. One of these limitations involves the evaluation of the quality of root canal filling and coronal restoration based on a 2D image of 3D structures. The radiographic appearance of the filled root canal space has been considered a method to evaluate its quality of sealing. Radiographic images have been used to indicate the presence of periapical infection or coronal leakage, consisting of a diagnostic resource often used in dental practice.

Pathological and clinical findings, often supported by radiographs, provide the basis for endodontic therapy. Images, however, are necessary in all phases of endodontic treatment (Estrela and Bueno, 2009). Since the discovery of X-rays by Roentgen in 1895, radiology has witnessed the constant development of new technologies. The angle variations proposed by Clark and the development of panoramic radiography produced novel applications in endodontics.

Several advanced radiographic techniques for the detection of bone lesions have been used in dentistry, namely, digital radiography, densitometry methods, CBCT, magnetic resonance imaging, ultrasound, and nuclear techniques (Arai et al., 1999; Cotti, 2010; Cotton et al., 2007; Estrela et al., 2008b; Gao et al., 2009; Hounsfield, 1973; Huumonen and Ørstavik, 2002; Lofthag-Hansen et al., 2007; Mozzo et al., 1998; Nair and Nair, 2007; Nakata et al., 2006; Nielsen et al., 1995; Patel et al.,

2007; Velvart et al., 2001). With the advent of computed tomography (CT) (Hounsfield, 1973) and more recently CBCT (Arai et al., 1999; Mozzo et al., 1998), new parameters to evaluate the diagnosis and prognosis of a pathological condition might be included in endodontic practice. CBCT introduced 3D imaging into dentistry (Arai et al., 1999; Mozzo et al., 1998) and brought benefits to specialties that had not yet enjoyed the advantages of medical CT due to its lack of specificity. CT is an important, nondestructive, and noninvasive diagnostic imaging tool (Arai et al., 1999; Cotti, 2010; Cotton et al., 2007; Estrela et al., 2008b; Gao et al., 2009; Hounsfield, 1973; Lofthag-Hansen et al., 2007; Mozzo et al., 1998; Nair and Nair, 2007; Nakata et al., 2006; Nielsen et al., 1995; Patel et al., 2007; Velvart et al., 2001). CBCT has been successfully used in endodontics with different goals, including study of root canal anatomy, external and internal macromorphology in 3D reconstruction of the teeth, evaluation of root canal preparation, obturation, retreatment, coronal microleakage, detection of bone lesions, root resorptions, and experimental endodontology (Arai et al., 1999; Cotti, 2010; Cotton et al., 2007; Estrela et al., 2008b; Gao et al., 2009; Hounsfield, 1973; Huumonen and Ørstavik, 2002; Lofthag-Hansen et al., 2007; Mozzo et al., 1998; Nair and Nair, 2007; Nakata et al., 2006; Nielsen et al., 1995; Patel et al., 2007; Velvart et al., 2001).

Differences in apical periodontitis image interpretation by using CBCT, conventional periapical radiography, or digital radiography were recently studied (Estrela et al., 2008b). CBCT has provided promising results with a more accurate detection of apical periodontitis (Cotti, 2010; Cotton et al., 2007; Estrela et al., 2008b; Gao et al., 2009; Lofthag-Hansen et al., 2007; Nakata et al., 2006; Patel et al., 2007; Velvart et al., 2001).

The therapeutic protocol to treat diseases of endodontic origin has routinely been based on the evaluation of pathologic and clinical characteristics frequently complemented by radiographic findings. Radiographic imaging is the most commonly used diagnostic resource in endodontic diagnosis and treatment, and image distortions constitute a serious inconvenience.

The knowledge of prevalence and severity of apical periodontitis is often based on periapical

Table 21.1   Prevalence of apical periododntitis in endodontically treated and untreated teeth, identified by panoramic, periapical and CBCT images.

	Panoramic	Periapical	CBCT	P-value*
Treated teeth ($n = 1425$)				
Presence of AP	251 (17.6%)	503 (35.3%)	902 (63.3%)	$P < 0.001$
Absence of AP	1174 (82.4%)	922 (64.7%)	523 (36.7%)	
Nontreated teeth ($n = 83$)				
Presence of AP	18 (21.7%)	30 (36.1%)	62 (74.7%)	$P < 0.001$
Absence of AP	65 (78.3%)	53 (63.9%)	21 (25.3%)	

* Chi-square test.
Source: Estrela et al., *J Endod* 2008b).

radiography, whose accuracy has been questionable. Therefore, considering the limitations of conventional radiography for detection of periapical bone lesions, and with advanced imaging methods, CBCT might add benefits to endodontics and offer a higher quality of diagnosis, treatment planning, and prognosis.

A recent study (Estrela et al., 2008b) looked at the accuracy of CBCT imaging, panoramic, and periapical radiographs on detection of apical periodontitis. A total of 1508 teeth were selected. The periapical index (PAI) by Ørstavik et al. (1986) was used to determine the periapical status by performing a visual analysis of all digital images. Based on the differences between imaging methods (using 2D and 3D), the number of roots with apical periodontitis viewed by periapical radiographs and CBCT scans, it was considered the root associated with the largest lesion extension. The prevalence of apical periodontitis identified by periapical and panoramic radiographs and dental CBCT is shown in Table 21.1. The findings of this investigation demonstrated that the CBCT images have a high accuracy in the detection of apical periodontitis. CBCT images tend to offer greater scores than periapical and panoramic radiographs, suggesting that diagnosis of the graduation of apical periodontitis with conventional images is frequently underestimated. Apical periodontitis was correctly identified in 54.5% of the cases with periapical radiographs (sensitivity, 0.55) and in 27.8% with panoramic radiographs (sensitivity, 0.28). Accuracy of periapical radiographs was significantly higher than that of panoramic radiographs. Apical periodontitis was correctly identified with conventional methods when a severe condition was present.

The likelihood that apical periodontitis exists and is not identified by periapical or panoramic radiographs is considerably high (Figure 21.2). The difficulty to accurately detect apical periodontitis has been mentioned elsewhere (Bender, 1982; Huumonen and Ørstavik, 2002; Ørstavik et al., 1986). One important aspect to be considered is that it is necessary to have approximately 30–50% of mineral loss in order to visualize apical periodontitis (Bender, 1982; Bender and Seltzer, 1961a, 1961b). Morphological variations of the apical region, bone density, X-ray angulations, radiographic contrast, and actual location of the periapical lesion will influence the radiographic interpretation (Halse and Molven, 1986; Halse et al., 2002; Molven et al., 2002).

The limitations of radiographic assessment as a study method should not be overlooked, as they to reduce false-negative results. In view of the limitations of periapical radiography to visualize apical periodontitis, *a review of epidemiologic studies should be undertaken considering the quality of periapical aspects offered by CBCT images.* In addition, it will certainly reduce the influence on radiographic interpretation, with minor possibility of false-negative diagnosis. Apical periodontitis prevalence in endodontically treated teeth, when comparing the panoramic and periapical radiographs and CBCT images, was 17.6%, 35.3%, and 63.3%, respectively, in the study reported (Estrela et al., 2008b). A considerable discrepancy can be observed among the imaging methods used to identify apical periodontitis.

The truth is that most dentists do not have CBCT equipment in their dental offices. Thus, during endodontic treatment, it is important to choose a radiographic technique that minimizes image

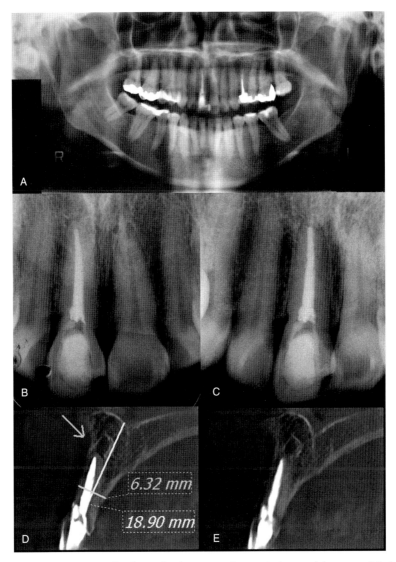

Figure 21.2   (a–e) Panoramic and periapical radiographs show normal periapical area of the upper right incisor. Apical periododntitis can be seen in the CBCT. (Estrela et al., *J Endod* 2008b).

distortions, such as the cone parallel technique, to obtain a high level of reproducibility and increase the diagnostic accuracy of the imaging method.

The use of conventional radiographic images for detection of apical periodontitis should be done with care because of the high possibility of a false-negative diagnosis. A great advantage of using CBCT in endodontics refers to its usefulness in aiding in the identification of periapical lesions and in a differential diagnosis using a noninvasive technique with high accuracy.

Recently, studies (Liang et al., 2011; Paula-Silva et al., 2009; Wu et al., 2009, 2011) discussed that traditional periapical radiographs are used to assess the outcome of root canal treatment with the absence of a periapical radiolucency being considered a confirmation of a healthy periapex. Based on new modalities of imaging diagnosis, the limitations of previously published systematic reviews evaluating the outcome of root canal treatment have been questioned. Wu et al. (2009) suggested that systematic reviews reporting the success rates of root canal treatment without referring to these limitations may mislead readers. The outcomes of root canal treatment should be reevaluated in long-term longitudinal studies using CBCT and stricter evaluation criteria.

Periapical index based on CBCT

It is natural that a new device with advanced potential to aid in diagnosis such as CBCT brings with it some challenges until we gain a better understanding of its properties and limitations. Developing new software could be valuable in the acquisition and reconstruction of CBCT scans.

Considering the great technological advances of recent years, CBCT has been used for several clinical and investigational purposes in endodontics (Arai et al., 1999; Cotti, 2010; Cotton et al., 2007; Estrela et al., 2008b; Gao et al., 2009; Lofthag-Hansen et al., 2007; Mozzo et al., 1998; Nair and Nair, 2007; Nakata et al., 2006; Nielsen et al., 1995; Patel et al., 2007; Velvart et al., 2001).

Previous studies (Brynolf, 1967; Ørstavik et al., 1986; Reit and Grøndahl, 1983) have referred to the periapical index (PAI) as a scoring system for radiographic assessment of apical periodontitis. The PAI represents an ordinal scale of five scores ranging from no disease to severe periodontitis with exacerbating features, and is based on reference radiographs with confirmed histological diagnosis as originally published by Brynolf (1967). Ørstavik et al. (1986) applied the PAI to both clinical trials and epidemiological surveys, and it may be transformed into success and failure criteria by defining cutoff points on the scale for a dichotomous outcome assessment (Huumonen and Ørstavik, 2002).

Therefore, with the possibility of detection of apical periodontitis by using new emerging 3D imaging modalities, the development of a new periapical index (Estrela et al., 2008a) was suggested when using CBCT technology.

Thus, a new periapical index (Estrela et al., 2008a) was recently proposed based on CBCT for identification of apical periodontitis. The CBCT periapical index (CBCTPAI) was developed based

Table 21.2 Cone beam computed tomography periapical index (CBCTPAI) scores.

Score	Quantitative bone alterations in mineral structures
0	Intact periapical bone structures
1	Diameter of periapical bone structure loss >0.5–1 mm
2	Diameter of periapical bone structure loss >1–2 mm
3	Diameter of periapical bone structure loss >2–4 mm
4	Diameter of periapical bone structure loss >4–8 mm
5	Diameter of periapical bone structure loss >8 mm
Score (n) + E*	Expansion of periapical cortical bone
Score (n) + D*	Destruction of periapical cortical bone

* Chi-square test.
Source: Estrela et al., J Endod 2008a

on criteria established from measurements corresponding to periapical radiolucency interpreted on CBCT scans. Radiolucent images suggestive of periapical lesions were measured using the working tools of Planimp® software on CBCT scans in three dimensions: buccopalatal, mesiodistal, and diagonal. The CBCTPAI was determined by the largest lesion extension. A 6-point (0–5) scoring system was used with two additional variables: expansion of cortical bone and destruction of cortical bone (Table 21.2, Figures 21.3–21.5). A total of 1014 images (periapical radiographs and CBCT scans) originally taken from 596 patients were evaluated using the CBCTPAI criteria (Table 21.2). Apical periodontitis was identified in 39.5% and 60.9% of cases by radiography and CBCT scans, respectively.

The CBCTPAI offers an accurate diagnostic method for use with high-resolution images, which can reduce the incidence of false-negative diagnosis, minimize observer interference, and increase the reliability of epidemiological studies, especially those referring to apical periodontitis prevalence and severity.

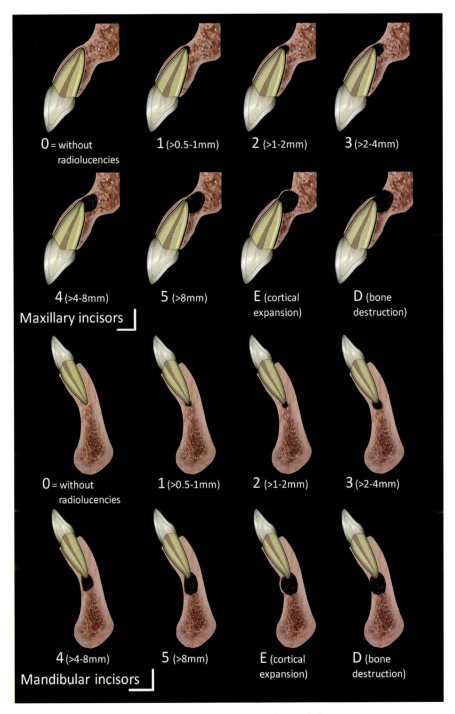

Figure 21.3 Schematic representations of incisors CBCTPAI. (Estrela et al., *J Endod* 2008a).

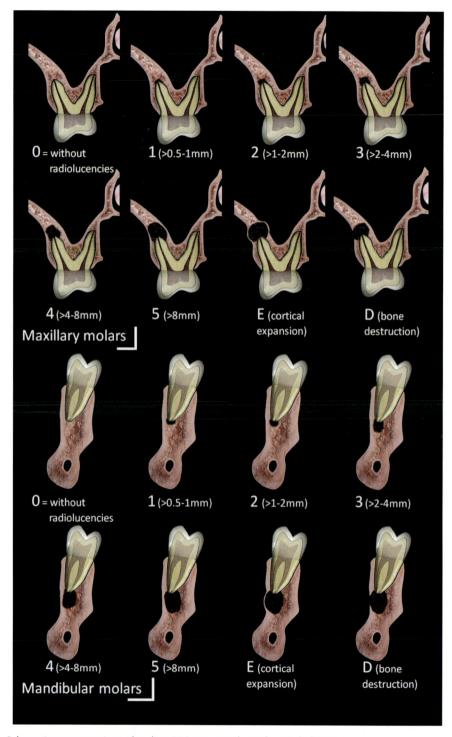

Figure 21.4   Schematic representations of molars CBCTPA. (Estrela et al., *J Endod* 2008a).

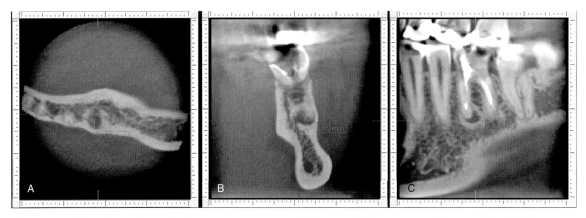

Figure 21.5   Clinical case of mandibular molar showing the axial (A), sagital (B), and coronal (C) planes. The CBCTPAI was determined by the largest extension of the lesion. (Estrela et al., *J Endod* 2008a).

The accuracy of CBCT scans compared to periapical radiographic images are in accordance with the findings of previous studies (Cotti, 2010; Cotton et al., 2007; Estrela et al., 2008b; Gao et al., 2009; Liang et al., 2011; Lofthag-Hansen et al., 2007; Nair and Nair, 2007; Nakata et al., 2006; Nielsen et al., 1995; Patel et al., 2007; Paula-Silva et al., 2009; Scarfe et al., 2007; Simon et al., 2006; Trope et al., 1989; Velvart et al., 2001; Wu et al., 2009, 2011). Lofthag-Hansen et al. (2007) compared intraoral periapical radiography and a 3D imaging system (3D Accuitomo) for the diagnosis of apical pathology in 36 patients (46 teeth). When both diagnostic methods were analyzed by all observers, they agreed that the CBCT images provided clinically relevant additional information not found with periapical radiography. The capacity of computer tomography to evaluate a region of interest in three dimensions might benefit both novice and experienced clinicians alike. The advantages include increased accuracy and higher resolution. In addition, it has been reported that CT scans can determine the difference in density between the cystic cavity content and the granulomatous tissue, favoring the choice for a noninvasive diagnosis method (Simon et al., 2006; Trope et al., 1989). Simon et al. (2006) compared the differential diagnosis of large periapical lesions (granuloma versus cyst) to traditional biopsy using CBCT. These results suggest that CBCT may provide a faster method to differentially diagnose a solid- from a fluid-filled lesion or cavity, without invasive surgery and/or waiting a long time to see if nonsurgical therapy is effective.

The use of conventional radiography for detection of apical periodontitis should be done with care because of the great possibility of false-negative diagnosis. The benefits of using CBCT in endodontics refer to its high accuracy in detecting periapical lesions even in its earliest stages and aiding in differential diagnosis as a noninvasive technique (Estrela et al., 2008a, 2008b).

The CBCTPAI proposed has some advantages for clinical applications. CBCTPAI scores are calculated by analysis of the lesion in three dimensions, with CT slices being obtained in mesiodistal, buccopalatal, and diagonal directions. The measurement of lesion depth contributes significantly to the diagnosis and consequently, to improve case prognosis.

The addition of the variables *expansion and destruction of cortical bone* to CBCTPAI scoring system permits the analysis of two possible sequels to apical periodontitis that may be missed by periapical radiography. Detection of these conditions will alter the diagnostic hypothesis and the treatment plan. The goal of this new index is therefore to offer a method based on the interpretation of high-resolution images that can provide a more precise measurement of apical periodontitis extension, minimizing observer interference and increasing the reliability of research results.

The limitations of periapical radiography to identify apical periodontitis support the need to review the epidemiological studies conducted in different populations worldwide. A considerable discrepancy among the imaging methods used to diagnose apical periodontitis, especially with a new baseline value, certainly may reduce the influence of radiographic interpretation and the possibility of false-negative diagnosis.

The CBCTPAI (Estrela et al., 2008a) offers an accurate diagnostic method for use with high-resolution images, which can reduce the incidence of false-negative diagnosis, minimize observer interference, and increase the reliability of epidemiological studies, especially those referring to apical periodontitis prevalence and severity.

Biotechnology has brought important changes to today's thinking, and the contemporary world has witnessed the benefits brought by computer-based sciences to several fields of knowledge and health sciences, including dental specialities.

Detection of inflammatory root resorption using CBCT

Root resorption is either a physiologic or pathologic condition associated with tooth structure loss caused by clastic cells. Permanent root resorption is invariably a local pathological condition caused by orthodontic treatment, traumatic dental injury, apical periodontitis, intracoronal bleaching, autotransplantation, dentigerous cyst, neoplasia, or idiopathic factors (Andreasen and Andreasen, 2001; Consolaro, 2005; Cortes and Bastos, 2009; Gunraj, 1999; Ne et al., 1999; Pierce, 1989; Trope et al., 2002). The external or internal superficial protective cell layer might be damaged, and inflammatory or replacement root resorption might affect any part of the root (Ne et al., 1999).

Several aspects of inflammatory root resorption, such as prevalence, etiologic factors, and classification based on dental surface, progression, extension, and pathologic mechanisms, have been extensively discussed (Andreasen and Andreasen, 2001; Andreasen et al., 1987; Consolaro, 2005; Cortes and Bastos, 2009; Eraso et al., 2007; Gunraj, 1999; Leach et al., 2001; Levander and Malmgren, 1988; Mattar, 2002; Mol et al., 2004; Ne et al., 1999; Pierce, 1989; Trope et al., 2002). However, inflammatory root resorption is an asymptomatic lesion that is difficult to diagnose and treat (Andreasen and Andreasen, 2001; Consolaro, 2005; Cortes and Bastos, 2009; Trope et al., 2002). The criterion standard for the diagnosis of inflammatory root resorption is microscopic analysis (Laux et al., 2000), and inflammatory root resorption might be classified as active, arrested, or repaired according to microscopic findings. The prevalence of each stage affects prognosis and treatment (Andreasen and Andreasen, 2001). Conventional radiographic images are frequently used to detect and follow up inflammatory root resorption (Andreasen and Andreasen, 2001; Andreasen et al., 1987; Consolaro, 2005; Cortes and Bastos, 2009; Gunraj, 1999; Ne et al., 1999; Pierce, 1989; Trope et al., 2002).

A root resorption index extensively used to determine the degree of apical root resorption during orthodontic treatment was described by Levander and Malmgren (1988). This index evaluated the levels of loss of apical root structure and scored it from 1–4: (1) irregular outline of apical surface, (2) up to 2 mm reduction of root length, (3) root reduction of 2 mm to one-third of the root, and (4) root length reduction larger than one-third of the root. The root form, classified as normal, short, blunt, apically bent, or pipette-shaped, can affect the degree of root resorption.

Patel et al. (2009) reported that a diagnostic test for root resorption should be able to suitably identify the presence or absence of different types of root resorption (validity) and should be repeatable to generate the same results. The authors verified that CBCT showed superior diagnostic accuracy in a better possibility of correct management of root resorption.

A method to measure inflammatory root resorption (Estrela et al., 2009a) by using CBCT scans was recently suggested. Inflammatory root resorption sites were classified according to root third and root surface, and inflammatory root resorption extension was measured on the axial, transverse, and tangent views of 3D CBCT scans. The method to evaluate inflammatory root resorption by using CBCT is similar to the one that was described in a previous study (Estrela et al., 2008a) of periapical indices and CBCT scans. The study criteria were established according to the analysis of inflammatory root resorption sites: root thirds—apical, middle, and cervical; root

Table 21.3   Site and extension of inflammatory root resorption according to CBCT scores.

Thirds/Surfaces	Mesial (1)	Distal (2)	Buccal (3)	Palatal (4)	Root apex (5)	Score—Extension of root resorption (RR)
Apical (1)	1	2	3	4	5	0: Intact structure
						1: >0.5–1 mm
						2: >1–3 mm
						3: >3–4 mm
						4: >4 mm
Middle (2)	1	2	3	4	5	0: Intact structure
						1: >0.5–1 mm
						2: >1–3 mm
						3: >3–4 mm
						4: >4 mm
Cervical (3)	1	2	3	4	5	0: Intact structure
						1: >0.5–1 mm
						2: >1–3 mm
						3: >3–4 mm
						4: >4 mm

Source: Estrela et al., *J Endod* 2009a.

Note: RR may affect more than one-third or one root surface. However, for each RR diagnosed, each measurement should be evaluated according to the largest RR extension. RR depth and direction are essential details in imaging tests, and axial, transverse, and tangent planes may provide better information. For teeth with more than one root, each root should be evaluated separately. IRR extension may be the same, but the number of thirds or surfaces may be different in oblique RR, apical RR, or apical and oblique RR.

surfaces—mesial, distal, buccal, palatal, or lingual and root apex; and inflammatory root resorption extension (Table 21.3). Inflammatory root resorption was outlined and measured with the Planimp software and three dimensions of CBCT scans: axial, transverse, and tangent (Figure 21.6). The greatest extension of root resorption was measured, and a 5-point (0–4) scoring system was used for analysis (Table 21.3 and Figures 21.6 and 21.7). A total of 48 periapical radiographs and CBCT scans originally taken from 40 patients were evaluated. Based on this method, inflammatory root resorption was detected in 68.8% (83 root surfaces) of the radiographs and 100% (154 root surfaces) of the CBCT scans. The extension of inflammatory root resorption was >1–4 mm in 95.8% of the CBCT images and in 52.1% of the images obtained by using the conventional method. CBCT seems to be useful in the evaluation of inflammatory root resorption, and its diagnostic performance was better than that of periapical radiography.

Map-reading strategy to diagnose endodontic lesions associated with root perforations

In spite of the dental imaging technique, care should be taken to avoid misinterpretation. The presence of intracanal metallic posts (ICPs), for example, may lead to equivocated interpretations due to artifact formation in CBCT images. Metallic objects can be present in either the tooth of interest or an adjacent one, and hinder the analysis of CBCT images (Lofthag-Hansen et al., 2007), though in current days, the influence of this artifact has been reduced. The map-reading by dental structure images may favor their evaluations.

However, dimensions misdiagnosed may result from imaging artifacts. Metal or solid structures (higher density materials) may produce nonhomogeneous artifacts and affect image contrast.

Concerns about diagnostic errors have motivated authors to study alternatives to correct beam hardening artifacts during image acquisition,

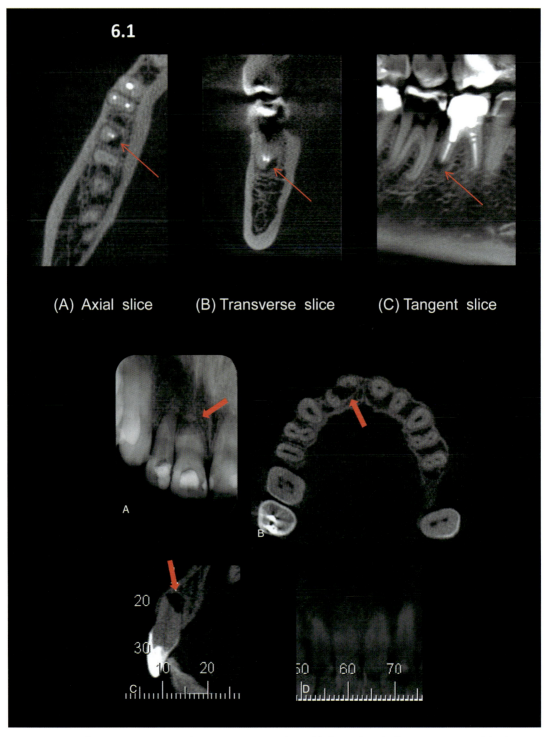

Figure 21.6 (1) Axial (A), transverse (B), and tangent (C) views of mandibular molar. The largest extension of the lesion was used for the inflammatory root resorption —CBCT method. (2) Clinical case of inflammatory root resorption of maxillary central incisor identified by radiography (A) and CBCT in axial (B), transverse (C), and tangent (D) views. (Estrela et al., *J Endod* 2009a).

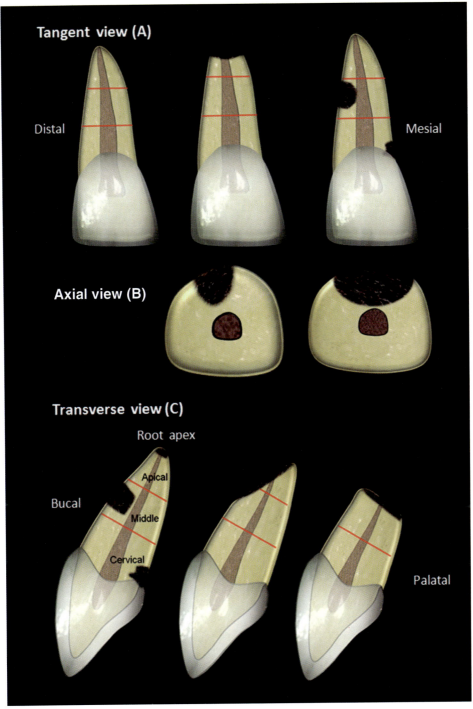

Figure 21.7 Schematic representation of IRR-CBCT method of maxillary incisor showing the tangent (A), axial (B), and transverse (C) views and the different surfaces with inflammatory root resorption. (Estrela et al., *J Endod* 2009a).

image reconstruction, or under other conditions (Arai et al., 1999; Estrela et al., 2009b; Haristoy et al., 2008; Herman, 1980; Hunter and McDavid, 2009; Huybrechts et al., 2009; Jian and Hongnian, 2006; Joseph and Spital, 1978; Katsumata et al., 2006, 2007, 2009; Ketcham and Carlson, 2001; Meganck et al., 2009; Mischkowski et al., 2007; Mozzo et al., 1998; Naumann et al., 2008).

Katsumata et al. (2006, 2007) reported that artifacts caused by halation or saturation from an imaging sensor decrease CT values on the buccal side of the jaws. In dental CBCT imaging, artifacts may change CT values of the soft tissues adjacent to the lingual and buccal sides of the jaws. The CT values of hard tissue structures may also be similarly affected.

CBCT images showing teeth with solid plastic or metal intracanal post (ICP) may project ghost images over the areas surrounding it and mask the actual root canal structures, which increases the risk of clinical misdiagnosis.

Root canal obturation is a major step in the last phase of endodontic treatment, which is completed with coronal restoration. However, endodontically treated teeth often have a substantial loss of dental structure and need an intracanal post (Estrela et al., 2009b).

Several types of intracanal posts have been recommended for dental reconstructions according to the analysis of important restoratives aspects: the possibility of endodontic post failure, which may result in loss of retention; the risk of root canal reinfection due to bacterial microleakage; the effect of intracanal post length on apical periodontitis; the retentive effect of adhesive systems for the different types of posts; the possibility of stress concentration; and the difference in modulus of elasticity between post and dentin (Demarchi and Sato, 2002; Naumann et al., 2008).

The effect caused by intracanal posts (glass-fiber post, carbon fiber root canal, prefabricated post—metal screws, silver alloy post, and gold alloy post) on the dimensions of CBCT images of endodontically treated teeth was recently evaluated (Estrela et al., 2011). The increase of intracanal posts dimensions in CBCT images ranged from 7.7% to 100%. Differences were significant between glass fiber post, carbon fiber post, and metal posts. Gold alloy and silver alloy posts had greater variations than glass fiber, carbon fiber, and metal posts. Gold alloy

and silver alloy post dimensions were greater on CBCT scans than on original specimens.

Thus, to determine the diagnostic hypothesis on the basis of periapical radiography is a great challenge for radiologists and endodontists. Visualization of 3D structures, available with CBCT, favors precise definition of the problem and treatment planning.

Performing exaggerated wear during preparation of intracanal post space is a common situation leading to perforation, which in some clinical situations requires special care to establish the hypothesis of diagnosis and therapeutic option.

However, diagnostic errors constitute a serious problem frequently detected in the presence of metallic or solid structure (with higher density), which produce image artifact, absence of homogeneity and definition on image contrasts. The problem with misdiagnosis encourages the search for alternatives to reduce the beam hardening effect during image acquisition and reconstruction or in other circumstances (Azevedo et al., 2008; Barrett and Keat, 2004; Duerinckx and Macovski, 1978; Haristoy et al., 2008; Herman, 1980; Hunter and McDavid, 2009; Huybrechts et al., 2009; Jian and Hongnian, 2006; Joseph and Spital, 1978; Katsumata et al., 2006, 2007, 2009; Ketcham and Carlson, 2001; Noujeim et al., 2009; Rao and Alfidi, 1981). Metallic artifacts associated with intracanal posts are potential risks of misdiagnosis, particularly when suggesting root perforation or destruction, and might also induce untrue images.

Bueno et al. (2011) suggested a map-reading strategy to diagnose root perforations near metallic intracanal posts by using CBCT. The incapacity to locate correctly the position of root perforation might lead to clinical failures. One strategy to minimize metallic artifact in root perforation associated with intracanal posts is to obtain sequential axial slices of each root, with an image navigation protocol from coronal to apical (or from apical to coronal), with axial slices of 0.2 mm/0.2 mm. This map-reading provides valuable information showing dynamic visualization toward the point of communication between the root canals and the periodontal space, associated with radiolucent areas, suggesting root perforation (Figure 21.8) (Bueno et al., 2011).

The accurate management of CBCT images might reveal abnormality that is unable to be

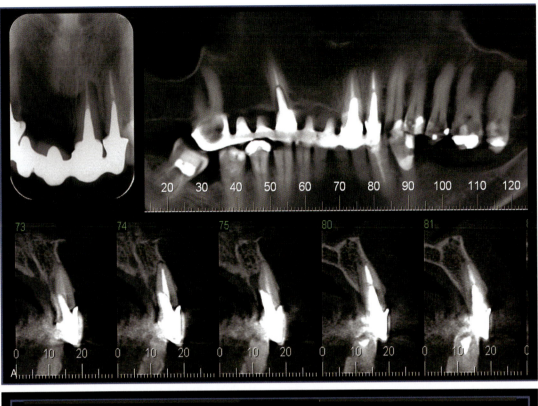

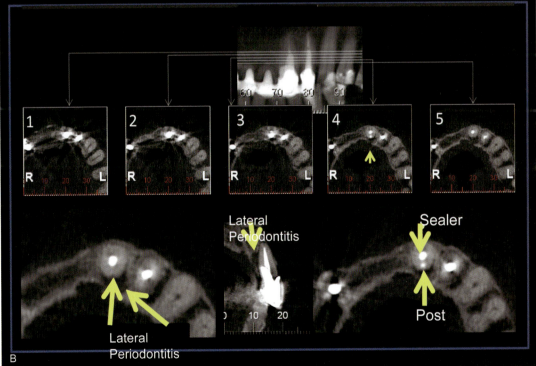

Figure 21.8 (A) Radiographic imaging of tooth #9 presented root canal filling until root apex, associated with ICP and absence of apical or lateral radiolucency. CBCT view shows in sagittal plane the ICP in palatal direction, presence of lateral radiolucency, associated with destruction of palatal wall. (B) (Tooth #9). Navigation in axial slices of 0.2 mm/0.2 mm involving the coronal to apical direction (and also in apical to coronal direction) provided important information regarding better visualization and localization, suggesting diagnosis of root perforation associated with lateral radiolucency.

detected in conventional periapical radiographs. The development of new software able to reduce metallic artifact in future reconstructions of CBCT images is necessary. The final diagnosis and choice of clinical therapeutics for these root perforations should always be made in conjunction with the clinical findings.

Apical periodontitis, dental granulomas, radicular cysts: Imaging methods and microscopic findings

Periapical radiographs provide important information about the development, reduction, and persistence of apical periodontitis (Bhaskar, 1966; Nair et al., 1996, 1999) as well as indispensable data to make decisions about treatment. Apical periodontitis often results from endodontic infection, which may lead to inflammatory and immunologic changes of periapical tissues seen on radiographs as bone radiolucencies (Nair et al., 1999).

The association of lesions with adjacent teeth may differentiate odontogenic from nonodontogenic lesions. Endodontic diagnosis is challenging and depends on the management of information obtained from the patient's history, clinical examination, previous conditions of pulp tissue, and analysis of radiographic findings.

Primary and secondary endodontic infections are commonly associated with clinically detected apical periodontitis or with periapical cysts or dental granulomas confirmed using histopathology (Bhaskar, 1966; Bueno and Estrela, 2009; Bueno et al., 2011; Nair et al., 1996, 1999; Torabinejad et al., 1985). The accurate diagnosis of apical periodontitis is an indispensable step in the decision about treatment for endodontic infections, and the definition of the probable cause of periapical disease should be part of the diagnostic process.

The definition of a diagnosis involves the establishment of a differential diagnosis, which should distinguish diseases of nonendodontic and endodontic origins. Radiolucent images in the mandibular or maxillary area surrounding the root apices might be a sign of nonendodontic disease and might lead to a misdiagnosis of apical periodontitis. This aspect may be associated with a vital pulp tooth or an endodontically treated tooth. Several pathoses may be misdiagnosed as apical periodontitis (Aggarwal et al., 2008; Bhaskar, 1966;

Bueno and Estrela, 2009; Harris and Brown, 1997; Neville et al., 2002; Regezi and Sciubba, 1999; Rosenberg et al., 2010; Sapp et al., 2004; Shear and Speight, 2007; Shrout et al., 1993; Stafne and Gibilisco, 1975; Zapata et al., 2011).

For example, unnecessary root canal treatment or retreatment may be prescribed because of the difficulty in defining diagnostic hypotheses when periapical radiographs show the superimposition of the incisor foramen over the apex of central incisors, which may mimic apical periodontitis, or when a nasopalatine duct cyst is directly or indirectly associated with endodontically treated central incisors (Figure 21.9) (Faitaroni et al., 2011). When the pulp is vital, a vitality test may be used to differentiate AP from nasopalatine duct cyst (Figure 21.10) (Faitaroni et al., 2011). However, when an area of periapical radiolucency is found in endodontically treated maxillary central incisors, nasopalatine duct cyst should be included in the differential diagnosis to avoid unnecessary endodontic retreatment (Figure 21.11) (Faitaroni et al., 2011). In these two clinical conditions, sagittal CBCT views show anatomical details of the lesion, which may help to establish a diagnostic hypothesis and to plan treatment. The use of cross-sectional imaging in the differential diagnosis of apical radiolucencies can reduce diagnostic uncertainty in the cases for which the analysis of radiolucency in the region of the apex of the upper first incisor fails to show typical radiologic features of apical pathology.

Cross-sectional images provide 3D information about the site of a cystic lesion of the anterior maxilla, and its association with adjacent anatomic structures helps to make a differential diagnosis and shows the best surgical access to the lesion (Harris and Brown, 1997). Rosenberg et al. (2010) studied the differentiation of radicular cysts from granulomas. CBCT images were compared with the existing standards, biopsy, and histopathology. Their results showed that surgical biopsy and histopathological examination remain the standard criteria to differentiate radicular cysts from granulomas.

The use of new diagnostic tools, such as CBCT imaging, may provide detailed high-resolution images of oral structures and help to make the initial diagnostic hypothesis and plan surgery. Histopathology remains mandatory for the diagnosis of periapical lesions. Thus, scientific consensus has

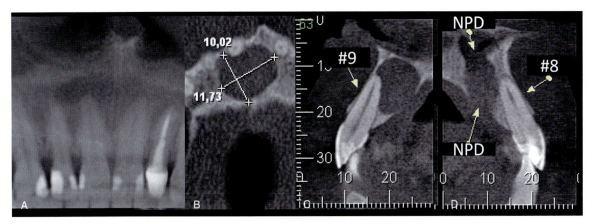

Figure 21.9   CBCT images of maxillary incisors (teeth #8-9) show well-circumscribed bone radiolucency in midline of anterior maxilla in anterior palatine foramen area. Clinical examination showed that anterior teeth were vital (pulp vitality test).

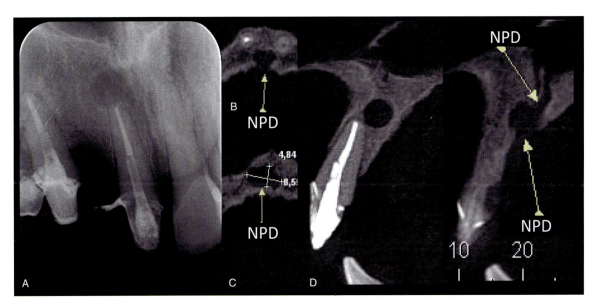

Figure 21.10   CBCT images of maxillary incisors (tooth #9) show well-circumscribed bone radiolucency in midline of anterior maxilla in anterior palatine foramen area. Clinical examination revealed asymptomatic, endodontically treated anterior teeth.

been reached to the fact that apical periodontitis is accurately identified by histological analysis.

Conclusions

Clinical and radiological criteria are often used to determine the status of endodontic treatment and

its correlation with apical periodontitis (Bueno and Estrela, 2009; Estrela et al., 2008b). Technological advances have added new imaging diagnostic tools to be used in dental radiology, such as CBCT (Arai et al., 1999; Cotti, 2010; Cotton et al., 2007; Estrela et al., 2008b; Gao et al., 2009; Hounsfield, 1973; Lofthag-Hansen et al., 2007; Mozzo et al., 1998; Nair and Nair, 2007; Nakata et al., 2006;

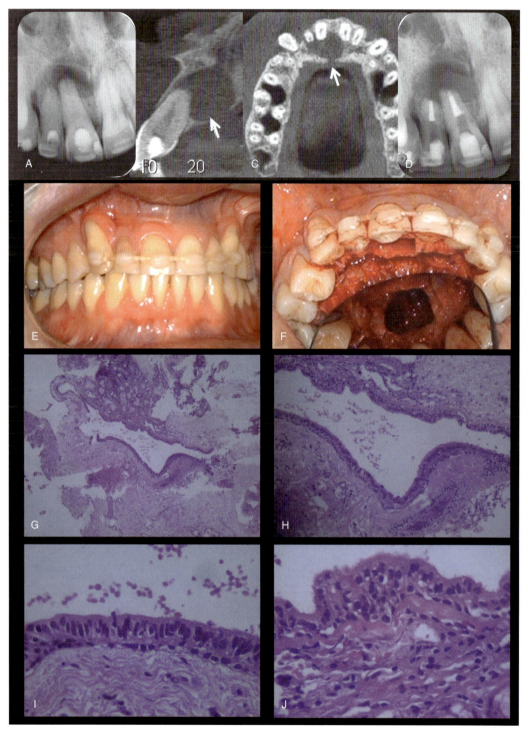

Figure 21.11 Nasopalatine duct cyst: histological sections show fragments of cystic capsule lined with stratified squamous epithelium in some areas and simple cuboidal epithelium in others. Cystic capsule, formed by dense connective tissue, shows interstitial hemorrhage and discrete mononuclear inflammatory infiltrate (hematoxylin and eosin; original magnification: G, X100; H, X200; I, X300; J, X400).

Nielsen et al., 1995; Patel et al., 2007; Velvart et al., 2001). They produce detailed high-resolution images of oral structures and detect bone lesions at an early stage. CBCT imaging should be considered in several clinical situations as a tool to make noninvasive diagnosis (Aggarwal et al., 2008; Cotti, 2010; Estrela et al., 2008b, 2009a).

Advanced imaging methods such as CBCT might add benefits to endodontics and offer a higher quality on diagnosis, treatment planning, and prognosis.

References

Aggarwal, V., Logani, A., and Shah, N. (2008) The evaluation of computed tomography scans and ultrasounds in the differential diagnosis of periapical lesions. *J Endod*, 34, 1312–1315.

Andreasen, F.M., Sewerin, I., Mandel, U., and Andreasen, J.O. (1987) Radiographic assessment of simulated root resorption cavities. *Endod Dent Traumatol*, 3, 21–27.

Andreasen, J.O. and Andreasen, F.M. (2001) *Essentials of Traumatic Injuries to the Teeth*, 2nd ed. Munksgaard, Copenhagen.

Arai, Y., Tammisalo, E., Iwai, K., Hashimoto, K., and Shinoda, K. (1999) Development of a compact computed tomographic apparatus for dental use. *Dentomaxillofac Radiol*, 28, 245–248.

Azevedo, B., Lee, R., Shintaku, W., Noujeim, M., and Nummikoski, P. (2008) Influence of the beam hardness on artifacts in cone-beam CT. *Oral Surg Oral Med Oral Pathol Oral Radiol Endod*, 105, e48.

Barrett, J.F. and Keat, N. (2004) Artifacts in CT: recognition and avoidance. *Radiographics*, 24, 1679–1691.

Bender, I.B. (1982) Factors influencing the radiographic appearance of bony lesions. *J Endod*, 8, 161–170.

Bender, I.B. and Seltzer, S. (1961a) Roentgenographic and direct observation of experimental lesions in bone I. *J Am Dent Assoc*, 62, 152–160.

Bender, I.B. and Seltzer, S. (1961b) Roentgenographic and direct observation of experimental lesions in bone II. *J Am Dent Assoc*, 62, 708–716.

Bhaskar, S.N. (1966) Periapical lesions—types, incidence, and clinical features. *Oral Surg Oral Med Oral Pathol*, 21, 657–671.

Brynolf, I. (1967) A histologic and roentgenologic study of the periapical region of human upper incisors. *Odontol Revy*, 18, 1–176.

Bueno, M.R. and Estrela, C. (2009) Cone beam computed tomography in endodontic diagnosis. In: C. Estrela, ed., *Endodontic Science*, 2nd ed., pp. 119–154. Artes Médicas, São Paulo.

Bueno, M.R., Carvalhosa, A.A.C., Castro, P.H.S., Pereira, K.C., Borges, F.T., and Estrela, C. (2008) Mesenchymal chondrosarcoma mimicking apical periodontitis. *J Endod*, 34, 1415–1419.

Bueno, M.R., Estrela, C., De Figueiredo, J.A., and Azevedo, B.C. (2011) Map-reading strategy to diagnose root perforations near metallic intracanal posts by using cone beam computed tomography. *J Endod*, 37, 85–90.

Consolaro, A. (2005) *Reabsorções dentárias nas especialidades clínicas*, 2nd ed. Dental Press, Maringá, Brazil.

Cortes, M.I.S. and Bastos, J.S. (2009) Biological and clinical aspects of traumatic injuries to the permanent teeth. In: C. Estrela, ed., *Endodontic Science*, 2nd ed., pp. 155–190. Artes Medicas, São Paulo.

Cotti, E. (2010) Advanced techniques for detecting lesions in bone. *Dent Clin North Am*, 54, 215–235.

Cotton, T.P., Geisler, T.M., Holden, D.T., Schwartz, S.A., and Schindler, W.G. (2007) Endodontic applications of cone beam volumetric tomography. *J Endod*, 33, 1121–1132.

Demarchi, M.G. and Sato, E.F. (2002) Leakage of interim post and cores used during laboratory fabrication of custom posts. *J Endod*, 28, 328–329.

Duerinckx, A.J. and Macovski, A. (1978) Polychromatic streak artifacts in computed tomography images. *J Comput Assist Tomogr*, 2, 481–487.

Eraso, F.E., Parks, E.T., Roberts, W.E., Hohlt, W.F., and Ofner, S. (2007) Density value means in the evaluation of external apical root resorption: an in vitro study for early detection in orthodontic case simulations. *Dentomaxillofac Radiol*, 36, 130–137.

Estrela, C. and Bueno, M.R. (2009) Epidemiology and therapy of apical periodontitis. In: C. Estrela, ed., *Endodontic Science*, 2nd ed., pp. 249–419. Artes Medicas, São Paulo.

Estrela, C., Bueno, M.R., Azevedo, B., Azevedo, J.R., and Pecora, J.D. (2008a) A new periapical index based on cone beam computed tomography. *J Endod*, 34, 1325–1331.

Estrela, C., Bueno, M.R., Leles, C.R., Azevedo, B., and Azevedo, J.R. (2008b) Accuracy of cone beam computed tomography and panoramic and periapical radiography for detection of apical periodontitis. *J Endod*, 34, 273–279.

Estrela, C., Bueno, M.R., Alencar, A.H., Mattar, R., Valladares-Neto, J., Azevedo, B.C., and Estrela, C.R.A. (2009a) Method to evaluate inflammatory root resorption using cone beam computed tomography. *J Endod*, 35, 1491–1497.

Estrela, C., Bueno, M.R., Porto, O.C.L., Rodrigues, C.D., and Pécora, J.D. (2009b) Influence of intracanal post on apical periodontitis identified by cone beam computed tomography. *Braz Dent J*, 20, 370–375.

Estrela, C., Decurcio, D.A., Silva, J.A., Mendonça, E.F., and Estrela, C.R.A. (2009c) Persistent apical periodontitis associated with calcifying odontogenic cyst. *Int Endod J*, 42, 539–545.

Estrela, C., Bueno, M.R., Silva, J.A., Leles, C.R., and Azevedo, B.C. (2011) Effect of intracanal posts on dimensions of cone beam computed tomography images of endodontically treated teeth. *Dent Press Endod*, 1, 16–21.

Faitaroni, L.A., Bueno, M.R., Carvalhosa, A.A., Ale, K.A.B., and Estrela, C. (2008) Ameloblastoma suggesting large apical periodontitis. *J Endod*, 34, 216–219.

Faitaroni, L.A., Bueno, M.R., Carvalhosa, A.A., Mendoza, E.F., and Estrela, C.C. (2011) Differential diagnosis of apical periodontitis and nasopalatine duct cyst. *J Endod*, 37, 403–410.

Gao, Y., Peters, O.A., Wu, H., and Zhou, X. (2009) An application framework of three-dimensional reconstruction and measurement for endodontic research. *J Endod*, 35, 269–274.

Gunraj, M. (1999) Dental root resorption. *Oral Surg Oral Med Oral Pathol Oral Radiol Endod*, 88, 647–653.

Halse, A. and Molven, O. (1986) A strategy for the diagnosis of periapical pathosis. *J Endod*, 12, 534–538.

Halse, A., Molven, O., and Fristad, I. (2002) Diagnosing periapical lesions: disagreement and borderline cases. *Int Endod J*, 35, 703–709.

Haristoy, R.A., Valiyaparambil, J.V., and Mallya, S.M. (2008) Correlation of CBCT gray scale values with bone densities. *Oral Surg Oral Med Oral Pathol Oral Radiol Endod*, 105, e28.

Harris, I.R. and Brown, J.E. (1997) Application of cross-sectional imaging in the differential diagnosis of apical radiolucency. *Int Endod J*, 30, 288–290.

Herman, G.T. (1980) *Image Reconstruction from Projections: The Fundamentals of Computerized Tomography*. Academic Publishers, New York.

Hounsfield, G.N. (1973) Computerised transverse axial scanning (tomography): I. Description of system. *Br J Radiol*, 46, 1016–1022.

Hunter, A. and McDavid, D. (2009) Analyzing the beam hardening artifact in the Planmeca ProMax. *Oral Surg Oral Med Oral Pathol Oral Radiol Endod*, 107, e28–e29.

Huumonen, S. and Ørstavik, D. (2002) Radiological aspects of apical periodontitis. *Endod Top*, 1, 3–25.

Huybrechts, B., Bud, M., Bergmans, L., Lambrechts, P., and Jacobs, R. (2009) Void detection in root fillings using intraoral analogue, intraoral digital and cone beam CT images. *Int Endod J*, 42, 675–685.

Jian, F. and Hongnian, L. (2006) Beam-hardening correction method based on original sonogram for X-CT. *Nucl Instrum Methods Phys Res A*, 556, 379–385.

Joseph, P.M. and Spital, R.D. (1978) Method for correcting bone induced artifacts in computed tomography scanners. *J Comput Assist Tomogr*, 2, 100–108.

Katsumata, A., Hirukawa, A., Noujeim, M., et al. (2006) Image artifact in dental cone-beam CT. *Oral Surg Oral Med Oral Pathol Oral Radiol Endod*, 101, 652–657.

Katsumata, A., Hirukawa, A., Okumura, S., et al. (2007) Effects of image artifacts on gray-value density in limited-volume cone-beam computerized tomography. *Oral Surg Oral Med Oral Pathol Oral Radiol Endod*, 104, 829–836.

Katsumata, A., Hirukawa, A., Okumura, S., et al. (2009) Relationship between density variability and imaging volume size in cone-beam computerized tomography scanning of the maxillofacial region: an in vitro study. *Oral Surg Oral Med Oral Pathol Oral Radiol Endod*, 107, 420–425.

Kerr, D.A., Ash, M.M., and Millard, H.D. (1978) *Oral Diagnosis*. Mosby, St. Louis, MO.

Ketcham, A. and Carlson, W.D. (2001) Acquisition, optimization and interpretation of X-ray computed tomography imagery: applications to the geosciences. *Comput Geosci*, 27, 381–400.

Laux, M., Abbott, P.V., Pajarola, G., and Nair, P.N.R. (2000) Apical inflammatory root resorption: a correlative radiographic and histological assessment. *Int Endod J*, 33, 483–493.

Leach, H.A., Ireland, A.J., and Whaites, E.J. (2001) Radiographic diagnosis of root resorption in relation to orthodontics. *Br Dent J*, 190, 16–22.

Levander, E. and Malmgren, O. (1988) Evaluation of the risk of root resorption during orthodontic treatment: a study of upper incisors. *Eur J Orthod*, 10, 30–38.

Liang, Y.-H., Li, G., Wesselink, P.R., and Wu, M.-K. (2011) Endodontic outcome predictors identified with periapical radiographs and cone-beam computed tomography scans. *J Endod*, 37, 326–331.

Lofthag-Hansen, S., Hummonen, S., Gröndahl, K., and Gröndahl, H.-G. (2007) Limited cone-beam computed tomography and intraoral radiography for the diagnosis of periapical pathology. *Oral Surg Oral Med Oral Pathol Oral Radiol Endod*, 103, 114–119.

Mattar, R. (2002) Reabsorção radicular pós traumatismo dentário: relação da presença, tipo, e grau com idade cronológica e idade óssea. Master's thesis. Campinas, Brazil: University São Leopoldo Mandic, 183.

Meganck, J.A., Kozloff, K.M., Thornton, M.M., Broski, S.M., and Goldstein, S.A. (2009) Beam hardening artifacts in micro-computed tomography scanning can be reduced by X-ray beam filtration and the resulting images can be used to accurately measure BMD. *Bone*, 45, 1104–1116.

Mischkowski, R.A., Pulsfort, R., Ritter, L., et al. (2007) Geometric accuracy of a newly developed cone-beam device for maxillofacial imaging. *Oral Surg Oral Med Oral Pathol Oral Radiol Endod*, 104, 551–559.

Mol, A., Mol, J.H., Chai-U-Dom, O., and Tyndall, D.A. (2004) Early detection and quantitative assessment of apical root resorption using crown-root ratio and turned-aperture computed tomography. *Oral Surg Oral Med Oral Pathol Oral Radiol Endod*, 97, 265.

Molven, O., Halse, A., and Fristad, I. (2002) Long-term reliability and observer comparisons in the radiographic diagnosis of periapical disease. *Int Endod J*, 35, 142–147.

Mozzo, P., Procacci, C., Tacconi, A., et al. (1998) A new volumetric CT machine for dental imaging based on the cone-beam technique: preliminary results. *Eur Radiol*, 8, 1558–1564.

Nair, M.K. and Nair, U.P. (2007) Digital and advanced imaging in endodontics: a review. *J Endod*, 33, 1–6.

Nair, P.N.R. (2004) Pathogenesis of apical periodontitis and the causes of endodontic failures. *Crit Rev Oral Biol Med*, 15, 348–381.

Nair, P.N.R. (2006) On the causes of persistent apical periodontitis: a review. *Int Endod J*, 39, 249–281.

Nair, P.N.R. (2009) Biology and pathology of apical periodontitis. In: C. Estrela, ed., *Endodontic Science*, 2nd ed., pp. 285–347. Artes Medicas, São Paulo.

Nair, P.N.R., Sjögren, U., Schumacher, E., and Sundqvist, G. (1993) Radicular cyst affecting a root-filled human tooth: a long-term post-treatment follow-up. *Int Endod J*, 26, 225–233.

Nair, P.N.R., Pajarola, G., and Schroeder, H.E. (1996) Types and incidence of human periapical lesions obtained with extracted teeth. *Oral Surg Oral Med Oral Pathol Oral Radiol Endod*, 81, 93–102.

Nair, P.N.R., Sjögren, U., Figdor, D., and Sundqvist, G. (1999) Persistent periapical radiolucencies of root-filled human teeth, failed endodontic treatments, and periapical scars. *Oral Surg Oral Med Oral Pathol Oral Radiol Endod*, 87, 617–627.

Nakata, K., Naitoh, M., Izumi, M., Inamoto, K., Ariji, E., and Nakamura, H. (2006) Effectiveness of dental computed tomography in diagnostic imaging of periradicular lesion of each root of a multirooted tooth: a case report. *J Endod*, 32, 583–587.

Naumann, M., Sterzenbach, G., Rosentritt, M., Beuer, F., and Frankenberger, R. (2008) Is adhesive cementation of endodontic posts necessary? *J Endod*, 34, 1006–1010.

Ne, R.F., Witherspoon, D.E., and Gutmann, J.L. (1999) Tooth resorption. *Quintessence Int*, 1999, 9–25.

Neville, B.W., Damm, D.D., Allen, C.M., et al. (2002) *Oral Maxillofacial Pathology*, 2nd ed. Saunders, Philadelphia.

Nielsen, R.B., Alyassin, A.M., Peters, D.D., Carnes, D.L., and Lancaster, J. (1995) Microcomputed tomography: an advanced system for detailed endodontic research. *J Endod*, 21, 561–568.

Noujeim, M., Prihoda, T.J., Langlais, R., and Nummikoski, P. (2009) Evaluation of high-resolution cone beam computed tomography in the detection of simulated interradicular bone lesions. *Dentomaxillofac Radiol*, 38, 156–162.

Ørstavik, D., Kerekes, K., and Eriksen, H.M. (1986) The periapical index: a scoring system for radiographic assessment of apical periodontitis. *Endod Dent Traumatol*, 2, 20–24.

Patel, S., Dawood, A., Pitt Ford, T., and Whaites, E. (2007) The potential applications of cone beam computed tomography in the management of endodontic problems. *Int Endod J*, 40, 818–823.

Patel, S., Dawood, A., Wilson, R., Horner, K., and Mannocci, F. (2009) The detection and management of root resorption lesions using intraoral radiography and conebeam computed tomography: an in vivo investigation. *Int Endod*, 42, 447–462.

Paula-Silva, F.W., Wu, M.K., Leonardo, M.R., Silva, L.A., and Wesselink, P.R. (2009) Accuracy of periapical radiography and cone-beam computed tomography scans in diagnosing apical periodontitis using histopathological findings as a gold standard. *J Endod*, 35, 1009–1012.

Pierce, A. (1989) Pathophysiological and therapeutic aspects of dentoalveolar resorption. *Aust Dent J*, 34, 437–448.

Rao, S.P. and Alfidi, R.J. (1981) The environmental density artifact: a beam-hardening effect in computed tomography. *Radiology*, 141, 223–227.

Regezi, J.A. and Sciubba, J.J. (1999) *Oral Pathology— Clinical Pathologic Correlations*, 3rd ed. Saunders, Philadelphia.

Reit, C. and Grøndahl, H.G. (1983) Application of statistical decision theory to radiographic diagnosis of endodontically treated teeth. *Scand J Dent Res*, 9, 213–218.

Rodrigues, C.D. and Estrela, C. (2008) Traumatic bone cyst suggestive of large apical periodontitis. *J Endod*, 34, 484–489.

Rosenberg, P.A., Frisbie, J., Lee, J., et al. (2010) Evaluation of pathologists (histopathology) and radiologists (cone beam computed tomography) differentiating radicular cysts from granulomas. *J Endod*, 36, 423–428.

Sapp, J.P., Eversole, L.R., and Wysocki, G.P. (2004) *Contemporary Oral and Maxillofacial Pathology*, 2nd ed. Mosby, St. Louis, MO.

Scarfe, W.C., Farman, A.G., and Sukovic, P. (2007) Clinical applications of cone-beam computed tomography in dental practice. *J Can Dent Assoc*, 72, 75–80.

Shear, M. and Speight, P. (2007) *Cysts of the Oral and Maxillofacial Regions*, 4th ed. Blackwell, London.

Shrout, M.K., Hall, J.M., and Hildebolt, C.E. (1993) Differentiation of periapical granulomas and radicular cysts by digital radiometric analysis. *Oral Surg Oral Med Oral Pathol*, 76, 356–361.

Simon, J.H.S., Enciso, R., Malfaz, J.M., et al. (2006) Differential diagnosis of large periapical lesions using cone beam computed tomography measurements and biopsy. *J Endod*, 32, 833–837.

Stafne, E.C. and Gibilisco, J.A. (1975) *Oral Roentgenographic Diagnosis*, 4th ed. Saunders, Philadelphia.

Torabinejad, M., Eby, W.C., and Naidorf, I.J. (1985) Inflammatory and immunological aspects of the pathogenesis of human periapical lesions. *J Endod*, 11, 479–484.

Trope, M., Pettigrew, J., Petras, J., Barnett, F., and Tronstad, L. (1989) Differentiation of radicular cyst and granulomas using computerized tomography. *Endod Dent Traumatol*, 5, 69–72.

Trope, M., Chivian, N., Sigurdsson, A., and Vann, W.F. (2002) Traumatic injuries. In: S. Cohen and R.C. Burns, eds., *Pathways of the Pulp*, 8th ed., pp. 603–649. Mosby, St. Louis, MO.

Van Der Stelt, P.F. (1985) Experimentally produced bone lesions. *Oral Surg Oral Med Oral Pathol Oral Radiol Endod*, 59, 306–312.

Velvart, P., Hecker, H., and Tillinger, G. (2001) Detection of the apical lesion and the mandibular canal in conventional radiography and computed tomography. *Oral Surg Oral Med Oral Pathol Oral Radiol Endod*, 92, 682–688.

Weber, A.L. (1993) Imaging of cysts and odontogenic tumors of the jaw: definition and classification. *Radiol Clin North Am*, 31, 101–120.

White, S.C., Atchison, K.A., Hewlett, E.R., and Flack, V.F. (1995) Efficacy of FDA guidelines for prescribing radiographs to detect dental and intraosseous conditions. *Oral Surg Oral Med Oral Pathol Oral Radiol Endod*, 80, 108–114.

Wood, N.K. and Goaz, P.W. (1991) *Differential Diagnosis of Oral and Maxillofacial Lesions*, 5th ed. Mosby, St. Louis, MO.

Wu, M.-K., Shemesh, H., and Wesselink, P.R. (2009) Limitations of previously published systematic reviews evaluating the outcome of endodontic treatment. *Int Endod J*, 42, 656–666.

Wu, M.-K., Wesselink, P.R., Shemesh, H., and Patel, S. (2011) Endodontic epidemiologic investigations and clinical outcome studies with cone-beam computed tomography. *J Endod*, 37(4), 513–516. doi: 10.1016/j.joen.2011.03.019.

Yoshiura, K., Weber, A.L., Runnels, S., et al. (2003) Cystic lesions of the mandible and maxilla. *Neuroimaging Clin N Am*, 13, 485–494.

Zapata, R.O., Bramante, C.M., Duarte, M.H., Fernandes, L.M.P.S.R., Camargo, E.J., Moraes, I.G., Bernardineli, N., Vivan, R.R., Capelozza, A.L.A., and Garcia, R.B. (2011) The influence of cone-beam computed tomography and periapical radiographic evaluation on the assessment of periapical bone destruction in dog's teeth. *Oral Surg Oral Med Oral Pathol Oral Radiol Endod*, 112(2), 272–279. doi: 10.1016/j.tripleo.2011.01.031

Part 6

Clinical Cases

Chapter 22   Clinical Cases

Chapter 23   Clinical Impact of Cone Beam Computed Tomography in Root Canal Treatment

22 Clinical Cases

Le O'Leary

Case 1

Diagnosis: Nasopalatine duct cyst

A 74-year-old Caucasian male with a noncontributory medical history, was referred for the evaluation of the left maxillary central incisor (MAX CI) because routine radiographic exam revealed a 7–8 mm corticated radiolucent lesion present at the root apex (Figure 22.1). The right and left maxillary lateral (MAX LI) and central incisors exhibit severe calcification in the coronal third of the canal system as seen in Figures 22.1 and 22.2. Clinical examination revealed the right and left MAX LI and MAX CI have buccal gingival recession of 2–3 mm from the cemento–enamel junction (CEJ). There was no periodontal probing >3 mm. The right and left MAX LI and MAX CI responded normally to the palpation, bite, percussion, and mobility tests. The tested teeth did not respond to the vitality test with the Endo Ice. The lack of response to the cold refrigerant was probably due to the calcification present in the coronal third of the canal system. The dilemma faced at this point is whether or not the left MAX CI was actually necrotic and warranted

endodontic treatment. A cone beam computed tomography (CBCT) scan of the area was taken. The Hitachi CB MercuRay was used with a field of view of 4 in. and a voxel resolution of 0.10. The axial view revealed the radiolucent lesion is lingual to the left MAX CI, and it is continuous with the incisive canal (Figure 22.3). The corresponding sagittal view revealed the lesion is positioned lingually to the root of the left MAX CI, extending along the whole length of the root. The lesion was within the confines of the bone, and it did spread lingually, resulting in a very thin lingual cortical plate in this area. The pattern of the lesion is not of endodontic origin; therefore, we recommended the patient sees an oral surgeon and have the area enucleated and biopsied. The oral surgeon excised the area and reported to the lab that the specimen is an asymptomatic mucus-filled intrabony lesion. Differential diagnosis was either a nasopalatine duct cyst or a lateral periodontal cyst. The microscopic description from the pathology report revealed the sections demonstrate a cyst having a thin layer of flattened to cuboidal epithelium. There was no appreciable atypia or evidence of malignancy. The final diagnosis was a nasopalatine duct cyst.

Endodontic Radiology, Second Edition. Edited by Bettina Basrani.
© 2012 John Wiley & Sons, Inc. Published 2012 by John Wiley & Sons, Inc.

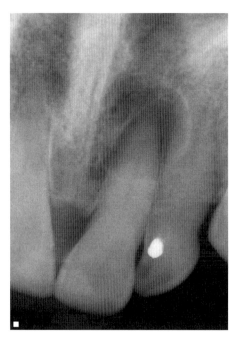

Figure 22.1 Periapical radiograph of the left MAX CI with a well circumscribed radiolucent lesion.

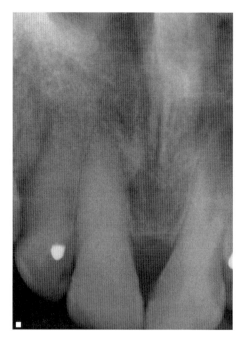

Figure 22.2 Periapical radiograph of the right MAX LI, right and left MAX CIs.

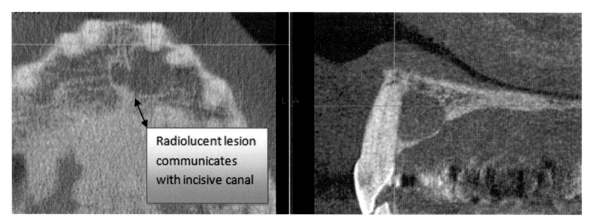

Figure 22.3 Left view is an axial view of the maxilla, the horizontal and vertical blue marker bars are located over the left maxillary central incisor, and this corresponds with the position of the same tooth in the sagittal view as seen on the right. The sagittal view reveals the radiolucent lesion is abutting against the lingual surface of the root of the left MAX CI. The axial view reveals the large radiolucent lesion, positioned lingually, and it communicates with the incisive canal (includes annotation on axial view).

Case 2

Retreatment of the right maxillary first molar (MAX 1st M)

A 17-year-old Asian female is presented with a dental history of nonsurgical endodontic treatment of the right maxillary first molar (MAX 1st M) at a young age, which was recently followed by a non-surgical endodontic retreatment of the same tooth by an endodontist. The reason for the retreatment of the tooth was infection noted around the root ends of the right MAX 1st M. Once the retreatment was completed, the patient saw a new general dentist to have the tooth crowned. Her dentist was concerned that the tooth may be fractured because the patient was still symptomatic. The patient was then referred to a different endodontist. The retreatment was completed 2 weeks prior to the patient's appointment with the new endodontist. The tooth was evaluated, and the only significant finding was sensitivity to percussion. The occlusion was within normal limits. There was no periodontal probing >3mm. The initial periapical radiograph of the right MAX 1st M revealed the root canal fillings of the mesial-buccal (MB) and distal-buccal (DB) canals were filled 1–1.5mm short of the radiographic apex (Figure 22.4). It was slightly difficult to determine the extent of the root canal filling of the palatal (P) root because of the superimposition of the zygoma and the maxillary sinus. One can discern that there are four canals treated in this tooth. Figure 22.5 is a periapical radiograph taken from a distal angle, and the MB1 and MB2 canals appear to join in the apical third. Figure 22.6 is a periapical radiograph taken at a slightly mesial foreshortened angle. From this angle, we were able to get separation of the MB1 and MB2 canals. The root canal fillings for MB1, MB2, DB, and P canals are all 1–2mm short of the radiographic apex. None of the periapical radiographs revealed obvious signs of periradicular lesions. The only radiograph that may show a slight hint of perira-dicular changes around the MB root is found in Figure 22.4. However, there is trabeculation through a slightly more radiolucent bone. This can be interpreted as an anatomical variation where the bone is thin or less dense. The tooth had a buildup with a core composite. Due to the limitations of two-dimensional views of periapical radiographs, a CBCT scan was taken of the area. The Hitachi CB MercuRay was used with a field of view of 4in. and a voxel resolution of 0.10. The sagittal view of the computed tomography (CT) images revealed the MB root of the MAX 1st M has a well-defined periradicular lesion, and the trans-axial or oblique view of this root revealed the MB1 root canal filling is slightly short, approximately 0.5mm, while the MB2 has a 2mm discrepancy (Figure 22.7). The DB root has a small radiolucent lesion (Figure 22.8), while the P root has a well-defined radiolucent lesion (Figure 22.9). The root canal fillings for both the P and DB roots are short of the radiographic apex, which concurs with the radiographic findings. An experienced user of the CT software is aware that several slices of the images must be reviewed to properly draw the appropriate conclusions as to the quality of the root canal fillings and the actual size and extent of pathology. The images selected were chosen to best represent the "true story" of the tooth; often the image slice is usually centered over the root of interest. The tooth was retreated in two appointments. Full working lengths (WLs) were achieved for all the canals. When the patient returned to have the tooth completed, drainage was observed from the MB and P canals. The patient had to commute for an hour and a half each way for her appointment and wanted to minimize her travel time. The best option to immediately address the draining canals was to seal the apical third of the canals with gray mineral trioxide aggregate (MTA). The canals were then backfilled with a flowable gutta-percha. The final radiographs revealed that the root canal fillings are to the radiographic apex (Figures 22.10 and 22.11).

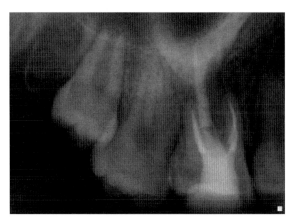

Figure 22.4 Preoperative radiograph of the right MAX 1st M revealed four canals were treated, and the root canal fillings of all the canals are approximately 1–2 mm short of the radiographic apex.

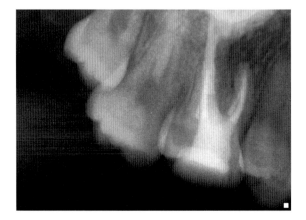

Figure 22.5 Preoperative radiograph of the right MAX 1st M taken from a distal angle.

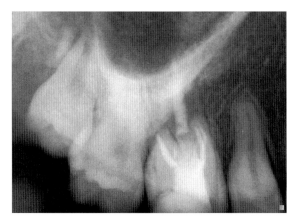

Figure 22.6 Pre-operative radiograph of the right MAX 1st M taken at a slightly mesial foreshortened angle revealed two distinct mesial-buccal (MB) canals.

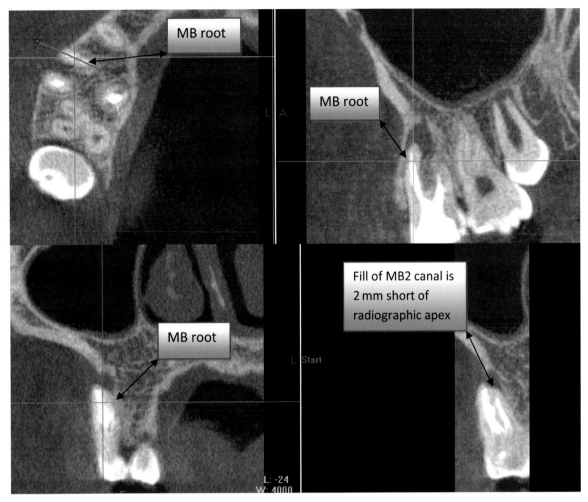

Figure 22.7 Upper left window is the axial view of the right MAX 1st M. Upper right window is the sagittal view of the same tooth, where a well-defined radiolucency can be observed around the mesial-buccal (MB) root of this tooth. A line was drawn over the MB root in the axial view to reflect the transaxial or oblique view of the MB root, which is displayed in the lower right window. The root canal filling of the MB2 canal is 2 mm short of the radiographic apex. Lower left window is the coronal view of the right MAX 1st M where the radiolucent lesion around the MB root has eroded the buccal cortical plate.

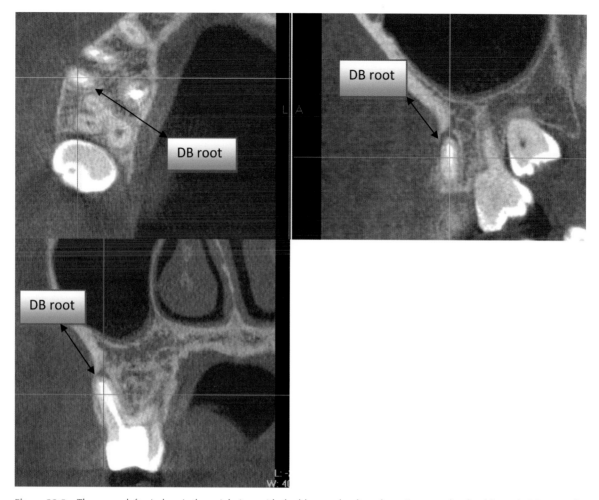

Figure 22.8 The upper left window is the axial view with the blue marker lines hovering over the distal-buccal (DB) root of the right MAX 1st M. By placing the blue marker lines over the area of interest in one view window, the other windows will correspond with the same area of interest in their specific view. Since the markers are over the DB root, the same markers that you see in the sagittal view (upper right window) are right over the DB root. This image reveals a very small radiolucent lesion around the DB root. The lower left window is the coronal view showing the position of the root of the tooth to the buccal cortical plate and the presence of a small radiolucent lesion.

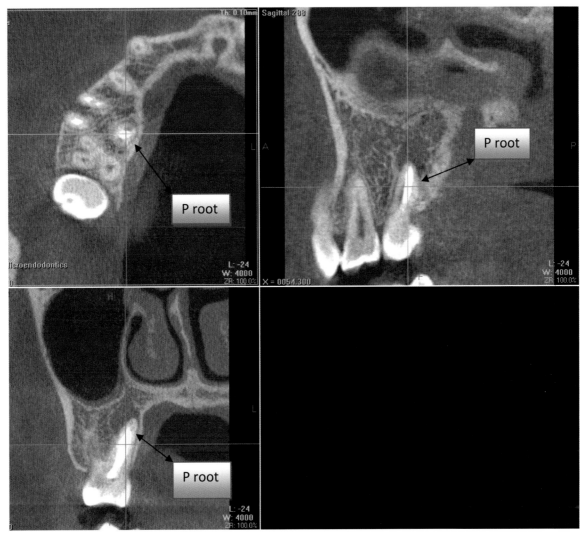

Figure 22.9   The upper left window is the axial view of the right MAX 1st M and the blue marker lines are over the palatal (P) root. This corresponds with the position of the right MAX 1st M in the sagittal view as seen in the upper right window, and a well-defined radiolucency is present around the root end of the P root. The lower left window is the coronal view which reveals the lesion is within the bony housing.

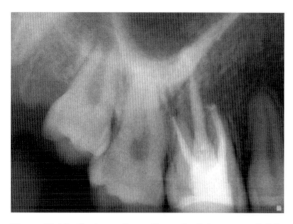

Figure 22.10   Postoperative radiograph of the retreated right MAX 1st M.

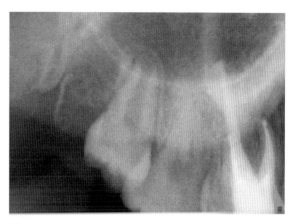

Figure 22.11   Postoperative radiograph of the right MAX 1st M taken from a distal angle.

Case 3

Missed canal: Distal-buccal root of the left maxillary second molar (MAX 1st M) has a second untreated DB canal

A healthy 39-year-old Asian man is presented with a failing root canal treatment of the left maxillary second molar (MAX 1st M). The root canal treatment was done by an endodontist in Michigan, and the patient was aware of an untreated canal due to calcification. Radiographic examination revealed the distal-buccal (DB) canal of the MAX 1st M was never negotiated, and as a result, there is a periapical lesion around the root end of this tooth (Figure 22.12). An angled periapical radiograph revealed the mesial-buccal (MB) root has two canals and the root canal fillings are slightly short of the radiographic apex (Figure 22.13). A CBCT scan was recommended. The Hitachi CB MercuRay was used with a field of view of 4 in. and a voxel resolution of 0.10. The axial view of the CT image shows the DB

root has two canals (upper left window of Figure 22.14). A transaxial or oblique view of the DB root, represented by the blue line drawn over the axial view, reveals two distinct canals along the length of the root (lower right window of Figure 22.14). A magnified view of this view can be seen in Figure 22.15. The tooth was retreated, and the DB canals were located, biomechanically prepared, and filled with gutta-percha (Figure 22.16). The DB2 canal was very calcified. Fortunately, the axial view of the CT images was helpful in determining the position of this canal in relation to the DB1 canal, because the DB1 was the first one to be found. The "road map" of the CT scan was very helpful in locating the DB2 canal; based on the axial view, the canal was 2–3 mm lingually from the DB1 and more distally positioned. An angled postoperative periapical radiograph displays both DB canals are filled (Figure 22.17). Clinically, the canals configuration of the DB root is a type II Weine's classification of canals (starts out as two separate canals and joins as one in the apical third of the root).

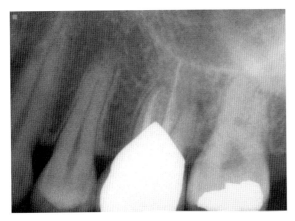

Figure 22.12 Preoperative radiograph of the MAX 1st M.

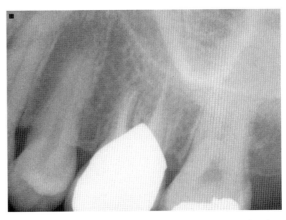

Figure 22.13 Preoperative radiograph taken from a distal angle.

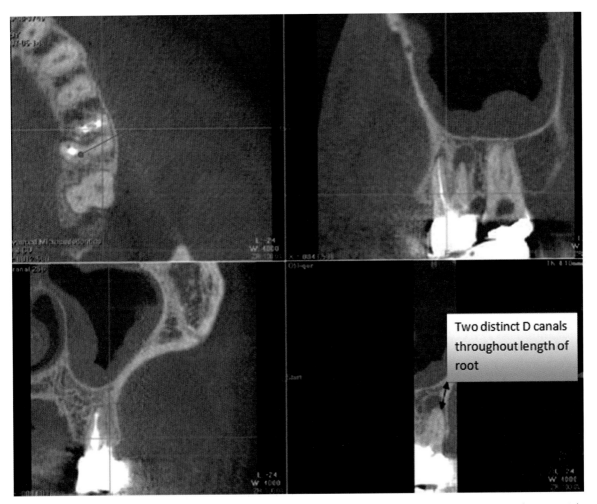

Two distinct D canals throughout length of root

Figure 22.14 In the axial view (upper left window), a blue line was drawn over the DB root, which represents the transaxial or oblique view, projected in the lower right window. It reveals the two distinct distal canals throughout the length of the root (includes annotation in oblique view). Sagittal view (upper right window) revealed radiolucent lesions around the mesial-buccal (MB) and DB roots.

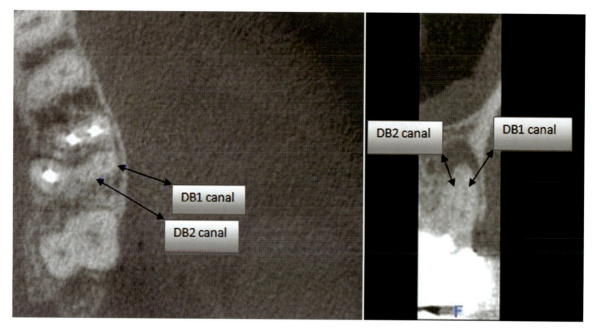

Figure 22.15 Magnified axial (left) and transaxial or oblique (right) view of the DB root (includes annotations on both views).

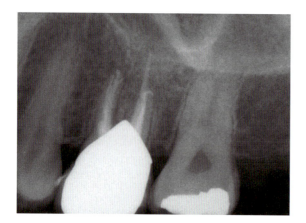

Figure 22.16 Postoperative radiograph.

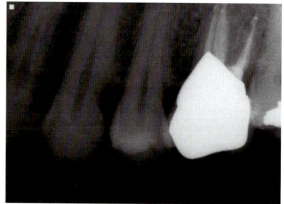

Figure 22.17 Angled postoperative radiograph showing the filled DB canals.

Case 4

Horizontal root fracture

The patient is an 85-year-old Caucasian male with a medical history of non-Hodgkin's lymphoma, heart bypass surgery, and high blood pressure. The patient had been experiencing pressure in the upper right area for a couple of months. He rated his pain scale as 2 out of 10. The patient was not able to recall when the root canal treatment was done. Clinical exam revealed the right maxillary first molar (MAX 1st M) was sensitive to palpation and percussion tests. The tooth exhibited a mobility of 1 with a type II furcal involvement. Periodontal pockets were noted in the following areas: buccal (B): 6 mm; lingual (L): 6 mm; mesial-buccal (MB); and mesial lingual (ML): 8 mm. Radiograph revealed a large radiolucent lesion around the MB root (Figure 22.18) and furcal breakdown (Figure 22.19). The palatal (P) root is not discernible on the radiograph, therefore, there is a possibility that this tooth has had a palatal root amputation. The patient did not have a good memory of his dental history and was unable to confirm if this procedure was performed on the tooth. The canals were undershaped, and the root canal fillings were short of the radiographic apices. There is a possibility of a missed MB2 canal. Based on the radiographic and clinical findings, the periradicular lesion is an endo-perio lesion. A CBCT scan was taken. The Hitachi CB MercuRay was used with a field of view of 4 in. and a voxel resolution of 0.10. The CT images revealed a large radiolucent lesion around the MB root end of the MAX 1st M, and there is an oblique horizontal root fracture of the MB root (Figure 22.20). The images also confirmed that there is no palatal root. Several image slices from the sagittal view also revealed the radiolucent lesion around the MB root of the MAX 1st M extending to include the root apex of the right maxillary second premolar (MAX 2nd PM). Clinically, the MAX 2nd PM was nonresponsive to the vitality test. The treatment plan was to extract the right MAX 1st M and start nonsurgical endodontic treatment on the right MAX 2nd PM.

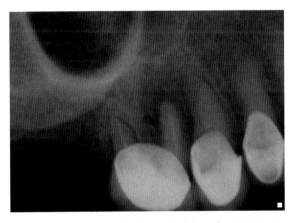

Figure 22.18 Periapical radiograph of the right MAX 1st M demonstrating a radiolucent lesion around the apex of the mesial-buccal (MB) root.

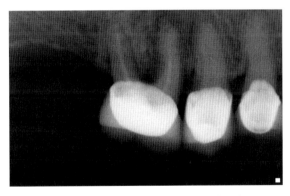

Figure 22.19 Periapical radiograph showing furcal breakdown of the right MAX 1st M.

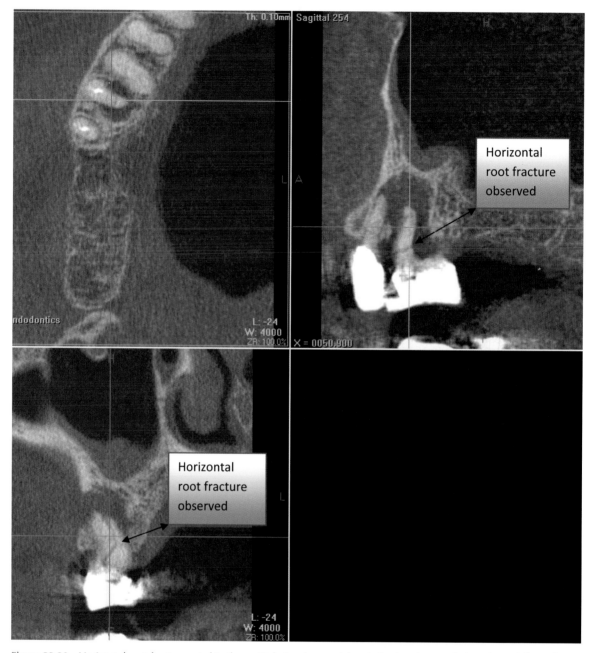

Figure 22.20 Horizontal root fracture noted in the sagittal view (upper right window) and coronal view (lower left window).

Case 5

Impacted molar

A 57-year-old Caucasian female with a medical history of high blood pressure and an allergy to Sulfa, presented with a chief complaint of chewing sensitivity, pressure, and spontaneous pain for 2 days. The discomfort was localized to the area of right mandibular first (MAND 1st M) and second molar (MAND 2nd M). Dental history revealed that the crown and the previous root canal treatment on the right MAND 2nd M were done 30 years ago by a general dentist in Nevada. A preoperative radiograph revealed the canals of the mesial (M) and distal (D) roots of the right MAND 2nd M were poorly instrumented and obturated approximately 2–4 mm short of the radiographic apices (Figure 22.21). There appeared to be a separated instrument in the M root because the root canal filling in the apical third appeared to be more radiopaque than the remaining filling. No periradicular pathology was noted around the root end of the right MAND 2nd M. The impacted wisdom tooth has a radiolucent halo around the clinical crown, and it is in close proximity to the distal lateral root surface of the right MAND 2nd M. Taking into consideration that there was no periradicular pathology present around the root end of a 30-year-old root canal treated tooth, there is a possibility that the symptoms can be associated with the impacted tooth (Figure 22.22). It is very easy to assume that the root canal treatment is failing because of the undershaped and short root canal fillings of the canal system. Most root canal treatments would have failed or showed signs or symptoms of failure earlier than this. A CBCT was recommended for thorough diagnosis (Figure 22.23). The Hitachi CB MercuRay was used with a field of view of 4 in. and a voxel resolution of 0.10. CT images revealed a large radiolucent area over the clinical crown of the right mandibular third molar (MAND 3rd M), and there is external resorption or possible decay of the clinical crown and bone loss extending to the distal lateral root surface of right MAND 2nd M (Figure 22.24). The pattern of the lesion is of a dentigerous cyst which is known to be developmental in origin, and it is often associated with the crown of an unerupted wisdom tooth. The infected wisdom tooth is exerting pressure on the right MAND 2nd M and surrounding nerve tissue in the bone, resulting in a symptomatic right MAND 2nd M. The wisdom tooth will need to be extracted to get resolution of the symptoms. This tooth is lying right above the inferior alveolar nerve, and the patient was advised that a possible complication associated in removal of this tooth is parasthesia of the jaw. Since the impacted molar is in close proximity to the right MAND 2nd M, the patient was informed that the right MAND 2nd M may also need to be extracted to get access to the impacted molar.

The patient was followed up 2 years after the diagnosis, and she reported she never had the right impacted MAND 3rd M extracted because she is currently asymptomatic, she was informed by an oral surgeon that there is a high possibility of parasthesia in the lower jaw if attempts were made to remove the right MAND 3rd M, and since the symptoms did resolve she decided to leave it alone.

Segmentation of the area of interest was done using the Simplant software. The inferior alveolar nerve and the impacted third molar were outlined to demonstrate their relationship with one another. Please refer to the Appendix (Figures A22.1–A22.3).

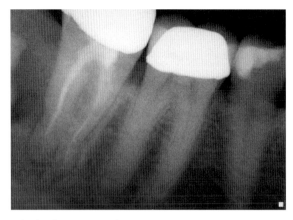

Figure 22.21 Periapical radiograph of right MAND 2nd M.

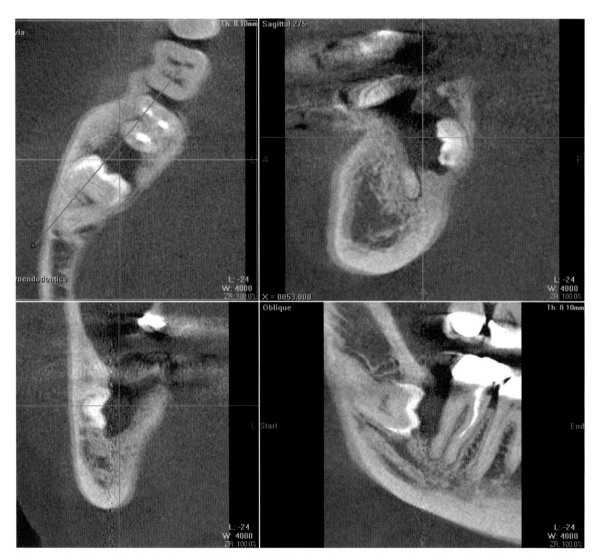

Figure 22.22 Upper left window is an axial view with the blue line drawn parallel to the arch, positioned over the mesial-buccal (MB) root of the MAND 2nd M, which is basically a sagittal view of the mandible which is more in line with the arch of the mandible. This view revealed a radiolucent halo around the clinical crown of the impacted MAND 3rd M. No periradicular pathology observed around the root apices of the MAND 2nd M.

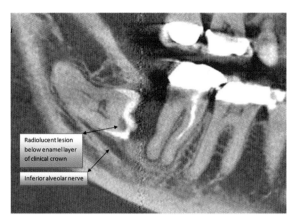

Figure 22.23 Magnified sagittal view created similarly as in Figure 22.22, but a different image slice depicting the position of the impacted MAND 3rd M, where the whole tooth with the root structure can be seen lying over the inferior alveolar nerve. This slice showed a radiolucent lesion below the enamel layer of the clinical crown of the tooth (includes two annotation boxes).

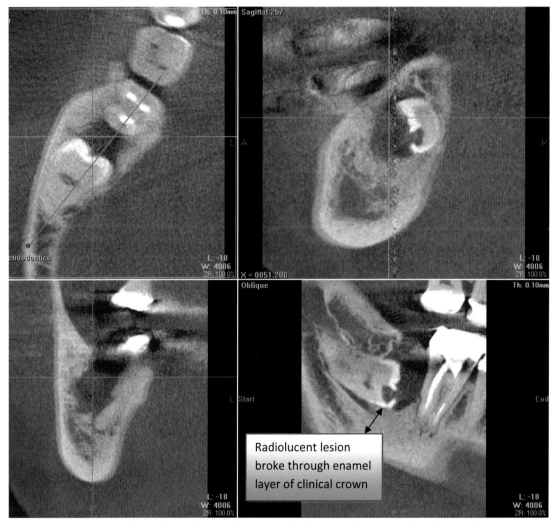

Figure 22.24 Upper left window is the axial view of the jaw with a blue line drawn more lingually from the one seen in Figure 22.22. The created sagittal view seen in the lower right hand window revealed the radiolucent lesion in the clinical crown has broken through the enamel layer of the tooth.

Case 6

External root resorption

A 52-year-old Caucasian female with a medical history of hormone replacement therapy and thyroid problems was referred for nonsurgical endodontic treatment of the right maxillary first molar (MAX 1st M). The patient had undergone periodontal treatment with this tooth for 2 years where the periodontist was trying to close the pocket and was not able to successfully treat the area. She then saw another periodontist who informed her a graft could be done, but would only be a temporary fix. Her other option was to extract the right MAX 2nd M to manage the pocket in between the teeth because the periodontist felt the periodontal problem stemmed from this tooth. Significant probing depths of 9 mm were noted in between the right MAX 1st M and maxillary second molar (MAX 2nd M). Clinical examination revealed that the right MAX 2nd M was slightly sensitive to bite, hyperresponsive to the cold test, and had a mobility of 2. The right MAX 1st M was sensitive to bite, nonresponsive to the cold test, and the mobility is within normal limits. Periapical radiograph revealed the tooth approximating the maxillary sinus floor (Figure 22.25). The buccal roots were fused and no obvious periradicular pathology noted. A CBCT was recommended for thorough diagnosis. The Hitachi CB MercuRay was used with a field of view of 4 in. and a voxel resolution of 0.10. CT images revealed external resorption of the distal buccal (DB) and palatal (P) roots of the MAX 1st M (Figure 22.26). There was a second area of external resorption in the lingual area of the P root (Figure 22.27). Based on the findings, the prognosis was deemed poor, and extraction was recommended. Nonsurgical root canal treatment was indicated for the right MAX 2nd M because the periodontal problem was due to the right MAX 1st M.

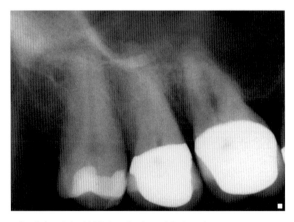

Figure 22.25   Periapical radiograph of the right MAX 1st, 2nd, and 3rd molars.

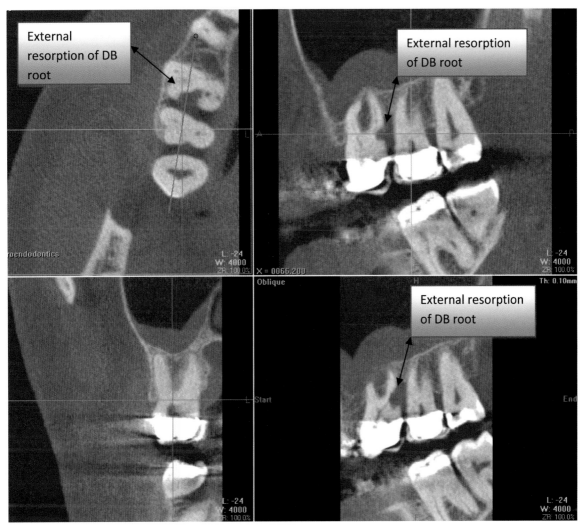

Figure 22.26 The axial view (upper left window) of the CT images revealed external resorption of the DB root, extending to the P root. The sagittal image (upper right window) showed the resorption of the DB root started in the coronal third of the root structure. Inflammation of the mucosal lining of the maxillary sinus is observed.

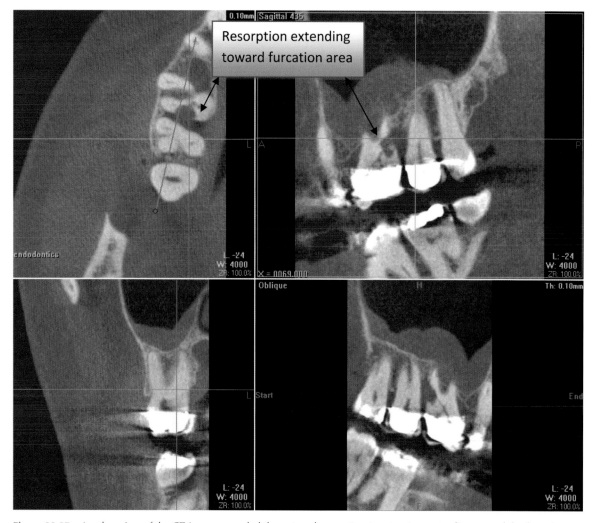

Figure 22.27 Another view of the CT images revealed the external resorption is extensive, extending toward the furcation area of tooth as seen in the axial (upper left window) and sagittal views (upper right window).

Case 7

Garre's osteomyelitis

A young healthy 12-year-old Caucasian female presented with swelling of the lower left border of the mandible. The patient was initially seen by a pedodontist, and she was later referred to an endodontist for the evaluation of the abscessed area. It was difficult to take any intraoral periapical radiographs of the area because the patient was crying and was in pain. Periapical radiographs revealed normal alveolar bone around the roots of the left mandibular first molar (MAND 1st M) (Figures 22.28 and 22.29). The tooth had no restoration. Clinical exam revealed the left MAND 1st M was vital. Palpation of the lingual gingival tissue of the unerupted mandibular 2nd M (MAND 2nd M) area elicited pain. The findings suggested that the swelling was nonendodontic in origin. Later, the patient was referred to our office for a CBCT scan. The Hitachi CB MercuRay was

used with a field of view of 9 in. and a voxel resolution of 0.29. An oral maxillofacial radiologist reviewed the scan and reported the following findings:

Axial, coronal, and sagittal multiplanar reconstructed images demonstrate Garre's osteomyelitis of the apical portion of nonerupted left MAND 2nd M and posteriorly included in the angle of the mandible (Figure 22.30). Noted especially is the "onion skin appearance" of the area in reaction to the inflammation and adjacent to the facial and lingual cortical borders of the mandible. Comparisons of the left and right posterior regions of the mandible accentuate the inflammatory reaction in the left posterior region. A single layer panoramic image of the region was created in the lower right window of the multiplanar reconstructed images to illustrate the difficulty illuminating osteomyelitis from this view (Figure 22.31).

The patient saw an oral surgeon and the MAND 2nd M was extracted, and the patient has been doing fine ever since.

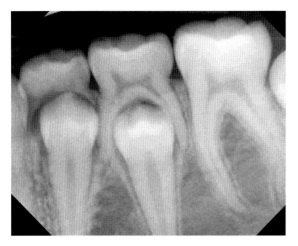

Figure 22.28   Periapical radiograph of the left MAND 1st M.

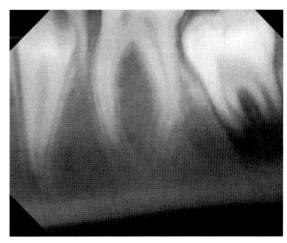

Figure 22.29   Periapical radiograph of the left MAND 1st M and unerupted MAND 2nd M.

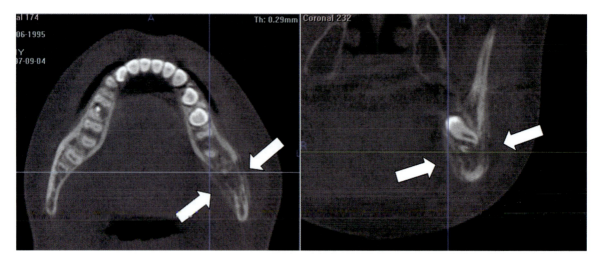

Figure 22.30 Axial and coronal views demonstrate the inflammatory process of the "Garre's osteomyelitis." The arrows are pointing to the "onion-skin" appearance (Courtesy of W. Bruce Howerton, Jr., DDS MS, Raleigh, NC).

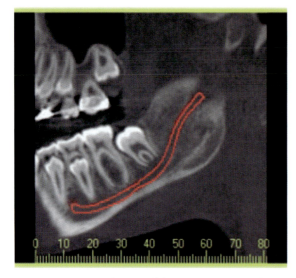

Figure 22.31 Sagittal image of the region (Courtesy of W. Bruce Howerton, Jr., DDS MS, Raleigh, NC).

APICAL SURGERY

Case 8

Apical surgery of the right mandibular first molar (MAND 1st M)

The patient is a 53-year-old Caucasian male with a medical history of diverticulitis, high blood pres-

sure, angina, sinus and respiratory trouble, and an allergy to erythromycin. The patient presented with a chief complaint of chewing sensitivity, constant pain, and pressure associated with the right mandibular first molar (MAND 1st M) for a week. The pain radiated to the ear and head area. The patient rated his pain scale as 10 out of 10. This tooth was endodontically treated by a general dentist 5 years ago. The right mandibular second molar implant was placed 3 years ago. Clinical examination revealed the MAND 1st M had a 3-mm gingival recession on the buccal (B) and 2 mm on the lingual (L). There was a small swelling of the buccal cervical gingival tissue of this tooth and was probably due to the infection draining through the sulcus. Clinically, the MAND 1st M was sensitive to the palpation, bite, and percussion tests. Radiographically, the root canal filling in the mesial (M) root of this tooth appeared to be clinically acceptable, and the root canal filling in the distal (D) root was slightly extruded (Figures 22.32 and 22.33). There is a moderately sized radiolucent lesion around the M root. No periradicular pathology was noted around the D root. A CBCT was taken (Figure 22.34). The Hitachi CB MercuRay was used with a field of view of 4 in. and a voxel resolution of 0.10. The CT images revealed a well-defined radiolucent lesion of approximately 5 mm in diameter present around the apical third of the M root. The D root exhibited a thickened periodontal ligament (PDL) space or very small radiolucent lesion right next to the extruded root canal filling material. Taking in consideration that the tooth has short roots, gingival recession, and the possibility of a root fracture, the prognosis was deemed as fair to guarded. Treatment options of extraction or apical surgery were discussed with the patient. The patient had reservations regarding the surgical procedure and wanted to consult with his general dentist. The patient was placed on antibiotics. A week later, the apical surgery was performed on this tooth. Upon reflection of a full triangular mucoperiosteal flap, pus drainage was observed. No cortical bony defect was present. The buccal cortical bone over the M root was soft to the pressure of the explorer. A round bur was used with light cutting strokes to remove the buccal cortical plate. Curettement of the tissue overlying the M root was carried out to get access to the root end. The root end was resected, retroprepped, and retrofilled with gray MTA. Prior to placing the retro-

filling material, methylene blue dye was applied to the M root to check for any root fracture. The bone over the D root end was removed to access the overfilled material. There was a small amount of granulation tissue present lingually to the root, and this was probably a foreign body reaction to the extruded material. When the tissue was curetted out, a small chunk of sealer also came out with it. Since the root of this tooth was already very short, the root end was not resected. The root was smoothed out with a diamond bur. This canal appeared to be filled with the plastic core "Thermafil" material because the gray core could be seen in the center of the canal. Methylene blue dye was also used on the D root to check for root fractures. The M and D osteotomies were grafted with a mixture of demineralized bone and clindamycin (aqueous form). Vicryl sutures were used to close the flap (Figure 22.35).

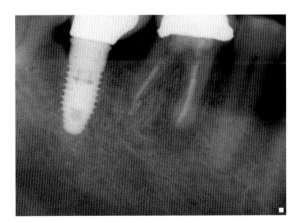

Figure 22.32 Preoperative radiograph of the right MAND 1st M.

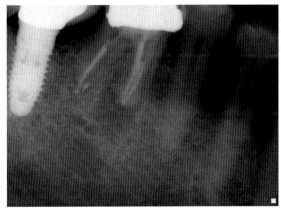

Figure 22.33 Preoperative angled radiograph of the right MAND 1st M.

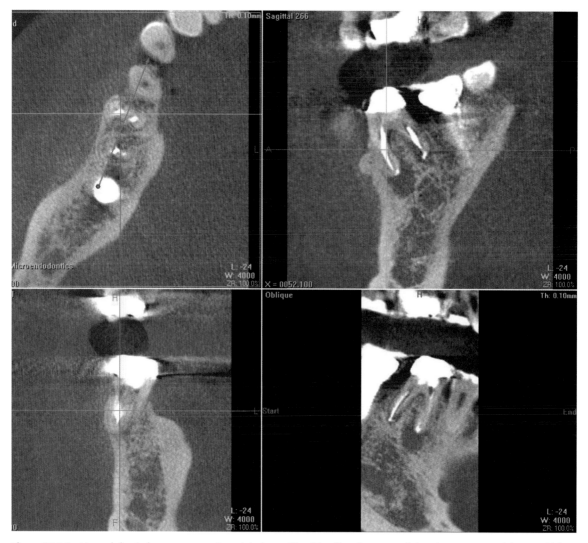

Figure 22.34 Upper left window represents the axial view with a blue line drawn parallel to the curvature of the mandible to create a transaxial or oblique view as seen in the lower right window. This view showed the radiolucent lesion around the M root with a thickened periodontal ligament, and this corresponds with the standard sagittal view as seen in the upper right window. Please keep in mind that this standard view is a mirror image of the jaw; therefore, if you were looking at this picture as a normal periapical radiograph, the tooth you are looking at would be considered as a *left* MAND 1st M.

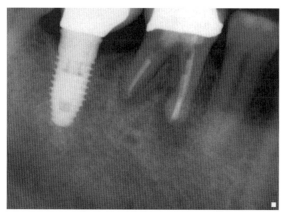

Figure 22.35 Postoperative radiograph.

Case 9

Apical surgery of the right maxillary canine (MAX C)

The patient, a healthy 44-year-old Caucasian woman, presented with discomfort on chewing and pressure sensitivity whenever her finger is pressed over the root of the right maxillary canine (MAX C). Other symptoms experienced in the areas are numbness, tightness, and occasional tingly sensation. This tooth was endodontically treated by a general dentist a year ago. A preoperative periapical radiograph revealed the root canal filling of the MAX C is slightly overextended with a thickened periodontal ligament (PDL) space in the apical third of the root (Figure 22.36). Palpation revealed a small bump over the root end of the right MAX C. A CBST scan was taken using the Hitachi CB MercuRay with a field of view of 4 in. and a voxel resolution of 0.10. The CT images revealed the root of the MAX C can be seen inclined slightly labially, and there is a lack of alveolar bone covering the root end of the tooth (Figures 22.37 and 22.38). This is often referred as a dehiscence of the root. The transaxial or oblique view reveals the extruded root canal filling material is beyond the confines of the bone (Figure 22.39). The patient was very nervous and therefore, she was orally sedated for the apical surgery procedure. A full triangular mucoperiosteal flap was reflected revealing an osseous fenestration with a soft tissue lesion at the root apex of the MAX C. The extruded root canal filling material can be seen intermixed with the granulation tissue. Curettage of the soft tissue lesion was carried out, and the tissue was submitted for a biopsy. The canal appeared to be filled with a plastic core carrier filling material (dark central core surrounded by an orange band of gutta-percha), often referred as a plastic "Thermafil." The root end was resected. Methylene blue dye was applied to the area, and there was no root fracture observed. There was a lateral canal present lingually from the main canal. The main canal and lateral canal were retroprepped and retrofilled with gray MTA (Figure 22.40). The area was grafted with demineralized bone prior to closure. The oral pathology report of the biopsied tissue revealed that it was a periapical granuloma. One year follow-up revealed good bone health around the root end of the tooth (Figure 22.41).

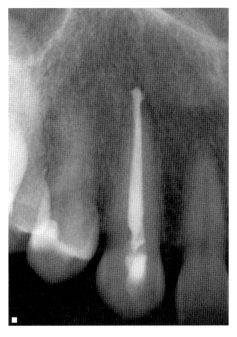

Figure 22.36   Preoperative radiograph of the right MAX C.

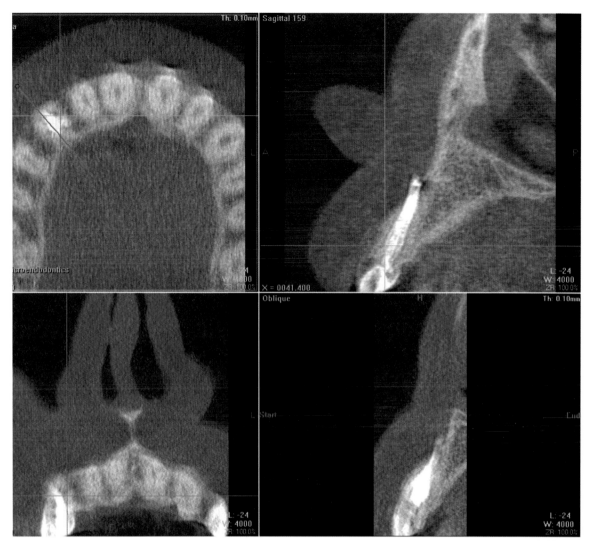

Figure 22.37 The different CT views of the tooth: axial (upper left window), sagittal (upper right window), coronal (lower left window), and transaxial or oblique (lower right window). The sagittal view shows a lack of buccal cortical plate overlying the root end of the MAX canine. In the axial view, the line drawn over the root creates the transaxial or oblique view image which revealed the absence of cortical bone coverage over the root apex; it looks more pronounced than the "standard" sagittal view.

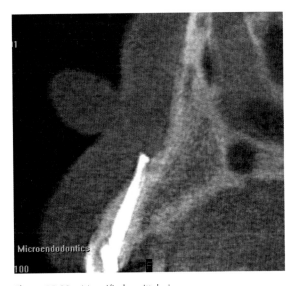

Figure 22.38 Magnified sagittal view.

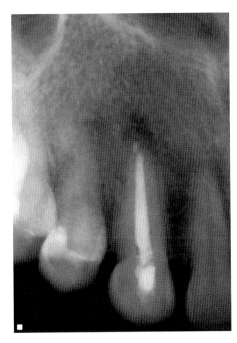

Figure 22.40 Postoperative radiograph with MTA retrograde fillings, the lateral canal filling can be seen as a stand-alone root canal filling from the main canal system (radio-opaque dot at the root end).

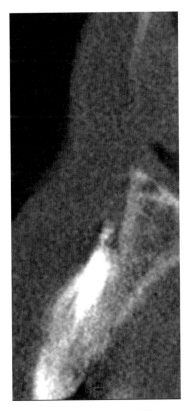

Figure 22.39 Magnified transaxial or oblique view.

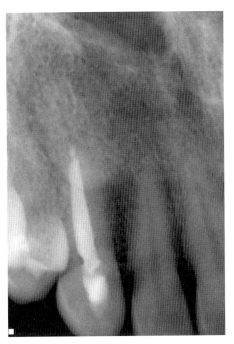

Figure 22.41 One year recall radiograph revealed excellent healing of the area.

Case 10

Apical surgery of the right maxillary first molar (MAX 1st M)

The patient is a 58-year-old Caucasian female with a medical history of Stage 4 breast cancer in remission. The patient was asymptomatic. Routine exam revealed a sinus tract on the buccal area of the right maxillary first molar (MAX 1st M) and second premolar (MAX 2nd PM). The right MAX 1st M was endodontically treated by an endodontist 10 years ago. The patient was unclear of the dental history of the endodontically treated MAX 2nd PM. Radiographic examination revealed the root canal fillings of both teeth are approximately 1–2.5 short of the radiographic apex (Figure 22.42). Clinical exam revealed the right MAX 1st M was sensitive to palpation and percussion, while the right MAX 2nd PM was sensitive to percussion and bite. Probing depths were within normal limits for both teeth. Radiographically, there are periradicular lesions around the mesial-buccal (MB) root of the MAX 1st M and the root end of the MAX 2nd PM. The possible reasons for the failing root canal treatments are missed canals, short root canal fillings and/or possible root fractures. A CBCT scan was taken (Figure 22.43). The Hitachi CB MercuRay was used with a field of view of 4 in. and a voxel resolution of 0.10. The CT images revealed a missed buccal canal for the MAX 2nd PM. The axial view also revealed the cross section of the MB root of the MAX 1st M is ovoid in shape, and this alludes to a possible missed MB2 canal since the root canal filling of the MB1 canal is off-centered. The radiolucent lesion around the MB root has eroded a small area of the floor of the maxillary sinus and also resulted in the inflammation of the mucosal lining of the maxillary sinus. The lesion was concentrated more around the MB root, but it did extend to the distal-buccal (DB) root. The patient was recommended nonsurgical endodontic retreatment of the affected teeth as a treatment option. The patient was advised of possible apical surgery if the area does not heal after or during the retreatments. Both teeth were retreated, and the results were the following: was able to gain lengths in all of the treated canals, located the B canal for the MAX 2nd PM, and unable to find the MB2 canal (this brought us to the conclusion that either the canal is very calcified or the true anatomy of this root only consists of one canal). At the time of the completion of the retreatment, the sinus tract did heal. Six months after the retreatment, the patient called to inform that the sinus tract had resurfaced, her breast cancer had returned, and she was back on chemotherapy. Clinical exam revealed the presence of a sinus tract in the B area of the MAX 1st M. Periapical radiograph revealed the radiolucent lesion around the MAX 2nd PM had healed, and this was also confirmed on the CT scan taken to evaluate the area (Figures 22.44 and 22.45). The second CT scan revealed that there was more erosion of the floor of the maxillary sinus when compared to the previous CT scan (Figure 22.46). There was also a loss of the buccal cortical plate overlying the MB root of the MAX 1st M. At this point, surgical intervention was indicated. The oncologist was consulted, and the patient had to postpone chemotherapy until after the surgery. All necessary lab tests were performed to ensure optimal healing for the patient postsurgically. A full triangular mucoperiosteal flap was reflected, and a cortical boney defect was present over the MB root, which confirmed the CT findings. The soft tissue was curetted out and submitted for a biopsy. Clinical impression of the soft tissue biopsy is of "an apical cyst." The soft tissue was mainly present around the MB root, and it did extend to the mesial lateral root surface of the DB root. Fortunately, it did not spread to the apical third of the DB root which would necessitate another retrofilling. The soft tissue was removed without invading the Schneiderian's membrane of the maxillary sinus. Since the defect was fairly large, the grayish tint of the membrane was visualized. Although it appeared as if the membrane of the sinus was intact, the patient could feel water from the handpiece draining down her throat during the root end preparation. In hindsight, a barrier should have been placed over the membrane prior to the root end preparation. The MB root was resected, and Methylene blue dye was used to check for root fractures. The root end was then retropepped and retrofilled with gray MTA. Gelfoam was placed over the sinus membrane, and it was used as a scaffold for the grafting material. Demineralized bone was used to graft the area. The oral pathology report of the biopsied tissue revealed that it was a periapical periodontal cyst.

The patient returned for a 1-year recall, and there was good healing of the bone on the periapical radiograph (Figures 22.47 and 22.48).

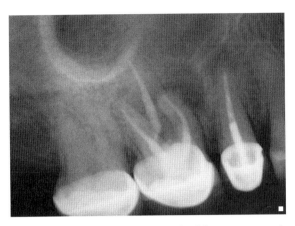

Figure 22.42 Preoperative radiograph of the retreatment of the right MAX 1st M and 2nd PM.

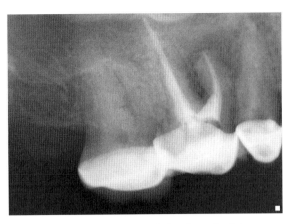

Figure 22.44 Postoperative angled radiograph of the retreatment of the right MAX 1st M. It showed the wide coronal dimension of the MB2 root due to area being trophed out in an attempt to locate the MB2 canal and it was subsequently filled with gutta-percha.

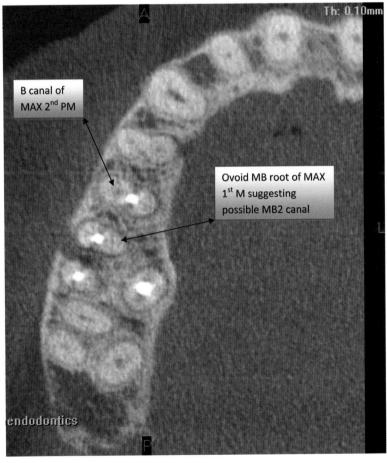

Figure 22.43 Axial view revealed an untreated B canal for the MAX 2nd PM. The cross section of the MB root of the MAX 1st M is ovoid with the root canal filling slightly off-centered, suggesting a possible untreated MB2 canal.

357

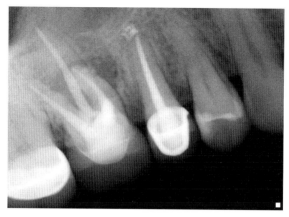

Figure 22.45 Postoperative radiograph of the completed retreatment of the right MAX 1st M and 2nd PM.

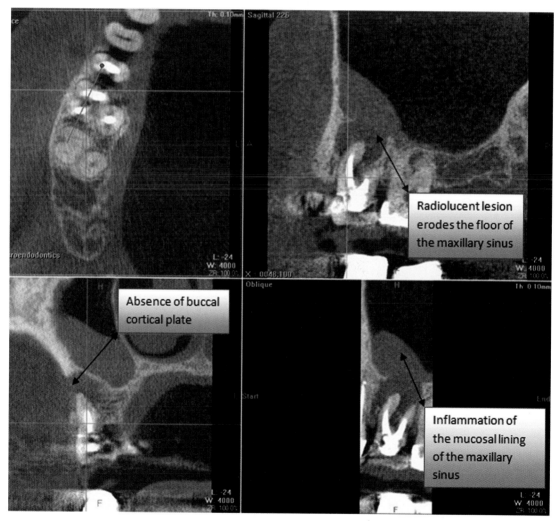

Radiolucent lesion erodes the floor of the maxillary sinus

Absence of buccal cortical plate

Inflammation of the mucosal lining of the maxillary sinus

Figure 22.46 Axial view (upper left window) has a blue line drawn parallel to the curvature of the arch and over the facial border of the MB and DB roots, which represents the transaxial or oblique view of the area as seen in the lower right window. In this created view there is a thin layer of bone between the radiolucent lesion and the floor of the sinus. The standard sagittal view, as seen in the upper right window, revealed the lesion has eroded the sinus floor causing a localized inflammation of the mucosal lining of the sinus.

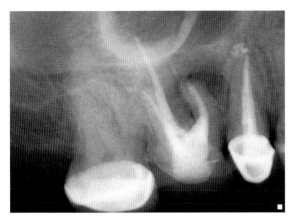

Figure 22.47 Postoperative surgical radiograph with MTA retrograde filling placed in the MB root.

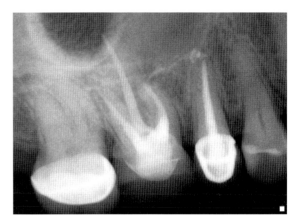

Figure 22.48 One year recall radiograph revealed the radiolucent lesion over the MB root has decreased in size.

Case 11

Apical surgery of the right maxillary lateral incisor (MLI), right and left maxillary central incisor (MCI)

A healthy 42-year-old Hispanic man presented with a chief complaint of "pressure in the gum area of my front teeth," pointing to the right maxillary lateral (MLI) and right and left central incisors (MCI). The patient reported a history of dental trauma to the area when he was 13-years-old by falling off a bike and hitting face first on the concrete road. Periapical radiograph revealed large periradicular lesions around the root end of the right MLI and right and left MCIs (Figure 22.49). The alveolar bone of the left MAX CI appeared normal (Figures 22.50–22.54). Clinical exam findings included the right MAX LI and MAX CI were sensitive to palpation and both teeth felt "different" upon percussion. The periodontal probing and mobility of the right and left MAX CI and right MAX LI were within normal limits. The Hitachi CB MercuRay was used to take a CBCT scan, with a field of view of 4 in. and a voxel resolution of 0.10. The findings of the oral maxillofacial radiologist report were as followed:

Axial, coronal, and sagittal multiplanar reconstructed images were evaluated to determine the presence and extent of rarefying osteitis in the maxillary anterior region. The screen capture for the right MAX LI demonstrates apical rarefying osteitis extending from the periapical region superiorly that does not include the inferior cortical border of the anterior region of the right maxillary sinus (Figure 22.55). The facial cortical border has been eroded, and a very thin border is seen along the palatal cortical border of the maxilla. Regarding the right MCI, the axial, coronal, and sagittal views demonstrate loss of facial cortical border and a very thin lingual cortical border, as the rarefying osteitis extends from the periapical region of the tooth superiorly and posteriorly, but does not include the inferior cortical border of the nasal cavity (Figure 22.56). After reviewing the screen capture of the left MCI, the rarefying osteitis extends laterally from the midline to include the apical region of this tooth. This is evident in the sagittal cross sections of the screen capture (Figure 22.57), and it should be noted the lesion was discernable on the CT images, but not on the periapical radiograph. It should be reiterated that the inferior cortical border of the nasal cavity and the right maxillary sinus are not involved.

Treatment options included periapical surgery and enucleation of the periradicular lesion including retrofill restorations. The radiologist considered the prognosis for the surgical treatment as guarded. A second option was extraction of the right MAX LI, right and left MAX CI, enucleation of the granulation tissue, placement of particulate graft material, and dental implant placements if adequate hard tissue is present. If hard tissue is not adequate, a bridge restoration may be an acceptable restoration in this region.

The patient wanted to save his teeth and chose the apical surgery route. A triangular full mucoperiosteal flap (right MAX C—left MAX LI) was reflected, and there was pus oozing from the area during the reflection process. All the surgically exposed teeth had crestal bone support, specifically the teeth of interests which consisted of the right MAX LI and right and left MAX CI. There was a large fenestration of the cortical bone present over the root apices of the right MAX LI and MAX CI. The cortical bone overlying the left MAX CI was soft to the touch with an explorer, and it was removed to extend the existing bony window and to further expose the underlying soft tissue lesion. This allowed adequate surgical access for the curettement of the soft tissue lesion, root-end section, and the placement of retrograde fillings. The lesion was curetted out and submitted for a biopsy. After the removal of the entire soft tissue lesion, the right maxillary anterior segment appeared fragile, and the affected teeth exhibited slight mobility because it was no longer supported by a mass of granulation tissue. The root end of the right MAX LI, right and left MAX CI were resected, retroprepped, and retrofilled with gray MTA (Figure 22.51). Methylene blue dye was used to check for root fractures. The area was grafted with demineralized bone and Bio-Gide® resorbable membrane. The oral pathology report of the biopsied tissue revealed that it was an apical periodontal cyst. The patient was followed up at 1 month, and he reported some numbness to the area. It was explained to the patient the lesion was very large to begin with, therefore the area is still recovering from the procedure, and it will take some time for the parasthesia to resolve. At 6 months recall, the numbness was barely noticeable and radiographically, the periapical lesion had decreased in size (Figure 22.52). At 1 year recall, the patient was doing well, and the periapical radiograph showed that the periapical lesion had further decreased in size (Figure 22.53). There is partial osseous repair of the area and the bone density is not fully reestablished to the same level as the adjacent "normal" bone. The patient returned for a 21-month recall, and currently resides in Florida. The patient was very dedicated on returning to our office for continued follow-up of the treated area. The periapical radiograph revealed the area has healed. Clinically, the teeth responded within normal limits to palpation, bite, percussion, and mobility tests. A CT scan was taken, and the images revealed healthy alveolar bone (Figures 22.58–22.60). The apical rarefactions around the right MLI to the right and left MCIs have healed up nicely.

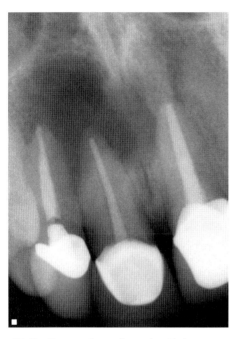

Figure 22.49 Preoperative radiograph with large radiolucent lesion around the root apices of the right MAX LI & MAX CI.

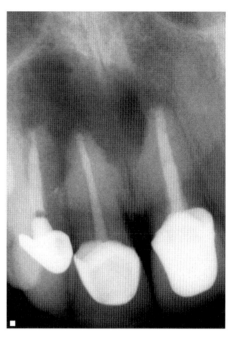

Figure 22.51 Postoperative radiograph of the surgical procedure.

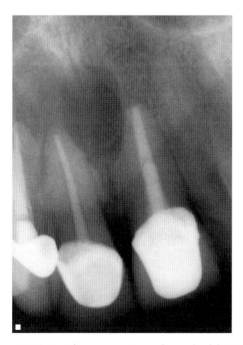

Figure 22.50 Another preoperative radiograph of the MAX CIs taken from a different angle.

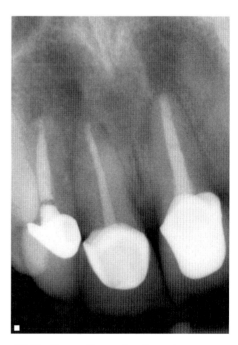

Figure 22.52 Six months recall radiograph.

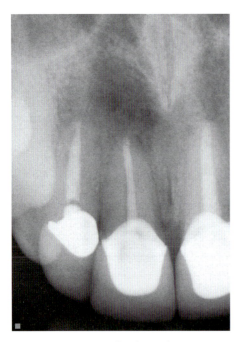

Figure 22.53 One year recall radiograph.

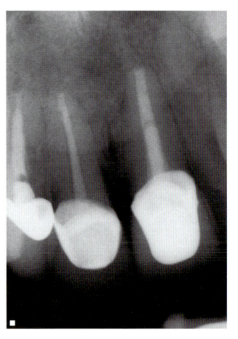

Figure 22.54 Twenty-one months recall radiograph.

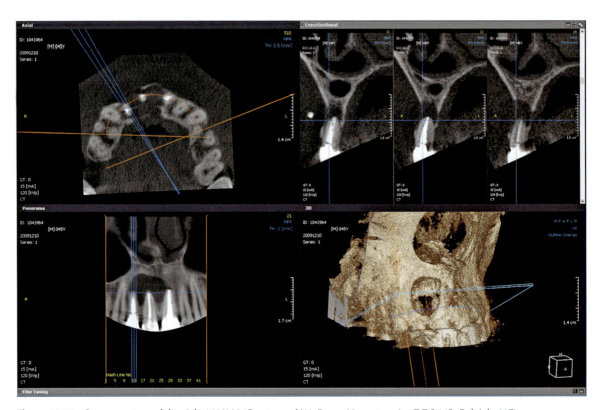

Figure 22.55 Screen capture of the right MAX LI (Courtesy of W. Bruce Howerton, Jr., DDS MS, Raleigh, NC).

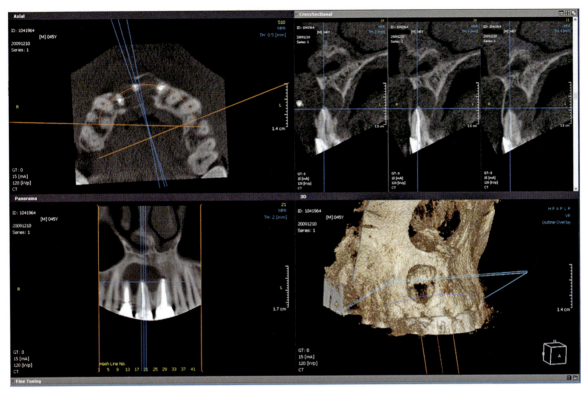

Figure 22.56 Screen capture of the right MAX CI (Courtesy of W. Bruce Howerton, Jr., DDS MS, Raleigh, NC).

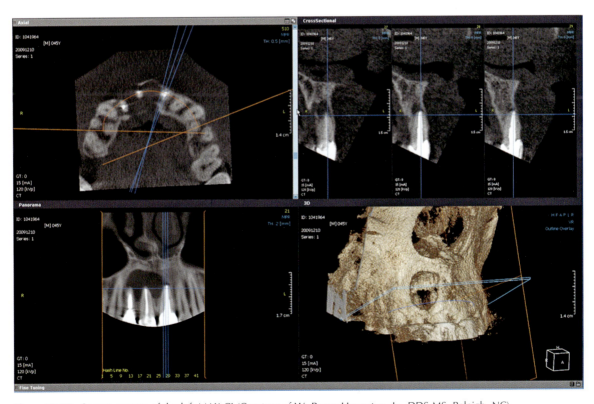

Figure 22.57 Screen capture of the left MAX CI (Courtesy of W. Bruce Howerton, Jr., DDS MS, Raleigh, NC).

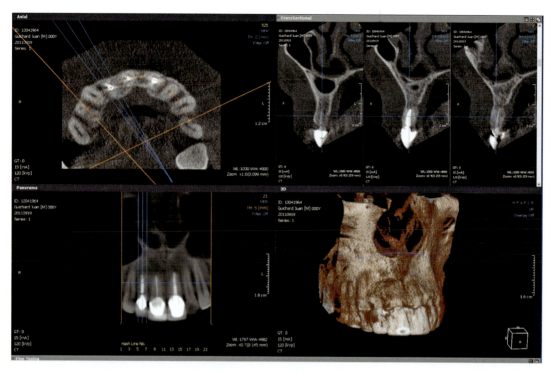

Figure 22.58 Twenty-one months recall screen capture of the right MAX LI demonstrates resolution at the root apex. The sagittal cross sections reveal the lingual cortical border has not reestablished its normal appearance; however, there is a marked improvement in comparison to the preoperative images (Courtesy of W. Bruce Howerton, Jr., DDS MS, Raleigh, NC).

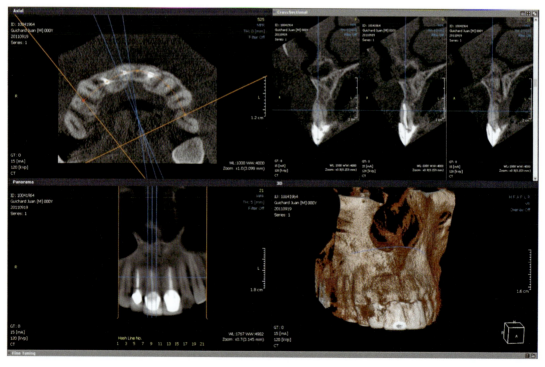

Figure 22.59 Twenty-one months recall screen capture of the right MAX CI showing resolution of the cortical border over the root apex. The far right sagittal cross section reveals a slight apical thickened PDL suggesting delayed healing or presence of a scar tissue (Courtesy of W. Bruce Howerton, Jr., DDS MS, Raleigh, NC).

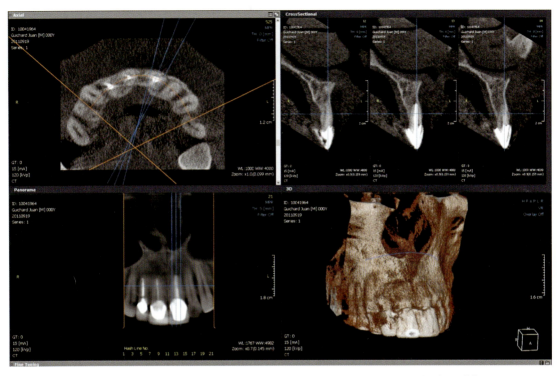

Figure 22.60 Twenty-one months recall screen capture of the left MAX CI suggests excellent healing of the area (Courtesy of W. Bruce Howerton, Jr., DDS MS, Raleigh, NC).

Suggested reading

Costa, F.F., Gaia, B.F., Umetsubo, O.S., and Paraiso Cavalcanti, M.G. (2011) Detection of horizontal root fracture with small-volume cone-beam computed tomography in the presence and absence of intracanal metallic post. *J Endod*, 37(10), 1456–1459.

Cotton, T.P., Geisler, T.M., Holden, D.T., Schwartz, S.A., and Schindler, W.G. (2007) Endodontic applications of cone-beam volumetric tomography. *J Endod*, 33(9), 1121–1132.

Kau, C.H. (2011) Cone beam CT of the head and neck: an anatomical atlas. March.

Maillet, M., Bowles, W.R., McClanahan, S.L., John, M.T., and Ahmad, M. (2011) Cone-beam computed tomography evaluation of maxillary sinusitis. *J Endod*, 37(6), 753–757.

Miles, D.A. (2008) Color atlas of cone beam volumetric imaging for dental applications. October.

Suter, V.G., Büttner, M., Altermatt, H.J., Reichart, P.A., and Bornstein, M.M. (2011) Expansive nasopalatine duct cysts with nasal involvement mimicking apical lesions of endodontic origin: a report of two cases. *J Endod*, 37(9), 1320–1326.

Zoller, J.E. (2008) Cone-beam volumetric imaging in dental, oral, and maxillofacial medicine: fundamental, diagnostics and treatment planning. July.

Appendix

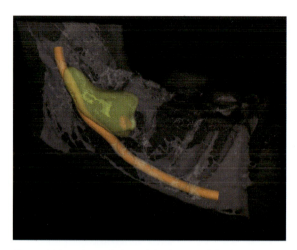

Figure A22.1   Buccal view of the impacted third molar to the inferior alveolar nerve.

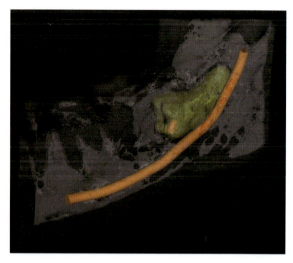

Figure A22.2   Lingual view of the impacted third molar to the inferior alveolar nerve.

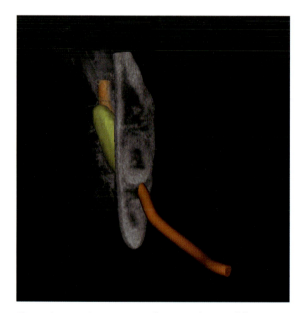

Figure A22.3   Cross section of a coronal view of the relationship of the impacted third molar tooth to the inferior alveolar nerve.

23 Clinical Impact of Cone Beam Computed Tomography in Root Canal Treatment

Carlos Bóveda Z.

Radiological examination is essential for diagnosis, treatment planning, management, and follow-up of endodontic disease. Until recently, this has been usually limited to two-dimensional periapical images. The interpretation of these images is difficult due to the limitations of its nature, where superimposition of the teeth and surrounding dentoalveolar structures reveals only limited aspects of the true three-dimensional configuration (Patel et al., 2007). Also, geometric distortion of the structures imaged is a common occurrence with conventional techniques (Grondahl and Huumonen, 2004). In consequence, essential images of the anatomy are not visible.

Clinical endodontics is heavily dependent on the ability of the practitioner to recognize and successfully deal with the complexities of root canal anatomy. An inability to detect, locate, and negotiate all root canals may lead to endodontic failure (Leonardo, 1998). As we know, anatomy varies significantly, even within the same tooth. A clear example is the mandibular first molar, the most endodontically treated tooth. Different studies show an incidence of a third root in around 13% of the cases. Three canals were present in 61.3%, 4 canals in 35.7%, and 5 canals in approximately 1%.

Root canal configuration of the mesial root revealed 2 canals in 94.4% and 3 canals in 2.3%. The presence of isthmus communications averaged 54.8% on the mesial and 20.2% on the distal root (Valencia de Pablo et al., 2010).

With a chance of there being unusual and atypical root shapes and numbers, there is a need to look further into what a clinician can see or imagine with conventional radiography. In terms of clinical approach, it means that each tooth requiring endodontic treatment needs to be searched clinically for all its possible anatomical variations. This usually results in extensive removal of tooth structure.

These limitations have been overcome with the use of cone beam computed tomography (CBCT) imaging, by providing high-quality three-dimensional views of the tooth and surrounding structures, with interrelational images in three orthogonal planes (axial, sagittal, and coronal). This enables the practitioner to visualize selected slices, evaluating endodontic anatomy and disease in a new way (Cotton et al., 2007). Most softwares provide multiplanar reformation (as oblique cross sections) useful for endodontic evaluation, where the reconstructed CBCT data can be reoriented

Endodontic Radiology, Second Edition. Edited by Bettina Basrani.
© 2012 John Wiley & Sons, Inc. Published 2012 by John Wiley & Sons, Inc.

and sectioned perpendicular to the plane of interest.

CBCT is changing the way the endodontic treatment is prepared and performed, as it has been validated as a tool to explore root canal anatomy. When reconstructions of root canal systems given by a CBCT (small field of view) equipment were compared with histological sections to evaluate the reliability of the reconstructions, strong to very strong correlation was found (Micheti et al., 2010). Small or limited field of view CBCT equipment are preferred for endodontic tasks because of the need for the highest possible resolution (less than 200 μm), the decreased radiation exposure to the patient, and to focus on the area of interest.

With high-resolution CBCT we are able to obtain a detailed identification of the root canal system, its variations, and anomalies; the position and size of the pulp chamber; calcifications; the number, position, size, extent, and curvatures of the roots and its canals; the tridimensional shape of each canal: whether it is round, oval, or has any other form at any specific level of the root; as well as the status of the surrounding bone.

All these information, combined with resources and technologies available in our field, such as magnification, increased illumination, ultraflexible instruments, and advanced irrigation have an impact on the approach and the procedures we use, as shown on the clinical cases that follow. They provide for significant smaller endodontic access cavities and more precise cleaning, shaping, and obturation maneuvers, preserving coronal and radicular tooth structure.

With the appropriate imaging technology, we should stop exploring every case searching for what "might be" in root canal anatomy and concentrate in what is "really present" in the tooth we are treating.

Case 1

Maxillary central incisor, necrotic. Front clinical view (Figure 23.1), a fistula was present. Comparison between pretreatment periapical X-ray (Figure 23.2) and CBCT slices, coronal (Figure 23.3), axial (Figure 23.4), and sagittal (Figure 23.5). A more incisal access cavity, as suggested by the CBCT reconstruction (Figure 23.6) resulted in an improved straight line access (Figures 23.7 and 23.8). Calcium hydoxide placed between visits (Figures 23.9 and 23.10). Final preparation (Figure 23.11) and obturation (Figures 23.12 and 23.13). Appearance of the procedure on a periapical X-ray (Figure 23.14) and CBCT slices, coronal (Figure 23.15), axial (Figure 23.16), and sagittal (Figure 23.17). Restored tooth, no fistula (Figure 23.18) (restoration by Dr. Tomás Seif R., Caracas, Venezuela).

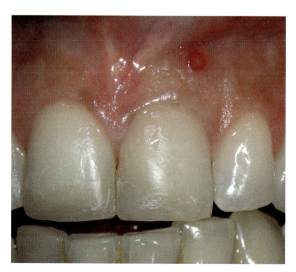

Figure 23.1 Front clinical view.

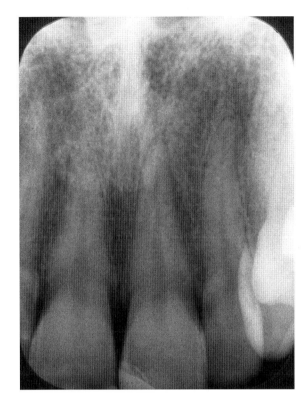

Figure 23.2   Pretreatment periapical X-ray.

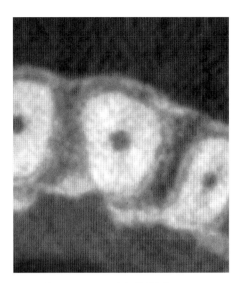

Figure 23.4   Pretreatment axial CBCT slice.

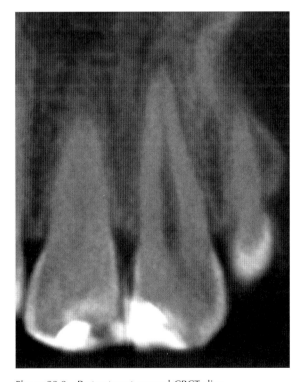

Figure 23.3   Pretreatment coronal CBCT slice.

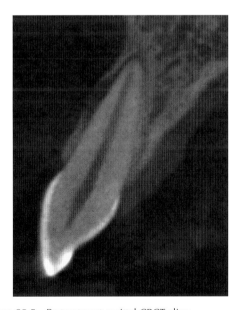

Figure 23.5   Pretreatment sagittal CBCT slice.

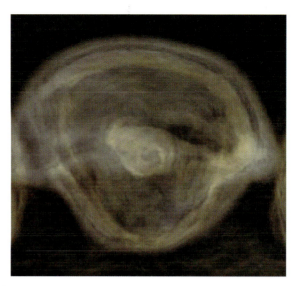

Figure 23.6 CBCT reconstruction.

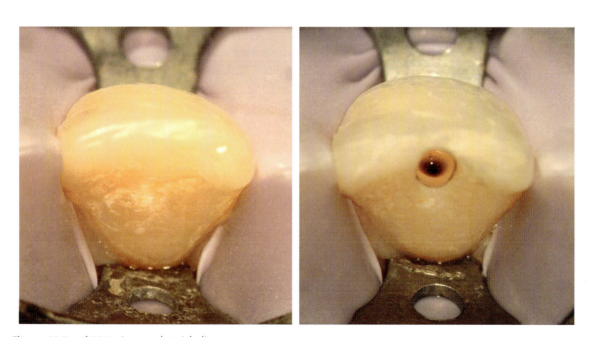

Figures 23.7 and 23.8 Improved straight line access.

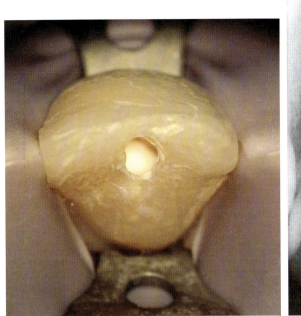 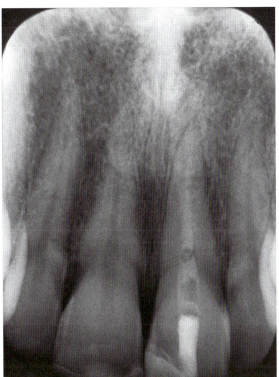

Figures 23.9 and 23.10 Calcium hydoxide placed between visits.

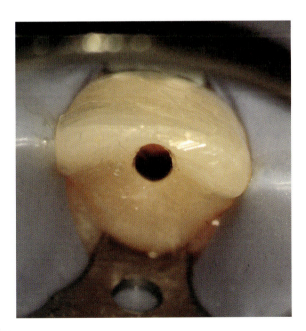

Figure 23.11 Final preparation.

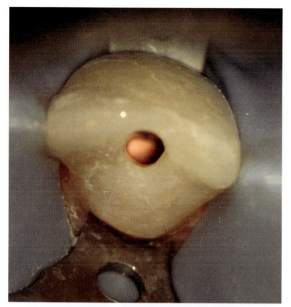

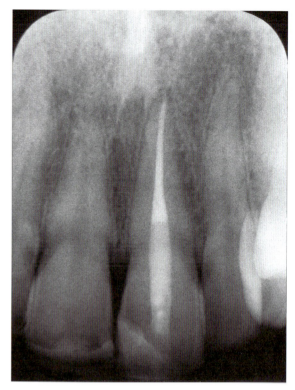

Figure 23.14   Appearance of the procedure on periapical X-ray.

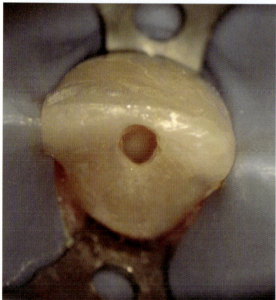

Figure 23.12 and 23.13   Obturation.

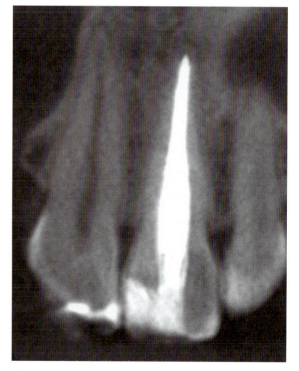

Figure 23.15   Appearance of the procedure on coronal CBCT slice.

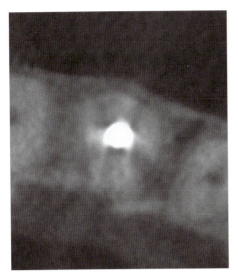

Figure 23.16 Appearance of the procedure on axial CBCT slice.

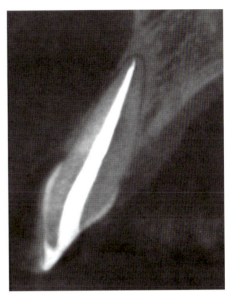

Figure 23.17 Appearance of the procedure on sagittal CBCT slice.

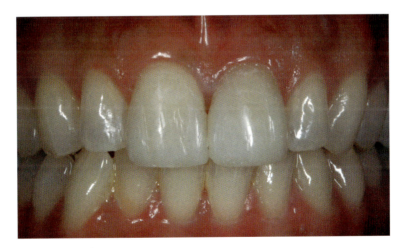

Figure 23.18 Restored tooth, no fistula.

Case 2

Maxillary central and lateral incisors, necrotic, trauma. As seen on pretreatment panoramic X-ray (Figure 23.19), periapical X-ray (Figure 23.20), and CBCT slices, coronal (Figure 23.21), axial (Figure 23.22), and sagittal (Figure 23.23 for the central incisor, Figure 23.24 for the lateral incisor). Note the unusual shapes of the canals, suggested on the X-ray but clearly seen on the CBCT slices. Appearance of the procedure on a periapical X-ray (Figure 23.25) and CBCT slices, coronal (Figure 23.26), axial (Figure 23.27), and sagittal (Figure 23.28 for the central incisor, Figure 23.29 for the lateral incisor).

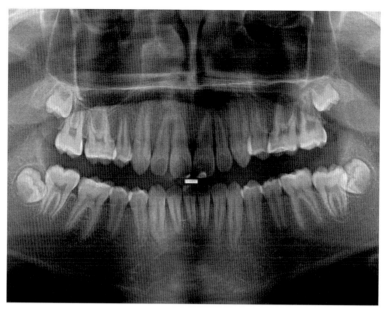

Figure 23.19 Pretreatment panoramic X-ray of maxillary central and lateral incisors, necrotic, trauma.

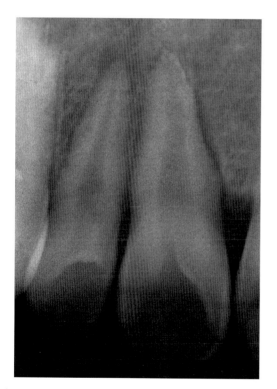

Figure 23.20 Pretreatment periapical X-ray.

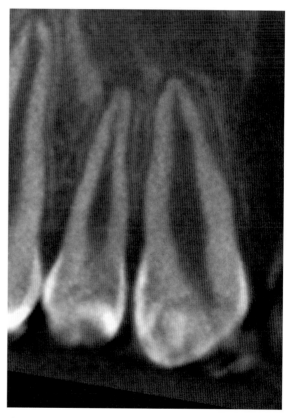

Figure 23.21 Pretreatment coronal CBCT slice.

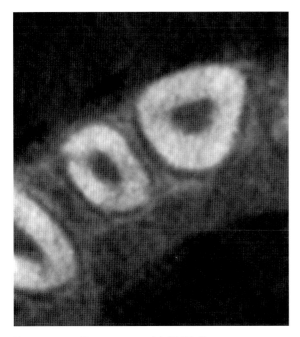

Figure 23.22 Pretreatment axial CBCT slice.

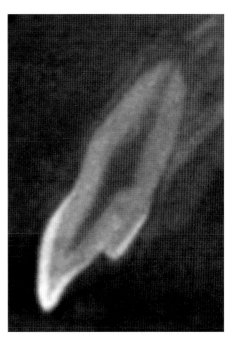

Figure 23.24 Pretreatment sagittal CBCT slice of the lateral incisor.

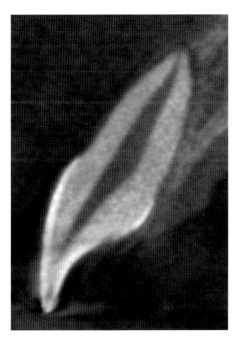

Figure 23.23 Pretreatment sagittal CBCT slice of central incisor.

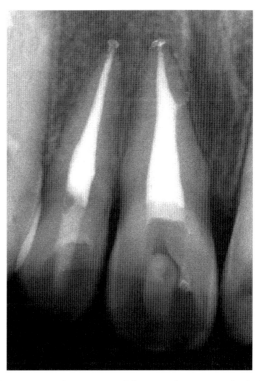

Figure 23.25 Appearance of the procedure on a periapical X-ray.

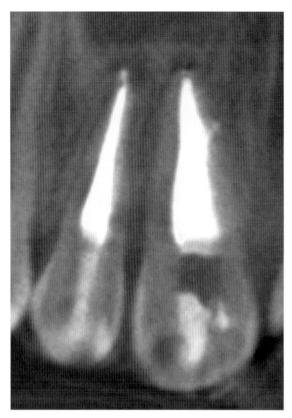

Figure 23.26 Appearance of the procedure on coronal CBCT slice.

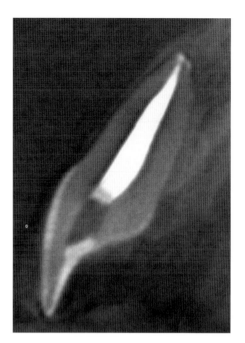

Figure 23.28 Appearance of the procedure on sagittal CBCT slice of the central incisor.

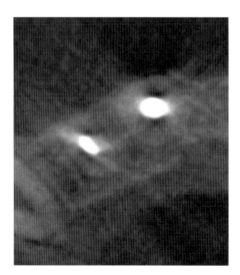

Figure 23.27 Appearance of the procedure on axial CBCT slice.

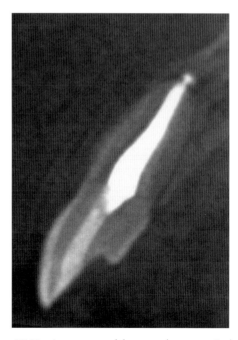

Figure 23.29 Appearance of the procedure on sagittal CBCT slice of the lateral incisor.

Case 3

Maxillary canine, irreversible pulpitis. As seen on pretreatment panoramic X-ray (Figure 23.30), periapical X-ray (Figure 23.31), and CBCT slices, coronal (Figure 23.32), sagittal (Figure 23.33), and axial (Figure 23.34). Appearance of the procedure on a panoramic X-ray (Figure 23.35), periapical X-ray (Figure 23.36), and CBCT slices, coronal (Figure 23.37), sagittal (Figure 23.38), and axial (Figure 23.39). Again, a more incisal approach results in tooth structure preservation.

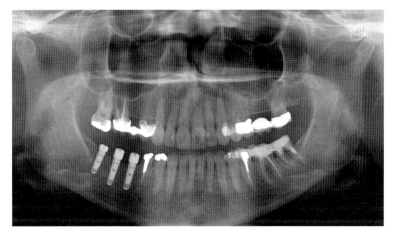

Figure 23.30   Pretreatment panoramic X-ray.

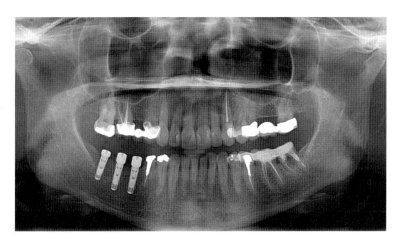

Figure 23.31   Appearance of the procedure on a panoramic X-ray.

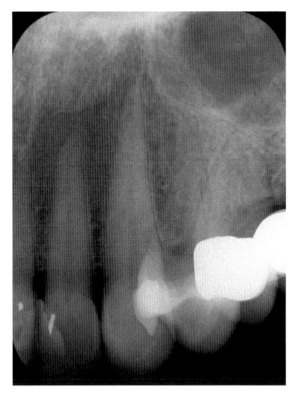

Figure 23.32   Pretreatment periapical X-ray.

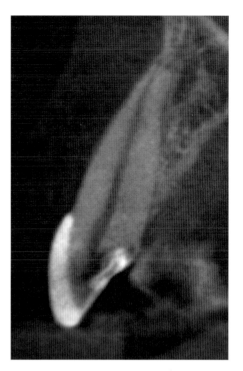

Figure 23.34   Pretreatment sagittal CBCT slice.

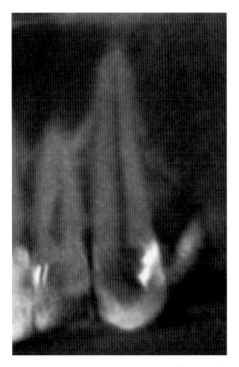

Figure 23.33   Case 3: Pretreatment coronal CBCT slice.

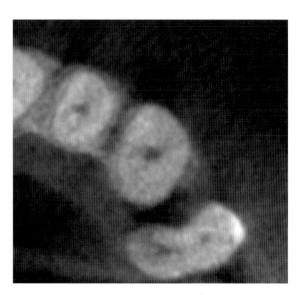

Figure 23.35   Pretreatment axial CBCT slice.

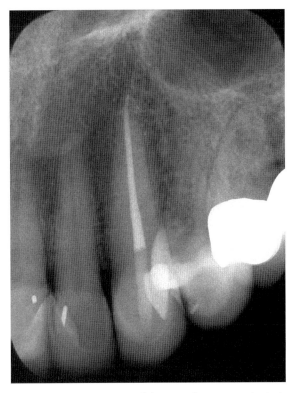

Figure 23.36 Appearance of the procedure on a periapical X-ray.

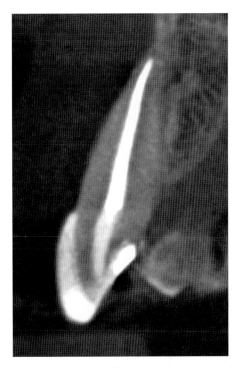

Figure 23.38 Appearance of the procedure on sagittal CBCT slice.

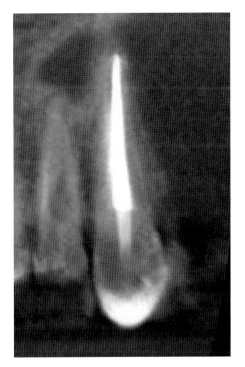

Figure 23.37 Appearance of the procedure on coronal CBCT slice.

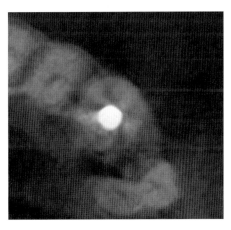

Figure 23.39 Appearance of the procedure on axial CBCT slice.

Case 4

Maxillary first bicuspid, irreversible pulpitis, caries. Comparison between pretreatment periapical X-ray (Figure 23.40) and CBCT slices, sagittal (Figure 23.41), axial, different levels (Figures 23.42–23.44), and coronal (Figure 23.45). Clinical approach: Isolation (Figure 23.46) CBCT reconstruction, occlusal view (Figure 23.47). Outline of a conventional approach as suggested for the location of the canals (Figure 23.48). Actual approach (Figures 23.49 and 23.50). Comparison on the outline of the conventional approach and the actual approach (Figure 23.51). This reduced access cavity impedes the simultaneous views and handling of both canals; however, it is enough for accessing as single canals. Occlusal view of the buccal canal (Figure 23.52) and palatal canal (Figure 23.53). Obturation (Figures 23.54–23.56). Restored tooth (Figure 23.57) (restoration by Dr. Tomás Seif R., Caracas, Venezuela). Appearance of the procedure on a periapical X-ray (Figure 23.58) and CBCT slices, axial, different levels (Figures 23.59 and 23.60), and coronal (Figure 23.61)

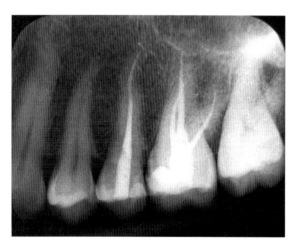

Figure 23.40 Pretreatment periapical X-ray.

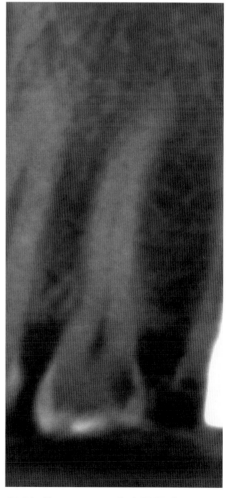

Figure 23.41 Pretreatment sagittal CBCT slice.

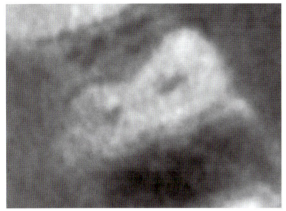

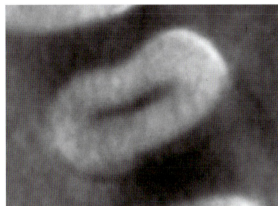

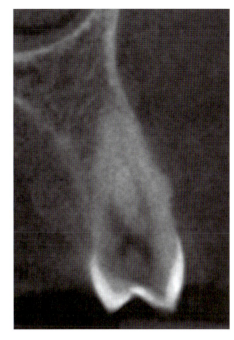

Figure 23.45 Pretreatment coronal CBCT slice.

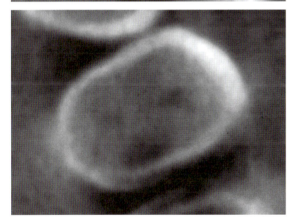

Figures 23.42–23.44 Pretreatment axial CBCT slices of different levels.

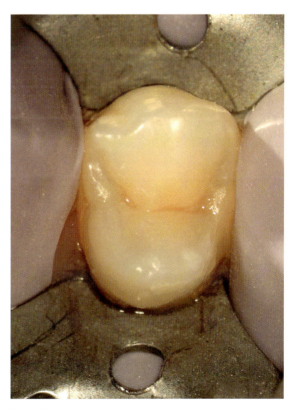

Figure 23.46 Isolation.

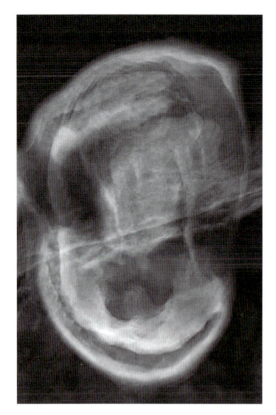

Figure 23.47 CBCT occlusal view.

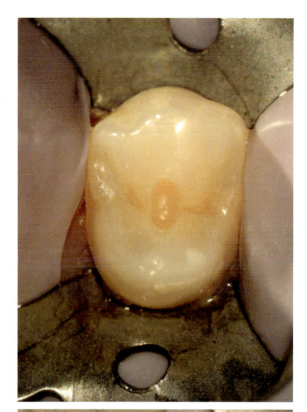

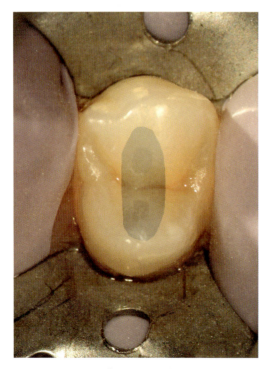

Figure 23.48 Suggested conventional approach for the location of the canals.

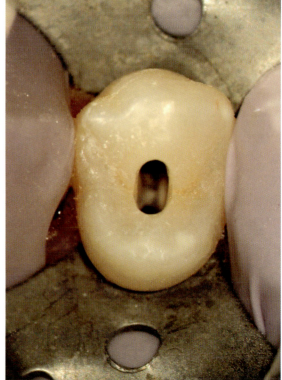

Figures 23.49 and 23.50 Actual approach for the location of the canals.

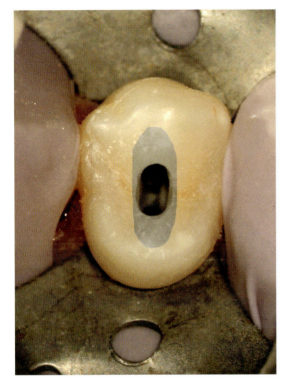

Figure 23.51 Comparison on the outline of the conventional approach and the actual approach.

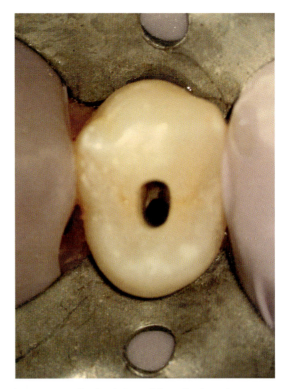

Figure 23.53 Occlusal view of the palatal canal.

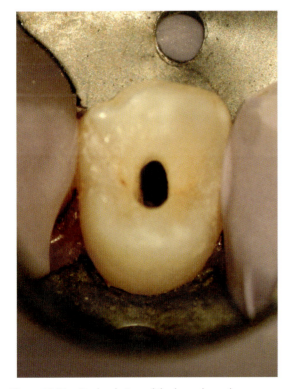

Figure 23.52 Occlusal view of the buccal canal.

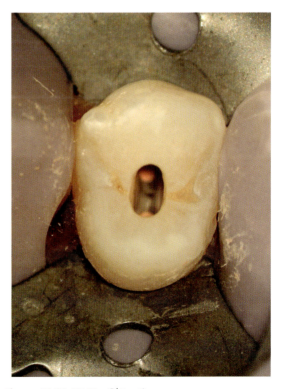

Figures 23.54–23.56 Obturation.

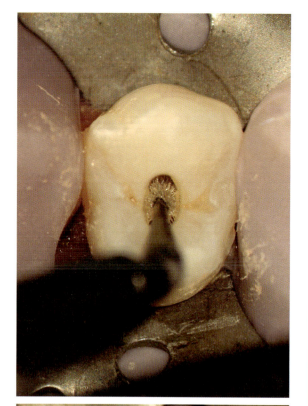

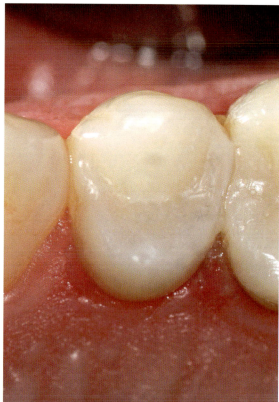

Figure 23.57 Restored tooth.

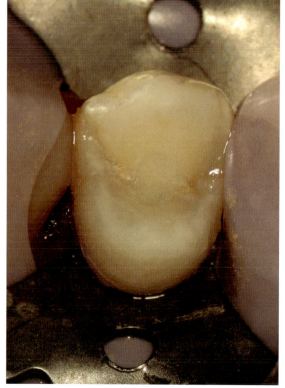

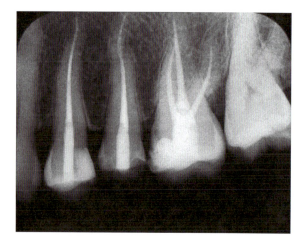

Figure 23.58 Appearance of the procedure on a periapical X-ray.

Figures 23.54–23.56 *(Continued)*

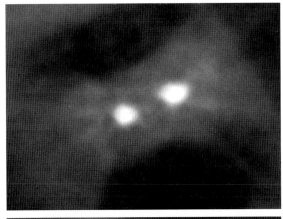

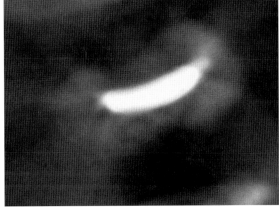

Figures 23.59 and 23.60   Appearance of the procedure on axial CBCT slices at different levels.

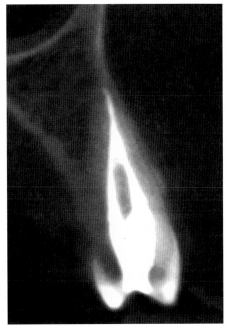

Figure 23.61   Appearance of the procedure on coronal CBCT slice.

Case 5

Maxillary first molar, irreversible pulpitis. Comparison between pretreatment periapical X-ray (Figures 23.62 and 23.63) and CBCT slices, sagittal (Figure 23.64), coronal (Figure 23.65), and axial, different levels (Figures 23.66–23.68). Note the certainty of the four canal configuration, as two canals are clearly seen on the MB root. Clinical approach: Isolation (Figure 23.69) Outline of a conventional approach as suggested for the location of the canals (Figure 23.70). Actual approach (Figure 23.71). Comparison on the outline of a conventional approach and the actual access cavity (Figure 23.72). Obturation (Figures 23.73 and 23.74). Access cavity seal (Figure 23.75). Appearance of the procedure on a periapical X-ray (Figure 23.76) and CBCT slices, sagittal (Figure 23.77), axial (Figure 23.78), and coronal (Figure 23.79).

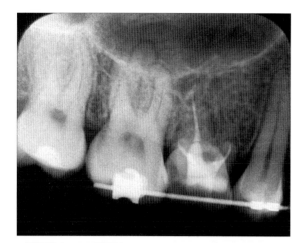

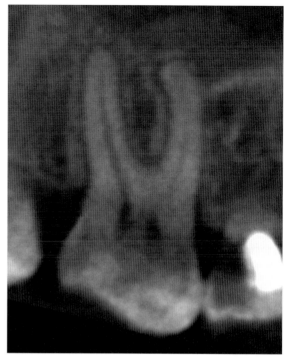

Figure 23.64   Pretreatment sagittal CBCT slice.

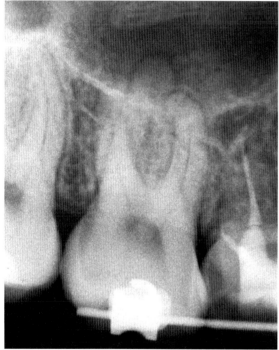

Figures 23.62 and 23.63   Pretreatment periapical X-ray.

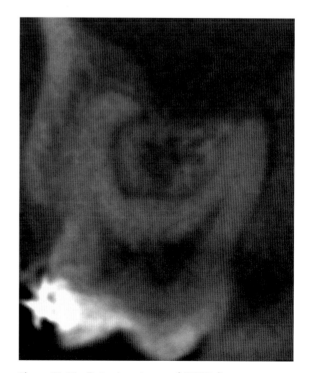

Figure 23.65   Pretreatment coronal CBCT slice.

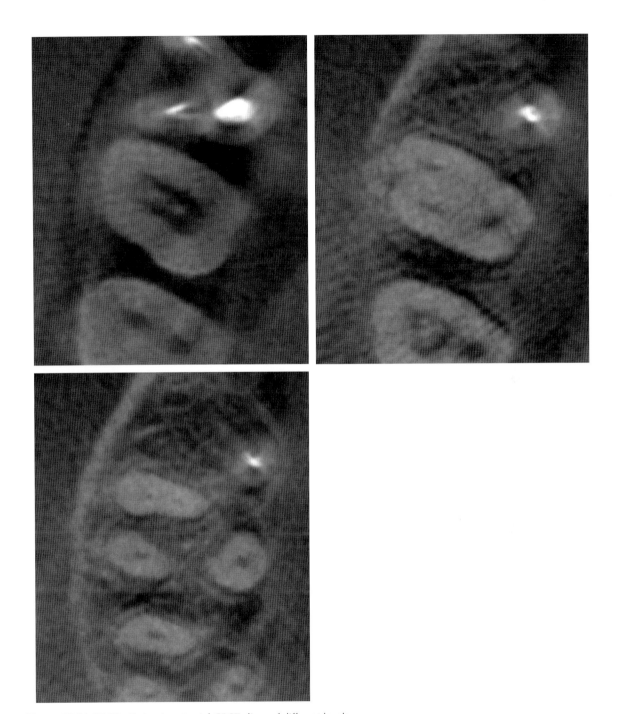

Figures 23.66–23.68 Pretreatment axial CBCT slices of different levels.

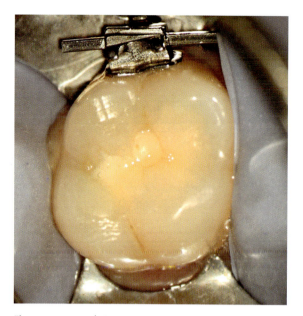

Figure 23.69 Isolation.

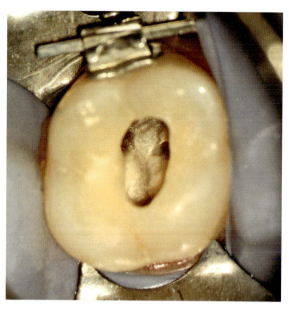

Figure 23.71 Actual approach for the location of the canals.

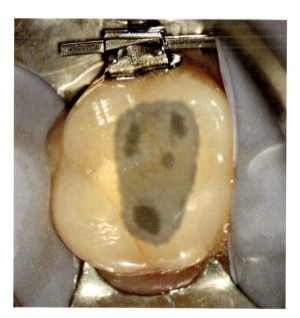

Figure 23.70 Suggested conventional approach for the location of the canals.

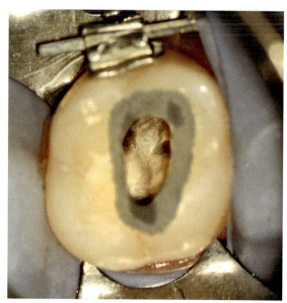

Figure 23.72 Comparison on the outline of a conventional approach and the actual access cavity.

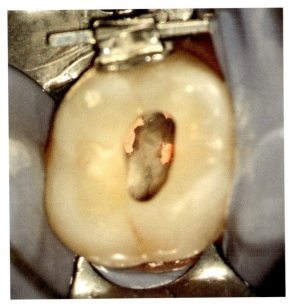

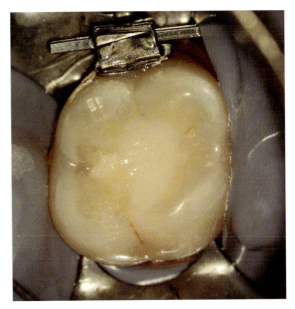

Figure 23.75 Access cavity seal.

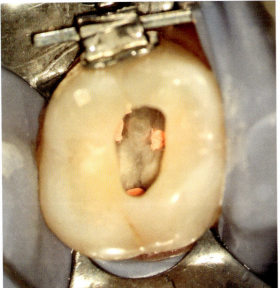

Figures 23.73 and 23.74 Obturation.

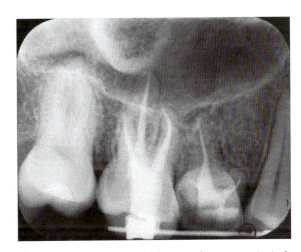

Figure 23.76 Appearance of the procedure on a periapical X-ray.

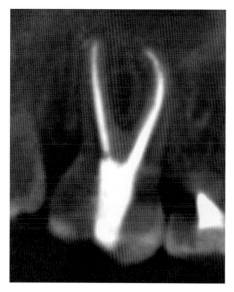

Figure 23.77   Appearance of the procedure on sagittal CBCT slice.

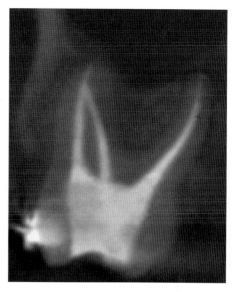

Figure 23.79   Appearance of the procedure on coronal CBCT slice.

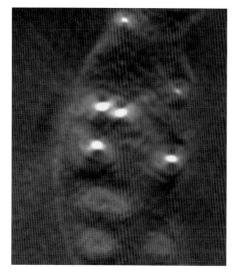

Figure 23.78   Appearance of the procedure on axial CBCT slice.

Case 6

Mandibular lateral incisors, irreversible pulpitis, restorative etiology. Comparison between pretreatment periapical X-rays (Figures 23.80 and 23.81) and CBCT slices, sagittal (Figures 23.82 and 23.83). Note the two canal configuration of both teeth, detailed by the oblique reformation of the CBCT data for each tooth, as the original position of these teeth in the CBCT scan does not necessarily match a perpendicular approach to the view of interest. Volume reconstruction of the entire data (Figure 23.84). Appearance of the procedure on a periapical X-rays (Figures 23.85 and 23.86) and CBCT slices, sagittal (Figures 23.87 and 23.88).

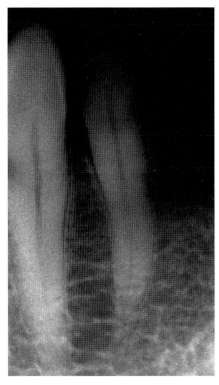

Figure 23.80 Pretreatment periapical X-ray, mandibular right lateral incisor.

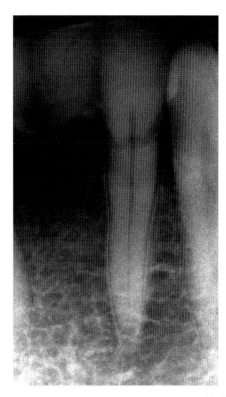

Figure 23.82 Pretreatment periapical X-ray, mandibular left lateral incisor.

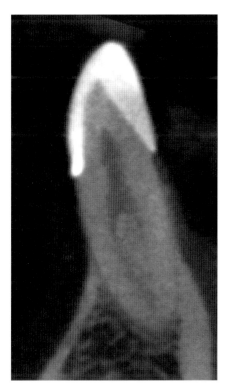

Figure 23.81 Pretreatment sagittal CBCT slice, mandibular right lateral incisor.

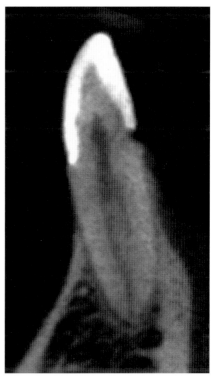

Figure 23.83 Pretreatment sagittal CBCT slice, mandibular left lateral incisor.

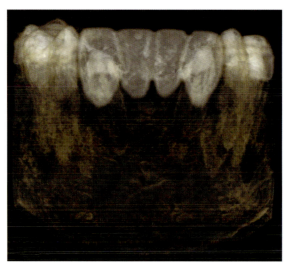

Figure 23.84 Volume reconstruction of the entire data.

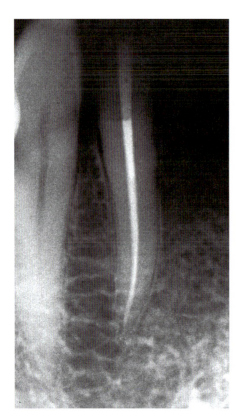

Figure 23.85 Appearance of the procedure on a periapical X-ray, mandibular right lateral incisor.

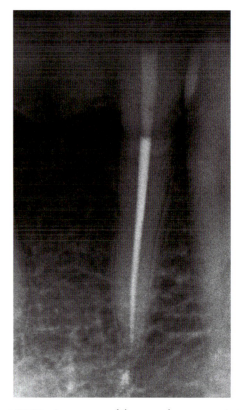

Figure 23.86 Appearance of the procedure on a periapical X-ray, mandibular left lateral incisor.

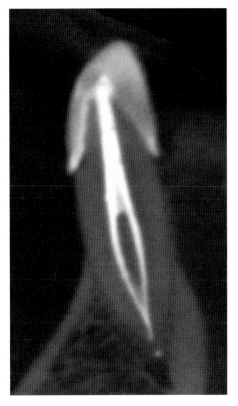

Figure 23.87   Appearance of the procedure on sagittal CBCT slice, mandibular right lateral incisor.

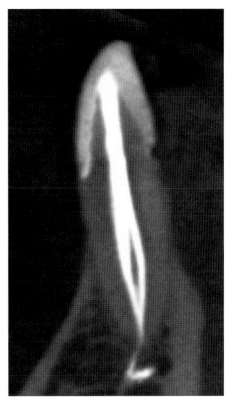

Figure 23.88   Appearance of the procedure on sagittal CBCT slice, mandibular left lateral incisor.

Case 7

Mandibular first bicuspid, necrotic, orthodontic etiology. Comparison between pretreatment panoramic X-ray (Figure 23.89), periapical X-ray (Figure 23.90), and CBCT slices, sagittal (Figure 23.91), coronal (Figure 23.92), and axial, different levels (Figures 23.93 and 23.94). Note the bifurca-tion of the canal, suggested on the X-ray but clearly seen on the CBCT slices. Clinical approach: Isolation (Figure 23.95), preparation (Figure 23.96), and obturation (Figure 23.97). Appearance of the procedure on a periapical X-ray (Figure 23.98) and CBCT slices, axial (Figure 23.99) and coronal (Figure 23.100).

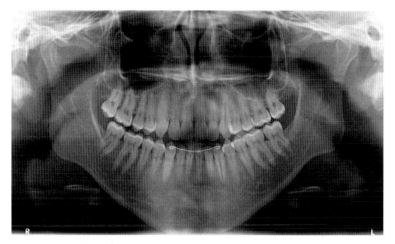

Figure 23.89   Pretreatment panoramic X-ray

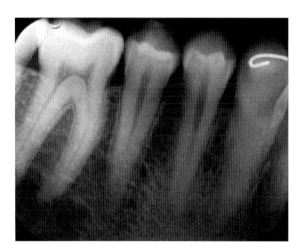

Figure 23.90   Pretreatment periapical X-ray.

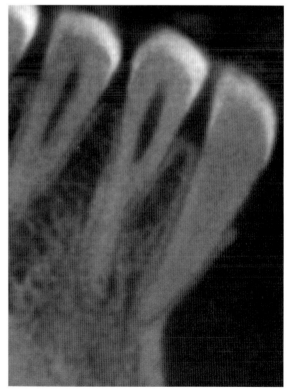

Figure 23.91   Pretreatment sagittal CBCT slice.

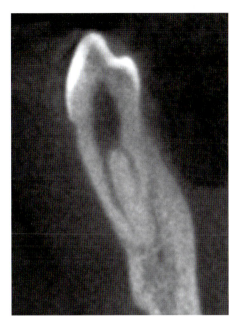

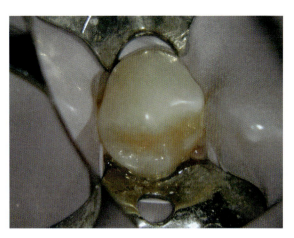

Figure 23.95   Isolation.

Figure 23.92   Pretreatment coronal CBCT slice.

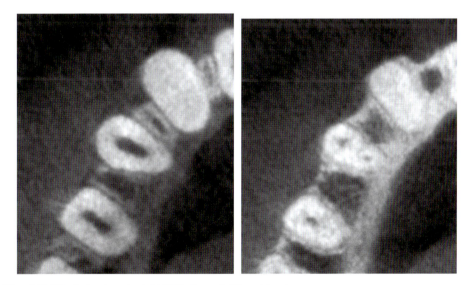

Figures 23.93 and 23.94   Pretreatment axial CBCT slices of different levels.

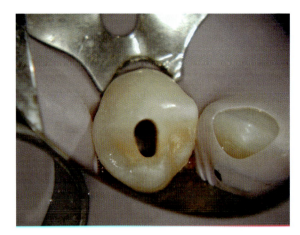

Figure 23.96 Preparation.

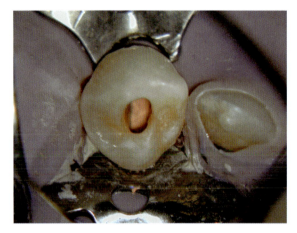

Figure 23.97 Obturation.

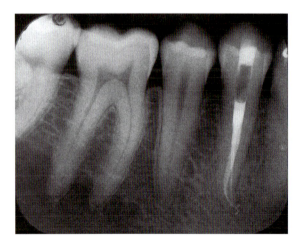

Figure 23.98 Appearance of the procedure on a periapical X-ray.

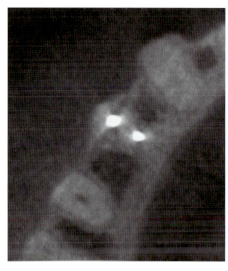

Figure 23.99 Appearance of the procedure on axial CBCT slice.

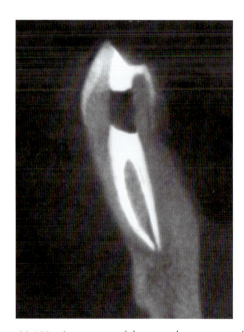

Figure 23.100 Appearance of the procedure on coronal CBCT slice.

Case 8

Mandibular first and second bicuspids, necrotics, orthodontic etiology. Comparison between pretreatment periapical X-ray (Figure 23.101) and CBCT slices, sagittal (Figure 23.102), coronal (Figure 23.103, first bicuspid, Figure 23.104, second bicuspid), and axial, different levels (Figures 23.105 and 23.106). Clinical approach: Access cavities (Figure 23.107, first bicuspid, Figure 23.108, second bicuspid). Evolution of the case with calcium hydroxide in it, periapical X-rays, at the time it was placed (Figure 23.109), 2-month period (Figure 23.110) and 4-month period (Figure 23.111). Obturation (Figure 23.112, first bicuspid, Figure 23.113, second bicuspid) Appearance of the procedure on a periapical X-ray (Figure 23.114) and CBCT slices, sagittal (Figure 23.115), coronal (Figure 23.116, first bicuspid, Figure 23.117, second bicuspid), axial, different levels (Figures 23.118 and 23.119). Restored teeth (restorations: Dr. Marines Senior D., Caracas, Venezuela) (Figure 23.120). Periapical X-ray, 6-month recall (Figure 23.121).

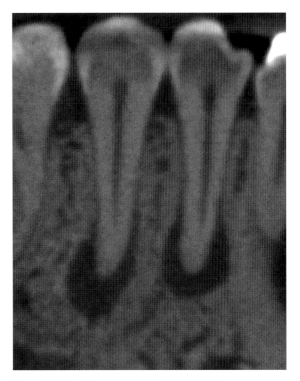

Figure 23.102   Pretreatment sagittal CBCT slice.

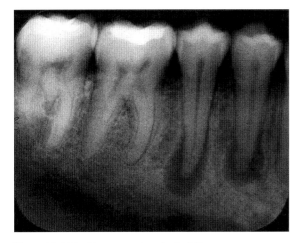

Figure 23.101   Pretreatment periapical X-ray.

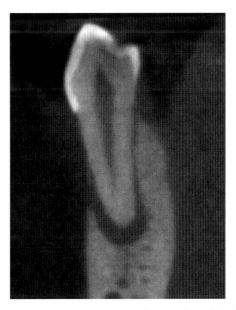

Figure 23.103   Pretreatment coronal CBCT slice of the first bicuspid.

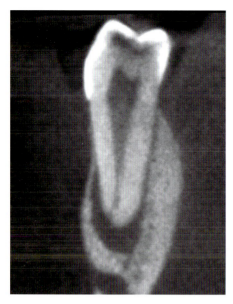

Figure 23.104 Pretreatment coronal CBCT slice of the second bicuspid.

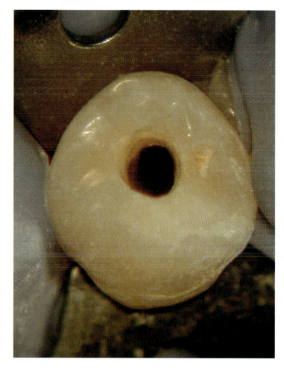

Figure 23.107 Access cavity, first bicuspid.

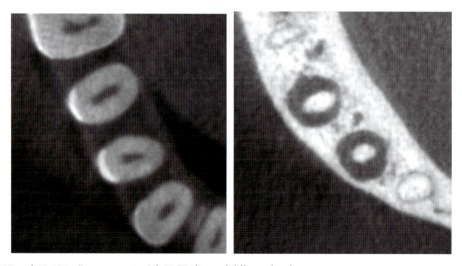

Figures 23.105 and 23.106 Pretreatment axial CBCT slices of different levels.

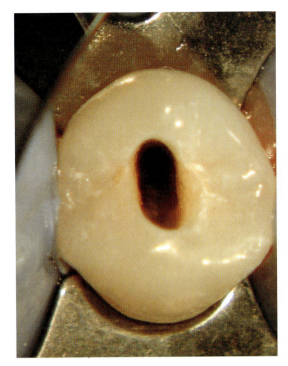

Figure 23.108 Access cavity, second bicuspid.

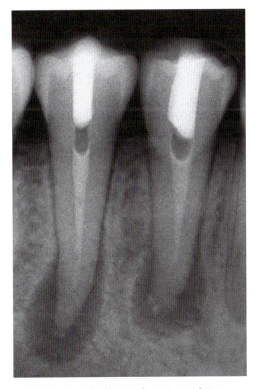

Figure 23.109 Periphical X-ray from time calcium hydroxide was placed.

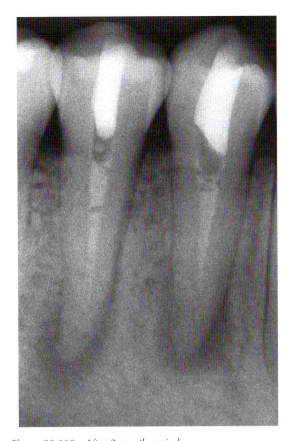

Figure 23.110 After 2-month period.

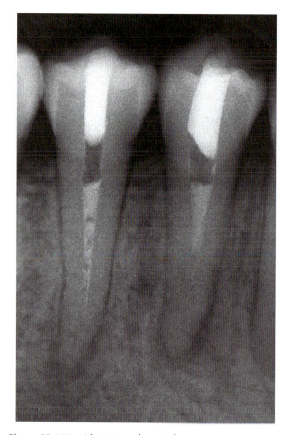

Figure 23.111   After 4-month period.

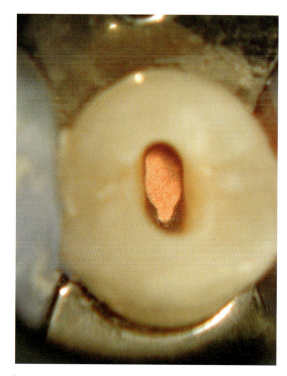

Figure 23.113   Obturation, second bicuspid.

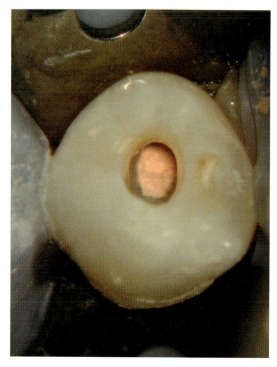

Figure 23.112   Obturation, first bicuspid.

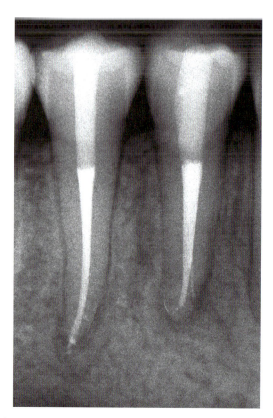

Figure 23.114   Appearance of the procedure on a periapical X-ray.

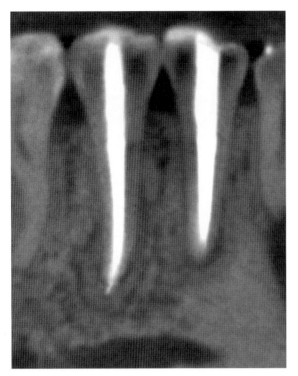

Figure 23.115 Appearance of the procedure on sagittal CBCT slice.

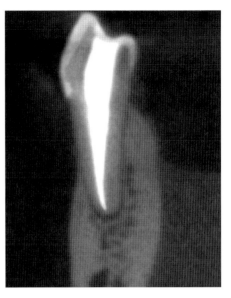

Figure 23.116 Appearance of the procedure on coronal CBCT slice of first bicuspid.

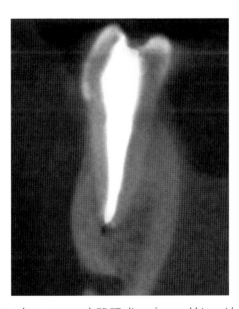

Figure 23.117 Appearance of the procedure on coronal CBCT slice of second bicuspid.

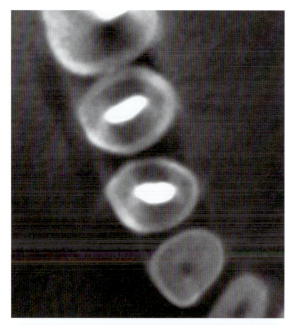

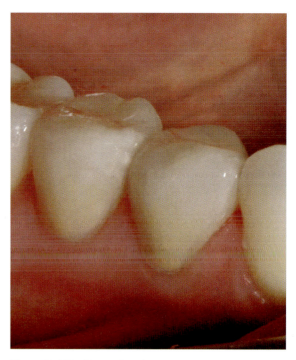

Figure 23.120   Restored teeth.

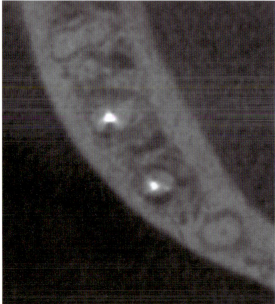

Figures 23.118 and 23.119   Appearance of the procedure on axial CBCT slices of different levels.

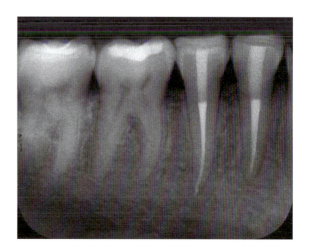

Figure 23.121   Periapical X-ray, 6-month recall.

Case 9

Mandibular first molar, irreversible pulpitis. Comparison between pretreatment periapical X-ray (Figure 23.122) and CBCT slices, sagittal (Figure 23.123), coronal (mesial root, Figure 23.124, distal root, Figure 23.125), and axial, pulp horns level (Figure 23.126), pulp chamber level (Figure 23.127), pulp floor level (Figure 23.128), radicular level (Figure 23.129). Note the round shape of mesial canals and the oval shape of the distal canal. Clinical approach: isolation (Figure 23.130) superimposition of the outline of the pulp chamber and location of the canals, describing the extension of a conventional access cavity (Figure 23.131). Actual access cavity (Figure 23.132). Again, this reduced access cavity impedes the simultaneous views and handling of all canals; however, it is enough for accessing them as single canals. Obturation (mesial canals, Figure 23.133, distal canal, Figure 23.134). Superimposition of the access cavity and the projected canals (Figure 23.135). Appearance of the procedure on a periapical X-ray (Figure 23.136). Restored tooth (Figure 23.137) (restoration: Dr. Mariela Febres Cordero, Caracas, Venezuela) and CBCT slices, axial, occlusal surface level (Figure 23.138), pulp chamber level (Figure 23.139), pulp floor level (Figure 23.140), sagittal (Figure 23.141), and coronal (mesial root, Figure 23.142, distal root, Figure 23.143).

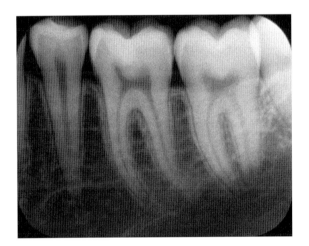

Figure 23.122   Pretreatment periapical X-ray.

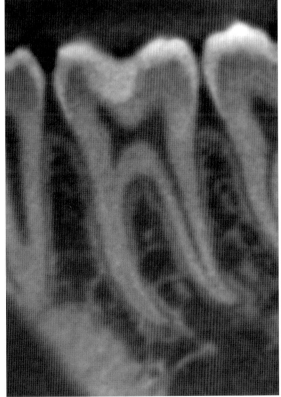

Figure 23.123   Pretreatment sagittal CBCT slice.

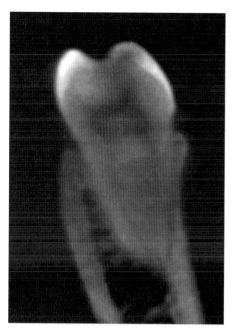

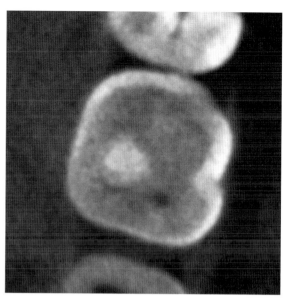

Figure 23.126 Pretreatment axial CBCT slice of pulp horns level.

Figure 23.124 Pretreatment coronal CBCT slice of the mesial root.

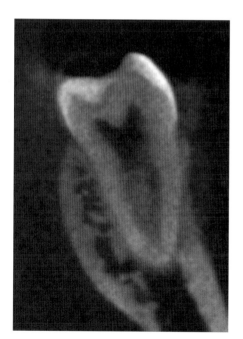

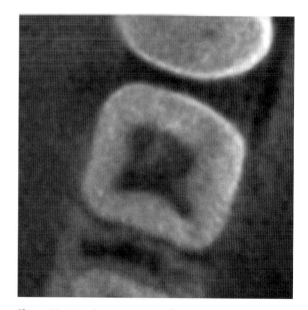

Figure 23.127 Pretreatment axial CBCT slice of pulp chamber level.

Figure 23.125 Pretreatment coronal CBCT slice of distal root.

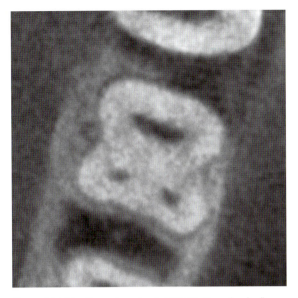

Figure 23.128 Pretreatment axial CBCT slice of pulp floor level.

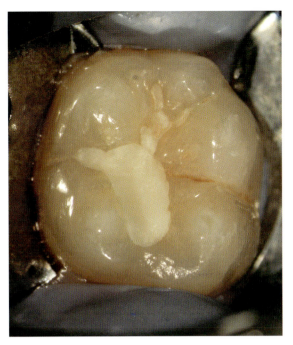

Figure 23.130 Isolation.

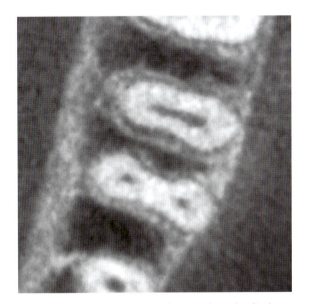

Figure 23.129 Pretreatment axial CBCT slice of radicular level.

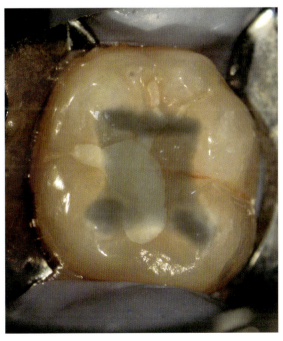

Figure 23.131 Extension of a conventional access cavity.

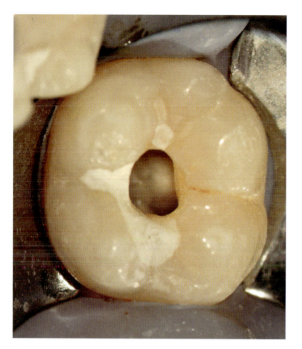

Figure 23.132 Actual access cavity.

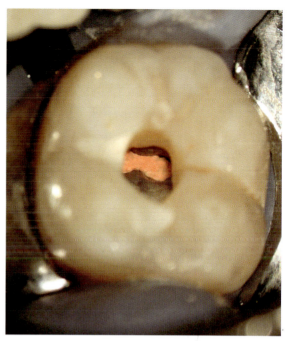

Figure 23.134 Obturation, distal canal.

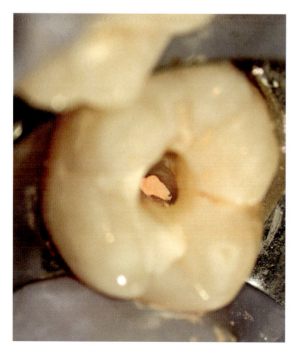

Figure 23.133 Obturation, mesial canals.

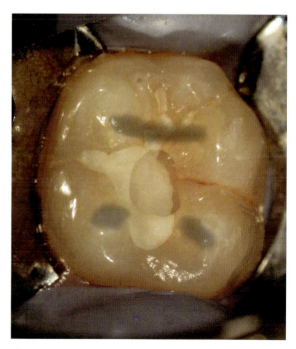

Figure 23.135 Superimposition of the access cavity and the projected canals.

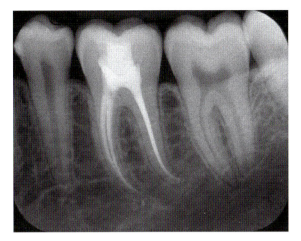

Figure 23.136 Appearance of the procedure on a periapical X-ray.

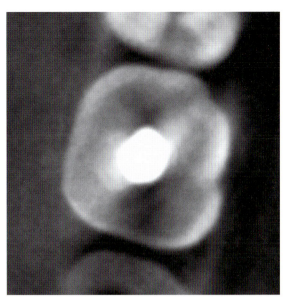

Figure 23.138 Appearance of the procedure on axial CBCT slice at occlusal surface level.

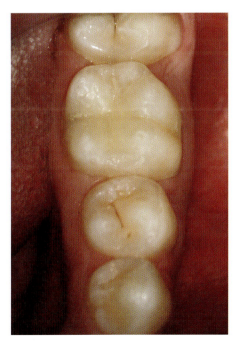

Figure 23.137 Restored tooth.

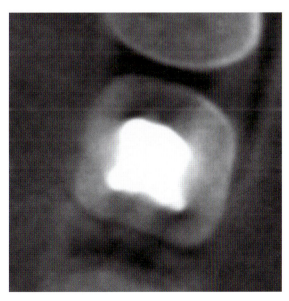

Figure 23.139 Appearance of the procedure on axial CBCT slice at pulp chamber level.

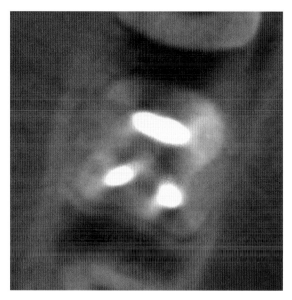

Figure 23.140 Appearance of the procedure on axial CBCT slice at pulp floor level.

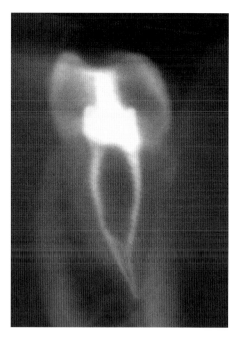

Figure 23.142 Appearance of the procedure on coronal CBCT slice at mesial root.

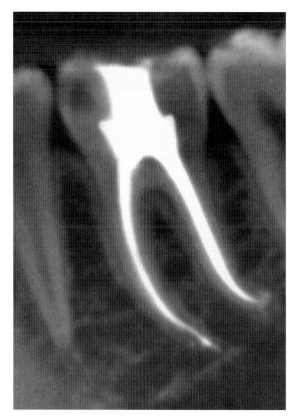

Figure 23.141 Appearance of the procedure on sagittal CBCT slice.

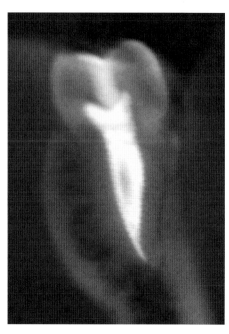

Figure 23.143 Appearance of the procedure on coronal CBCT slice at distal root.

Case 10

Mandibular second molar, irreversible pulpitis, caries. Comparison between pretreatment periapical X-ray (Figure 23.144) and CBCT slices, coronal (Figure 23.145) and axial (Figure 23.146). Note the proximity of the mesial canals, only distinguishable on the CBCT slices. Clinical approach (Figure 23.147). Higher magnification to see in detail the proximity and the isthmus in between mesial canals (Figure 23.148). Obturation (distal canal, Figure 23.149, mesial canals, Figure 23.150). Appearance of the procedure on a periapical X-ray (Figure 23.151) and CBCT slices, coronal (Figure 23.152) and axial (Figure 23.153).

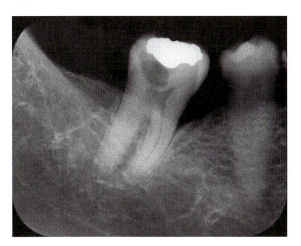

Figure 23.144   Pretreatment periapical X-ray.

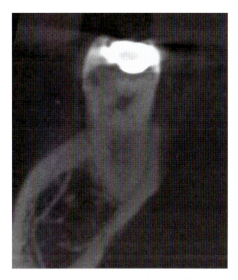

Figure 23.145   Pretreatment coronal CBCT slice.

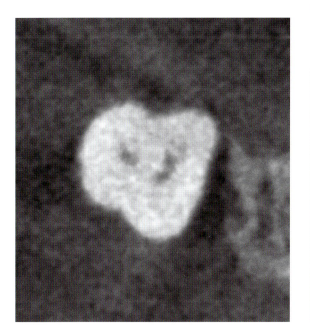

Figure 23.146   Pretreatment axial CBCT slice.

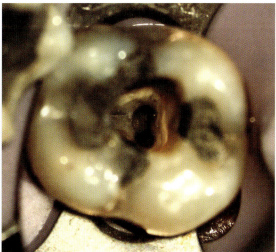

Figure 23.147   Clinical approach.

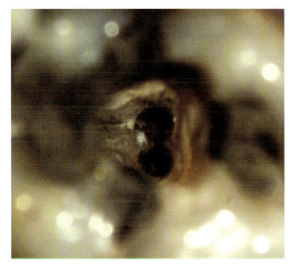

Figure 23.148 Higher magnification to see in detail the proximity and the isthmus in between mesial canals.

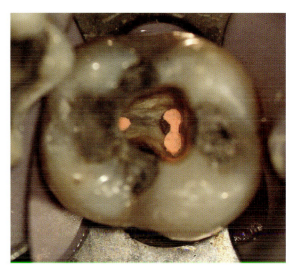

Figure 23.150 Obturation of mesial canals.

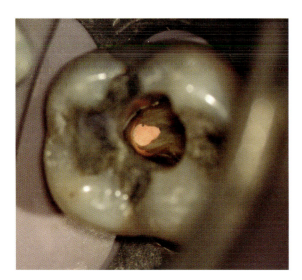

Figure 23.149 Obturation of distal canal.

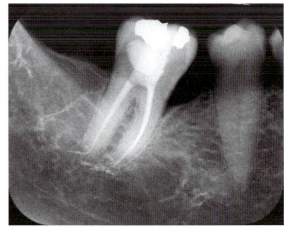

Figure 23.151 Appearance of the procedure on a periapical X-ray.

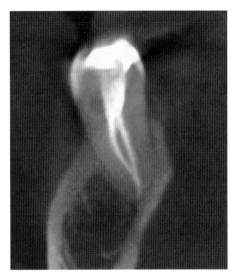

Figure 23.152   Appearance of the procedure on coronal CBCT slice.

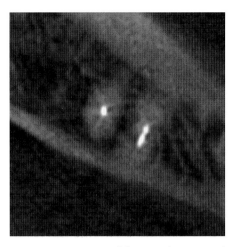

Figure 23.153   Appearance of the procedure on axial CBCT slice.

Case 11

Mandibular second molar, irreversible pulpitis. Comparison between pretreatment periapical X-ray (Figure 23.154) and CBCT slices, sagittal (Figure 23.155), coronal (Figure 23.156), and axial, (Figure 23.157). Note the atypical anatomy, from 1 ribbon C-shape canals (on the axial view) to 2 independent single S-shape canals (on the coronal view). Clinical approach: Isolation (Figure 23.158), access cavity (Figure 23.159), preparation (Figure 23.160), and obturation (Figure 23.161). Appearance of the procedure on a periapical X-ray (Figure 23.162) and CBCT slices, sagittal (Figure 23.163), coronal (Figure 23.164), and axial (Figure 23.165). Restored tooth (Figure 23.166) (restoration Dr. Raul Zajia B., Caracas, Venezuela). Periapical X-ray, 12-month period recall (Figure 23.167).

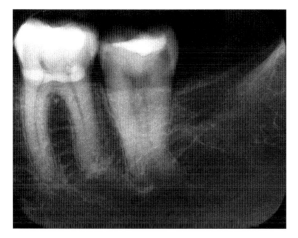

Figure 23.154 Pretreatment periapical X-ray.

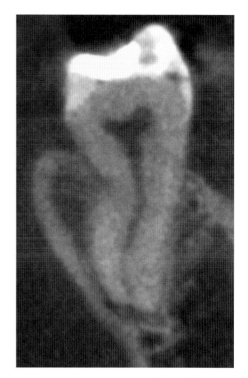

Figure 23.156 Pretreatment coronal CBCT slice.

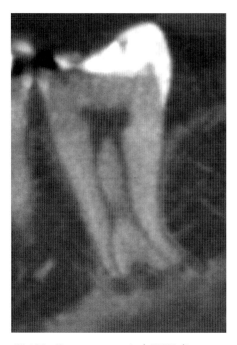

Figure 23.155 Pretreatment sagittal CBCT slice.

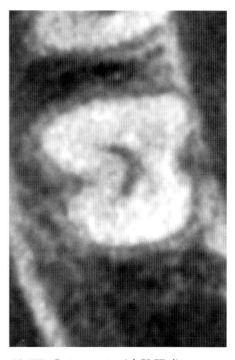

Figure 23.157 Pretreatment axial CBCT slice.

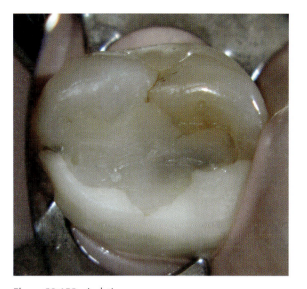

Figure 23.158 Isolation.

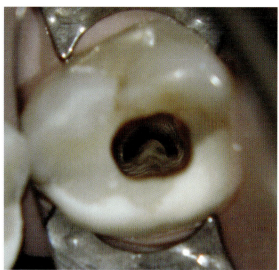

Figure 23.160 Preparation.

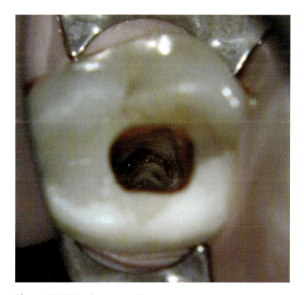

Figure 23.159 Access cavity.

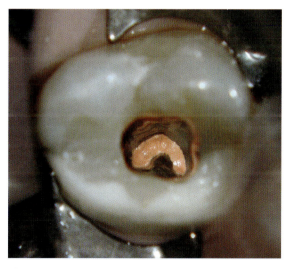

Figure 23.161 Obturation.

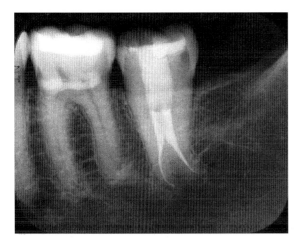

Figure 23.162 Appearance of the procedure on a periapical X-ray.

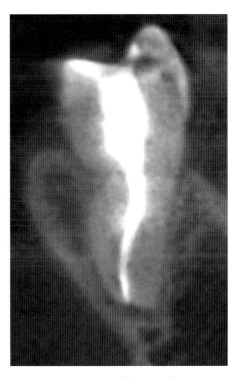

Figure 23.164 Appearance of the procedure on coronal CBCT slice.

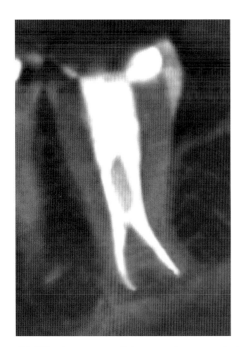

Figure 23.163 Appearance of the procedure on sagittal CBCT slice.

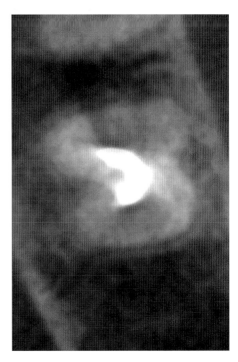

Figure 23.165 Appearance of the procedure on axial CBCT slice.

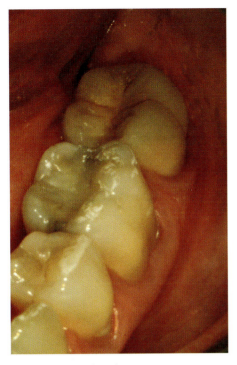

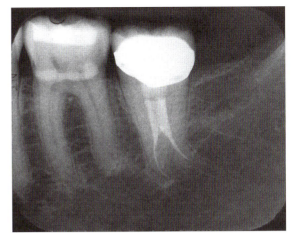

Figure 23.167   Periapical X-ray, 12-month period recall.

Figure 23.166   Restored tooth.

References

Cotton, T.P., et al. (2007) Endodontic applications of cone-beam volumetric tomography. *J Endod*, 33, 1121–1132.

Grondahl, H.G. and Huumonen, S. (2004) Radiographic manifestations of periapical inflammatory lesions. *Endod Top*, 8, 55–67.

Leonardo, M.R. (1998) Aspectos anatômicos da cavidade pulpar: relações com o tratamento de canais radiculares. In: M.R. Leonardo and J.M. Leal, eds., *Endodontia: tratamento de canais radiculares*, 3rd ed. p. 191. Panamericana, São Paulo.

Micheti, J., Maret, D., Mallet, J.P., and Diemer, F. (2010) Validation of cone beam computed tomography as a tool to explore root canal anatomy. *J Endod*, 36(7), 1187–1190.

Patel, S., Dawood, A., Ford, T.P., and Whaites, E. (2007) The potential applications of cone beam computed tomography in the management of endodontic problems. *Int Endod J*, 40(10), 818–830.

Valencia de Pablo, O., et al. (2010) Root anatomy and canal configuration of the permanent mandibular first molar: a systematic review. *J Endod*, 36, 1919–1931.

Index

Abfraction, 154, 157
Abrasion,
  as acquired pathological condition, 157
  dental floss injury, 157
Abscess
  periodontal, 170
  periradicular, 65, 111, 160, 170, 196, 307, 349
Access, 163, 185, 189, 201-208, 368-413
Accidents,
  automobile, 129
  during access, 204
Acquired abnormalities, dental anomalies and, 54
Acquired pathological conditions
  abrasion, 157
  attrition, 153-155
  erosion, 153, 155-157, 195, 296, 308, 356
  external resorption, 89–90, 109, 111, 115, 119, 198,
    316, 343, 346
  hypercementosis, 52, 152, 154, 163-164
  internal resorption, 95, 97–98, 158
  pulpal stones, 52, 163, 198
  secondary dentin, 50, 154
Acquisition,
  of diagnostic images, 18, 181, 317, 258, 331
  image, CBCT, and, 14, 183, 279, 304
Acquisition artifacts, 182, 244, 247, 288–289, 317, 320
Acute apical periodontitis, 252, 308
Acute bacterial infection, 252
Acute lesions, 252

ADA. *See also* American Dental Association 19
Advance images
  cone beam computed tomography, 304, 306-309,
    312-325, 331-415
  conventional tomography (CT), 13, 292
  extraoral radiograph and, 18, 34, 36, 147, 181
  micro-computed tomography, 277-283
  MRI, 14, 119, 121, 287, 296 301
  procedure for, 298
  ultrasound, 287, 291
Aging process, attrition related, 153
ALARA (as low as reasonably achievable), 19, 21, 39,
    184, 188
Altered morphology of teeth
  amelogeneisis imperfect, 72
  dens in dente, 61, 198
  dens invaginatus, 54, 75
  dentinogenesis imperfecta 73
  talon cusp, 74
  taurodontism, 67, 198
Alveolar bone, changes in morphology of, 81, 130,
    141, 160, 166, 167
  buccal or lingual cortical loss, 167
  horizontal bone loss, 168
  vertical bone defects, 168, 177
Alveolar crest, 166
  clinical features, 146
  definition, 146
  fractures of, 146

radiographic features,   146
Ameloblastoma,   115, 119, 160
    additional images of,   119
    clinical images of,   119
        CT of,   119
    definition of,   119
    differential diagnosis of,   119
    MRI of,   119
    radiographic features of,   119
        internal structure,   109, 119
        location,   119
        periphery,   119
Amelogenesis imperfecta,   72
    clinical features,   72
        hypocalcification,   72
        hypoplastic type,   72
    definition,   72
    differential diagnosis,   72
    radiographic features,   72
American Dental Association (ADA),   19
    dental radiography and,   6
Angulation guidelines,   22, 25
    for bisecting technique,   7, 20, 22-26, 33, 47, 181, 188,
        201
Angulation of tube head,   22, 47, 214
    bisecting angle, technique,   22, 47, 214
    paralleling angle technique,   25
Ankylosis,   161
    definition,   161
    differential diagnosis,   161
    radiographic features of,   161
    treatment,   161
Anomalies
    dental. See also dental anomalies,   54, 173
Anterior mandible,   48, 96, 108
    occlusal projection,   33
Anterior maxillary occlusal projection,   33
Apex, of teeth,   50-51, 84, 94, 102, 111, 130, 141, 170,
        194, 218
Apical periodontitis,   250-262, 296, 307
    epidemiology,   261
Apical periodontitis cyst,   93, 252, 293, 322, 356
Apical surgery,   67, 253, 350-360
Apron,   7, 19, 37, 39
Archiving, exporting and distribution (CBCT),   9,
        304-306
    relating to,   304-307
Artifacts, see also Image artifacts, CBCT and
    acquisition,   317
    beam-hardening,   244, 288, 320
    CT and,   182

Bacteria, dental caries relating to,   61, 81, 84, 126, 170,
        307
Bacterial plaque-associated gingivitis,   170, 173

Barrier-protected film or disposable container, use of,
        19
Barriers, infection control and,   19
BBC,   110, 113
Beam, X-ray. See also CBCT; X-ray beam,   14
Beam alignment,   20
    film placement and,   20
Benign ameloblastomas. See also ameloblastoma   119
Benign giant cell lesions,   115
Bisecting-angle projections, angulation guidelines for
        22, 25, 47, 214
Bisecting-angle technique,   18, 47
    of periapical radiography,   18, 22
        patient positioning,   19
        receptor-holding instruments,   19-20
        tube head, angulation of,   22, 47, 214
Bitewing examinations,   30
    horizontal bitewing receptors,   30
    vertical bitewing receptors,   31
Bitewing films,   31
Bitewing projections,   31
    caries relating to,   31
    molar,   31
    posterior,   31
    premolar,   31
Blurring. See also Radiographs, faulty causes of,
        blurring,   11, 26
Bone(s), see also Dense bone island
    cancellous,   103, 106, 108, 126, 166, 170
    periodontal loss of,   172
    quantity of, assessed for dental implants,   177
    resorption of,   149, 316
    trabecular pattern of,   103
Bone dysplasia,   123
    cement-osseous,   123
    fibrous,   123
Brightness and contrast,   13, 228
Buccal bifurcation cysts (BBC),   110, 113
Buccal object rule,   30, 207
Buccal roots,   201, 198, 346

Calcifications,   121, 163
Calcium,   210
Calcium hydroxide,   134, 158-160, 201, 210, 237, 368,
        397
Canines,   115, 155, 201
Caries. See also Dental caries,   7, 22, 228, 296, 409,
    bitewing projections and,   30
Cathode ray tube,   5
    display of,   5
Cathodes,   5
CBCT. See also Cone-beam computed tomography,   13,
        239, 293, 300, 303, 308-415
CCD. See also Charge-coupled device,   9, 19-21, 37,
        43-47

CEJ. *See also* Cementoenamel junction, 218
Cementoenamel junction (CEJ), 54, 61, 273, 331
Central incisor projection, maxillary, 22
Central X-ray beam, 22
  lateral skull projection and, 22
  mandibular oblique lateral projections and, 22
  mandibular ramus projection and, 22
Cervical root resorption, 158, 160-161
Chair, disinfecting and covering of, 19
Characteristics, 9
  digital detector, 9, 43
Charge-coupled device (CCD), 9, 19-21, 37,
    43-47
  occlusal radiography and, 33, 47
  panoramic imaging and, 36, 47
  periapical radiography and, 6, 22, 45
Chronic apical periodontitis, 250-262, 296, 307
Chronic lesions, 87
Clark's rule, 207, 309
Clinical examination, radiographic interpretation
    relating to, 13, 22
CMOS, 9, 19-21, 45-47
Collimation, 6, 10
  beam alignment and, 6, 10, 181
Combination crown and root fractures, 135, 148
  clinical features of, 135
  definition of, 135
  management of, 135
  radiographic features of, 135
Complementary metal oxide semiconductors (CMOS),
    9, 19-21, 45-47
Computed tomography, 13, 140, 180, 239, 250
  application, 13, 292
  artifacts and, 13, 317
  of cysts, 322
    nasoplatine duct, 322, 324, 331
    radicular, 93-95, 111, 322,
    residual, 295
  implants and, 182
  trauma and, 8, 130, 133, 239, 316
Concussion, 140
  clinical features of, 140
  definition of, 140
  management of, 140
  radiographic features of, 140
  teeth relating to, 140
Cone beamed–related artifacts, 244, 288, 320
Cone-beam computed tomography (CBCT), 141, 146,
    304, 307
  image artifacts and, 244, 288, 320
  implants and, 182
  limitations of, 244, 312
    poor soft tissue contrast, 10
  of mandible, for dental implants, 184
  of maxilla, for dental implants, 184

Congenital syphilis, 75
Contamination, 19
  infection control and, 19
  of processing equipment, prevention of, 13
Contrast. *See also* Images(s), characteristics,
    radiographic contrast, 10-12
  brightness and, 10
  gray scale, 10, 257
  insufficient, 10
  low, 10, 13, 228
Contrast agents,
  MRI and, 14, 298
Contrast resolution, 10
Conventional intraoral film, for radiographic
    examination, 10
Conventional radiographs, 6
Conventional tomography, 182
  for dental implants, 182
  for osseous structures,
Cortical border, of mandible, 103
Cross-contamination, 19
Cross-sectional mandibular occlusal projection, 33
Cross-sectional maxillary occlusal projection, 33
C-shape canal, 65, 202
CT. *See also* Computed tomography, 13
Cystic lesions, 293
Cyst(s). *See also* Bone, 113, 322
  apical periodontal, 114, 308
  incisive canal, 115
  nasopalatine canal, 180, 322, 324, 331,
  nonodontogenic, 90, 102, 322
  periapical, 252, 293, 322,
  squamous cell carcinoma, 102, 106, 117, 120

Dark spots or lines, 288
DBI, 126-127
Decay, 81, 259, 343
DEJ, 49
Dense bone island. *See also* DBI 126
Dens evaginatus, 54
  clinical features of, 54
  defferential diagnosis and, 54
  definition of, 54
  management of, 54
  radiographic features of, 54
  synonym for, 54
Dens invaginatu/dens in dente/dilated odontome
    54
  clinical features of, 54
  defferential diagnosis and, 54
  definition of, 54
  management of, 54
  radiographic features of, 54
  synonyms for, 54
Densitometer,

Density,
 of bone, trabecular pattern and,   83-85, 169, 180, 182,
  254-255, 258
 of film,   158, 161
 internal, trabecular pattern of bone and, changes in,
  109
 radiographic,   158, 161
Dental anomalies,   54
 acquired abnormalities,   54
 developmental abnormalities,   54
 disease detection/monitoring, dental radiographs
  and,   54
 radiographs and,   54
Dental caries,   7, 163
Dental conditions, periodontial disease associated with,
  168, 296
 local irritating factors,   167
 occlusal trauma,   167
Dental crown fractures,   130
 clinical features of,   130
 complicated,   130
 definition of,   130
 management of,   130
 radiographic features of,   130
 uncomplicated,   130
Dental exposure, PID and,   181
Dental exposure to radiation, reduction of,   182-184,
  197
 principles relating to,   25
  dose limitation,   7, 280, 302
  optimization,   326
Dental floss injury,   155
 clinical features of,   155
 differential diagnosis and,   155
 management of,   155
 radiographic features of,   155
Dental implants,   177
 bone quantity assessed for,   177
 diagnostic imaging for,   178
 imaging techniques for,   178
  conventional tomography,   179
  intraoral radiography,   181
  panoramic radiography,   181
  reformatted CBCT and MDCT,   183, 304
 intraoperative and postoperative assessments,
  177
 preoperative planning for,   178
  imaging stents,   178
Dental radiographs,   6-7, 10, 213
 ADA and,   19
 cost versus benefits of,   46, 129, 150, 181
 disease detection/monitoring and,   81
 examination relating to,   256
 guidelines for ordering of and patient examination
  relating to,

pregnancy,   39
 radiation therapy,   39
Dental radiography,
Dental radiology, for cancer survivor,   39
Dental root fractures,   130, 135, 337, 351, 356
 clinical features of,   138
 definition of,   138
 differential diagnosis and,   138
 management of,   138
 radiographic features of,   138
Dental X-ray beam,   6, 166, 182, 201, 214, 238, 304
Dental X-ray machine,   7, 21, 23-24, 214
Dentin   See also Secondary dentin,   49-52
Dentin dysplasia,   74
 clinical features of,   74
 coronal,   74
 definition of,   74
 differential diagnosis and,   74
 management of,   74
 radicular,   74
 radiographic features of,   74
Dentine,   49-50
Dentine-pulp complex,   50
Dentinoenamel junction (DEJ),   49
Dentinogenesis imperfecta   73
 clinical features of,   73
 definition of,   73
 differential diagnosis and,   73
 management of,   73
 radiographic features of,   73
 synonym for,   73
Dentistry,
 extraoral projection in,   18, 34, 36
 specific CBCT applications in,   14, 304, 307, 331,
  365
  endodontics   304, 330, 367
  implant site assessment and,   182, 179
  inferior alveolar canal, localization of,   180, 182
Detector sensitivity,
 CCD and,   9, 19-20, 47
 as digital detector characteristic,   45
 PSP and,   9, 12, 19, 20-21, 45
Detectors. See also Digital detector characteristics   9, 45
Developer,   11
Diagnosis   234, 261, 268, 287,
Diagnostic imaging
 for dental implants,   184
Diagnostic tools, for dental caries   7, 163
DICOM,   9
Digital, definition of   9
Digital detector characteristics,   9, 43, 183
 contrast resolution,   43
 latitude,   43
 sensitivity,   43
 spatial resolution,   43

Digital image receptor exposure, processing, and
        handling,   43
    damaged image receptors,   20, 43
    image processing, improper use of,   13, 43
    Images,   45
        distorted,   45
Digital image receptors,   9, 20, 45
    infection and,   45
    technology of,   45
        photostimulable phosphor,   45
        solid-state,   45
Digital images,   45
Digital image viewing,
    cathode ray tube display,   43
    electronic display considerations,   43
    image analysis,   45
    image processing,   13
Digital imaging,   45
    analog versus digital,   45
    clinical considerations of,   45
    digital detector characteristics,   45
    digital image receptors,   20
    digital image viewing,   13
    film or, intensifying screens and,   45
    film versus,   45
    image storage,   45
    psp and,   45
    for radiologic examination,   45
    solid-state detectors and,   45
    systems compatibility,   45
Digital imaging and communications in medicine
        (DICOM),   9
Digital subtraction radiography,   263
Dilaceration,   67
    clinical features of,   67
    definition of,   67
    differential diagnosis and,   67
    management of,   67
    radiographic features of,   67
Disease(s)
    caries and,   81
    dental anomalies and,   54
    implants and,   177
    inflammatory odontogenic,   81
    maxillary sinuses relating to,   81
    periapical,   81
    periodontal and,   166
    trauma and,   129
Disinfecting solution, infection control and,   19, 215
Disinfection, infection control and,   19
Distorted images,   10, 215, 309
Distortion,   10, 215, 309
    of image shape. See also Image shape distortion,
        215
    of image size,   215

Documentation,   113, 193, 213
Doppler ultrasound,   289
Dose,
    absorbed,   44
    patient exposure and,   21
    radiation, low, CBCT relating to,   14, 305
    risk and, in radiology,   44
DSR,   263
Dysplasia(s). See also Dentin dysplasia; Bone dysplasia,
        fibrous,   48, 74-75, 102
    bone,   123-125
Dystrophic calcification,   121, 163

EAL. See also electronic apex locator,   207,
        218
Electronic apex locator. See also EAL,   218
    advantages,   225
    digital radiography, and,   227
    limitation,   226
    perforations and,   228, 206
Elongation,   71, 215
Endodontic disease,   49, 81, 306, 367
Endodontics, radiographic techniques,   8, 18,
        261
Endodontic therapy,   8, 135, 224, 237, 309
Epidemiology, apical periodontitis, of,   261
Erosion,   155
    clinical features,   155
    definition,   155
    differential diagnosis,   156
    management,   156
    radiographic features,   156
Exposure. See also radiation,   182-184, 197
    to dental radiation. See also dental exposure to
        radiation, reduction of,   21, 182-184, 197
    digital image receptor relating to. See Digital image
        receptor exposure, processing and handling,   20,
        45
    PID and,   21
Exposure film,   10, 21
Exposure time,   7, 12, 20, 22, 43
    correct, establishment of,   22
    X-ray beam relating to,   22
External resorption,   149, 157, 198, 316, 343
    clinical features,   149, 157
    definition,   149, 157
    differential diagnosis,   149, 157
    management,   149, 157
    radiographic features,   149, 157
Extraoral films,   34
    panoramic views,   34
Extraoral radiography,   34

Field of view,   239, 304
Film contrast,   12

Film fog,   11
Film holder instruments,   6, 11, 21, 40
Film processor,   13
   automatic,   13
   infection control,   19
Films. *See also* X-ray film   13
   automatic processor of,   13
   barrier protected,   19
   bitewing,   30
   density of,   12
   digital imaging of,   45
   direct exposure,   12
   extraoral,   34
   film sensor and,   44
   F-speed,   12
   high contrast,   12
   panoramic,   34
   placement of, beam alignment and,   34
   processing,   34
Fog,   11
Food drug administration (FDA),   38
Foreshortening,   215
Fractures,   129-151, 230
   teeth,   129, 235
      apex locator and,   230
      clinical features,   135-151
      definition,   135-151
      differential diagnosis,   135-151
      management,   135-151
      radiographic features   135-151
F-speed film   181
Fusion,   61, 198, 202
   clinical features,   61
   definition,   61
   differential diagnosis,   61
   management,   61
   radiographic features,   61
   synonyms,   61

Gag reflex, radiographic examination and,   40, 226
Gemination,   63
   clinical features,   63
   definition,   63
   differential diagnosis,   63
   management,   63
   radiographic features,   63
   synonyms,   63
Granuloma,   111, 170, 252, 292, 306, 322
Gutta percha,   211, 270
      cone/cone fit radiograph,   211, 270
      tracing fistula,   108, 172

Hazards,   7
Hematogenous abnormalities,   119
Hertwig epithelial root sheath,   93, 111

History,   5
   apex locators, of,   218
   radiology, of,   5
Horizontal angulation of tube head,   24, 197, 214
Horizontal bitewing receptor,   31
Horizontal bone loss,   168
Horizontal root fracture,   230, 236, 341
Hypercementosis,   152, 154, 163
   clinical features,   163
   definition,   163
   differential diagnosis,   163
   management,   163
   radiographic features,   163
   synonyms,   163

Image(s),
   characteristics,   9
   CT and,   45
   digital,   45
   image quality,   9
   interpretation,   13,
   radiographic blurring,   10
   radiographic contrast,   10
   radiographic density,   10
   radiographic noise,   10
Image acquisition, CBCT, and,   14
Image analysis,
   diagnosis,   193, 317
   extraoral radiography,   34
   intraoral images relating to,   193
   radiographic interpretation and,   13, 22, 193
Image artifacts, CBCT, and. *See also* Artifacts   182, 244, 247, 288–289
   cone beam related,   317, 320
Image quality,   9, 13
Image receptor,   20
   blurring of,   10
   panoramic imaging and,   10
   patient placement and,   19
Image reconstruction
   CBCT and,   306, 320, 322, 368
   CT and,   306
   micro CT,   277
Image shape distortion   10, 18, 22, 181
   minimization of,   215
Image sharpness and resolution,   13, 215
Image size distortion,   215
Implants. *See also* dental implants,   177–188
   CBCT and,   184
   radiographs and,   181
Incisive canal,   115, 331
Incisive canal cyst,   115
Incisive foramen,   201
Incisors,   200–201

Indices, 259
        periapical index (PAI), 259
        periapical index based on CBCT (CBCT PAI),
            312
Infection (s)
        automatic film processor and, 13
        control of, 19
Inflammation, 52, 81, 251
Inflammatory process, 81
Initial radiograph, 184, 203
Injuries. *See also* abrasion, 157
        floss, 157
        tooth brush, 157
        traumatic, 157
Instruments, 19
        film holder, 6, 11, 21, 40
        receptor holder, 6, 11, 21, 40
Internal resorption 95, 157
    clinical features, 95, 157
    definition, 95, 157
    differential diagnosis, 95, 157
    management, 95, 157
    radiographic features, 95, 157
Interpretation, 13, 254, 288
Interproximal films/radiographs, 30
Intraoral film, conventional, 18
Intraoral images, 18
Intraoral radiographs, 18
        interproximal, 18
        occlusal, 18, 33
        periapical, 18, 22

Jaws, 91

Keratocystic tumor, 115
Kilovoltage (kVp), 6, 12, 44, 303

Lamina dura, 51, 85, 166
Lead collimation, 6, 10
Leaded aprons and collars, 7, 19, 37, 39
Lesions, *see also* Bone(s)
        acute, 252
        carious, 252
        chronic, 252
        radiolucent, 103
Low contrast, 10, 13, 228
Luxation, 143-144
    clinical features, 141
    definition, 141
    differential diagnosis, 141
    management, 141
    radiographic features, 141

Magnetic resonance images (MRI), 14, 287
        application of, 297

Magnification. *See also* image shape distortion, 10, 18,
            22, 181
Mandible, 25
        CBCT, 349
Master apical file radiograph 211, 270
Maxilla, 25
        CBCT for, 349
Maxillary sinusitis, 90
Micro-computed tomography (Micro CT), 278-284
        applications, 279
        limitations, 280
Microdens, 198
Microdontia, 67
Molars, 201
        impacted, 106, 343
        roots of, 105, 201
        surgery of, 350
Monitoring healing, 251
Morphology of teeth, 201
Multirooted teeth, 201

Nasal cavity, 90
Nasal fossa, 90
Nasopalatine canal, 190
Nasopalatine duct cyst, 322, 331
Necrosis, 96, 111, 140, 147, 161, 170
Nutrient canals, 90

Object localization, 287
        tube shift technique, 287
Occlusal films, 34-36
Occlusal plane, panoramic, 36
Occlusal radiographs, 36
Occlusal view, intraoral X-ray film related, 33-37
Odontogenic cyst, 326
Osteitis, 111
Osteomyelitis, 107, 124, 126, 298, 349

PAI, 259
Palatal root, 30, 215
Palatine torus, 41
Panoramic equipment, 36
Panoramic images, 36
        machines, 6, 36
        technique, 36
Panoramic radiographs, 38
Paralleling technique, 7, 47, 181, 193
Patient
        examination, 19
        exposure, 19
        with mental or physical disabilities, 41
        preparation, 19
        selection criteria, 19
PCD, 124
PDL, 130, 140, 154, 167, 219

Perforation,   198, 204, 208, 228, 317
Periapical abscess,   65, 111, 160, 170, 196, 307, 349
Periapical projection,   138
Periapical cemento dysplasia (PCD),   124
Peripaical cyst,   93, 252, 293, 322, 356
Periapical disease,   81, 307
Periapical films,   18, 22
Periapical granuloma,   81, 111, 170, 252, 292, 306,
     322
Periapical index (PAI),   259
Peripical inflammatory lesions,   81
     clinical features,   81
     definition,   81
     differential diagnosis,   81
     radiographic interpretation,   18, 13, 254, 288
Periapical radiographs,   22, 122, 130
Periapical radiography,   18, 22
     bisecting angle,   22, 47
     bitewing,   30
     CCD and,   20
     CMSO and,   20
     exposure,   20
     paralleling techniques,   18
Periapical views, of intraoral films,   18, 22
Periodontal bone loss, pattern of,   168
Periodontal cyst,   114, 331
     apical,   114
     lateral,   114
Periodontal disease,   167
     assessment,   167
     normal anatomy,   167
     periodontitis,   167
     radiographs,   167
Periodontal ligament (PDL),   130, 140, 154, 167, 219
Periodontum,   51, 167
Physical disabilities, patients with   41
PID. See also Position indicating device,   32
Plastic wrap, infection control and,   34, 215
Position and head alignment, of patient,   19
Position indicating device (PID),   32
     dental exposure and,   32
     infection control and,   34
Preclinical endodontics,   269
Processing solutions,   12
Processor automatic,   12
Pulp,   50
     canal of,   50
     chamber of,   50
Pulp necrosis,   96, 111, 140, 147, 161, 170
Pulp stone,   52, 163
     clinical features,   163
     definition,   163
     differential diagnosis,   163
     management of,   163
     radiographic features,   163

Quality
     of diagnosis images,   10
     image,   10
Quality criteria,   10

Radiation. See also dose,   7, 280, 302
     characteristics,   19
     kilovoltage,   6, 12, 44, 303
     lead apron and collars,   7, 19, 37, 39
     patients,   19
     protection,   7
     therapy,   39
Radicular cysts,   93, 322
     clinical features,   93
     definition,   93
     differential diagnosis,   93
     management of,   93
     radiographic features,   93
Radiographic abnormalities,   101
Radiographic anatomy,   269
Radiographic assessment, of endodontic conditions,…
     255
Radiographic examination
     extraoral,   36
     gag reflex,   40
     intraoral,   18
     pregnancy and,   39
Radiographic infection control,   19
Radiographic interpretation,   13
     clinical examination and,   13, 254, 288
     image analysis,   13, 254, 288
Radiographic report,   213
Radiographic techniques for endodontics,   8, 213
Radiographs. See also dental radiographs   6-7, 10,
     213
     extraoral radiographs,   34
     dental anomalies,   54
     faulty, causes of,   10
          blurring,   10
          dark,   10
          fog,   10–11
          partial image,   10
     interproximal,   30
     intraoral,   18
     occlusal,   33, 47
     panoramic,   36
     periodontal disease and,   167
Radiography
     dental,   6-7, 10, 213
     dose and risks,   7, 280, 302
     extraoral,   34
     occlusal,   18, 33, 47
     panoramic. See also panoramic radiographs,
          36
     periapical,   18, 22

Radiologic examination
  with conventional intraoral films, 18
  with digital imaging, 43-47
Radiology, 5
Radiolucent, 101
  lesion, 101
  presentation, 101
Radiopaque, 101
  presentation, 101
Rarefying osteitis, 103, 111
Recall, 213
Receptor, 19
  bitewing, 18
  definition, 19
  holding instruments, 20
  image, 19
Resolution,
  contrast, 10, 13, 228
  image sharpness, 10
Resonance. *See also* Magnetic resonance images, 14,
    287
Resorption,
  bone, 149, 316
  cervical, 158, 160-161
  erosion, 149
  external, 149, 157, 159-160, 198, 230, 316, 346
  internal, 95, 97–98, 158
Restorative materials
  calcium hydroxide, 134, 158-160, 201, 210, 237, 368,
    397
Retreatment 231, 333
  gutta percha, 211, 270
Root canal
Roots, 193
  buccal, 193, 336
  of molars, 193, 336
  palatal, 193, 336
  vertical fracture of, 67, 173, 231, 235

Scanners
  cone beam, 14
  micro-CT, 279
  MRI, 297
Scar, bone or fibrous, 121
Secondary dentin, 154
Sensors, 44, 304
  film, 19
  infection control, 19
Size and cost of CBCT, 14, 46, 183
Solid malignancies, 120
Solutions
  changing, 12
  developing, 12
  fixing, 12
  processing, 12

Surgery, apical, 67, 253, 350-360
Syphilis, congenital, 75

Talon cusp, 74
  clinical features of, 74
  definition of, 74
  differential diagnosis and, 74
  management of, 74
  radiographic features of, 74
Taurodontism, 67, 198
  clinical features of, 67
  definition of, 67
  differential diagnosis and, 67
  management of, 67
  radiographic features of, 67
Teeth. *See also* altered morphology of teeth
  apex, 50-51, 84, 94, 102, 111, 130, 141, 170, 194, 218
  CCD relating to, 20, 43
  cementum, 52
  dentin, 49
  enamel, 49
  lamina dura, periodontal membrane space, and
    intraosseous lesions relating to, 52, 167
  multirooted, 201
  number of, 201
  osteopetrosis relating to, 50
  pulp,
    canal, 50
    chamber, 204
  root canal, 204
  size of, 204
  trauma to, 129
Teeth and facial structures, trauma to applied radiology
    for, 146
  CT of, 146
  fractures, 146, 337
    of alveolar processes, 146, 337
    combination crown and root, 140
    dental crown, 140
    dental root, 140
    le fort, 146
    mandibular, 147
    monitoring healing of, 148
    radiographic signs of, 146
    vertical root, 67, 173, 231, 235
  injuries
    avulsion, 144
    concussion, 198, 140
    facial bones, 140
    luxation, 140
Tooth
  microflora, dental caries relating to, 61, 81, 84, 126,
    170, 307
  mobility of, periodontal disease and, 168
Toothbrush abrasion, 157

Toothbrush injury,   155
   clinical features of,   155
   radiographic features of,   155
Torus mandibularis
   clinical features of,   41
   definition of,   41
   radiographic features of,   41
      internal structures,   41
      location,   41
      periphery and shape,   41
   synonym for,   41
Trabecular pattern,   97, 170
   bone density and,   83-85, 169, 180, 182, 254-255, 258
   of bone, internal density and   183-185, 169, 180, 182, 254-255, 258
Trauma
   CBCT and,   129-152, 337
   CT and,   129-152
   dental radiographs and,   129-152
   occlusal, periodontal disease and,   168
   to teeth,   129-152
Traumatic injuries to teeth and facial structures,   129-152
Tube current (mA),   44
Tube head, angulation of,   22, 47, 214
   bisecting-angle technique,   7, 20, 22-26, 33, 47, 181, 188, 201
      horizontal,   24, 197, 214
      vertical,   24, 197, 214
   paralleling technique,   24, 197, 214
Tube head stability,   24

Ultrasonography (US)   14, 288
   for salivary gland disease,   297
Uncomplicated dental crown fractures,   130

Vertical angulation, of tube head,   24, 197, 214
Vertical bitewing receptors,   30–31
Vertical bone defects,   168

Vertical root fractures,   67, 173, 231, 235
   clinical features of,   235-248
   definition of,   235-248
   management of,   235-248
   radiographic features of,   235-248
View-boxes, cleaning of   13
Voxel   331
   size,   14, 239, 304,

Working length,   207-208, 210, 218, 224, 270, 333
   definition,   218
   methods,   219
   radiograph,   207-208, 219, 270
Working surfaces, disinfecting and covering of   19, 216-217
World Health Organization,   13, 115, 130

X-ray   6-9, 26, 43, 45, 256, 301,309, 373, 393
   angulations,   309-10
   beam,   6-7, 12, 14, 19, 21, 24-29, 32, 36, 37, 43- 44, 47,108, 166, 182-3, 201,214-5, 238, 304
      dental. *See also* Dental X-ray,   6, 10, 24, 26, 39, 40, 214
      factors in controlling of,   21
         collimation,   6, 10, 44, 181, 304
         exposure time,   7, 12, 20, 22, 43, 44, 244,
   exposure,   6-7
   film,   6, 40
   generation,   44,
      patient positioning,   182
   machine,   6, 11-2, 21, 43-4, 214
   penetration,   6
   Rinn® XCP,   28, 31
   source,   37, 279
   tube,
   6, 12, 21, 23, 27, 30, 42-3, 186, 201

Zygomatic process/ bone/zygomatic arch,   20, 30, 201, 220

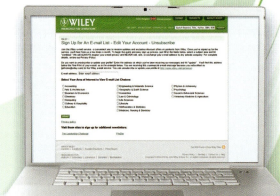
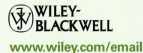